SKILLS PERFORMANCE CHECKLISTS

to accompany

CLINICAL NURSING SKILLS & TECHNIQUES

FOURTH EDITION

PATRICIA A. CASTALDI, RN, BSN, MSN

Associate Dean

Elizabeth General Medical Center School of Nursing

Elizabeth, New Jersey

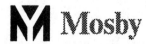 Mosby

St. Louis Baltimore Boston Carlsbad Chicago Naples New York Philadelphia Portland
London Madrid Mexico City Singapore Sydney Tokyo Toronto Wiesbaden

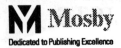

Mosby

Dedicated to Publishing Excellence

A Times Mirror
Company

Vice President and Publisher   Nancy L. Coon
Senior Editor   Susan Epstein
Senior Developmental Editor   Beverly J. Copland
Project Manager   Gayle May Morris
Manufacturing Manager   Linda Ierardi
Cover Design   E. Rohne Rudder

Printed in the United States of America
Composition by Graphic World
Printing/binding by Plus Communications

Mosby–Year Book, Inc.
11830 Westline Industrial Drive
St. Louis, Missouri 63146

International Standard Book Number 0-8151-4306-0

97 98 99 00 01 / 9 8 7 6 5 4 3 2 1

The checklists in this book were developed to provide an evaluation tool to determine your competence in performing the skills presented in *Clinical Nursing Skills and Techniques.* Instructors can check "Satisfactory," "Unsatisfactory," or "Needs Practice" for each step. Specific instructions or feedback can be provided in the "Comments" column or at the end of the checklist. These chestlists can also be used for independent self-evaluation of competency.

While we understand that each Instructor may require slightly different steps in the evaluation of the performance of a specific skill, these checklists have been streamlined to include only the critical steps needed to satisfactorily master the skill. They are not intended to replace the text, which describes and illustrates in detail each step of the nursing skill.

These checklists will be a valuable time saver for Instructors or a handy tool for self-evaluation. Each checklist begins on a separate page and is perforated for easy removal.

SKILLS PERFORMANCE CHECKLISTS

Student _____   Date _____

Instructor _____   Date _____

PERFORMANCE CHECKLIST 1-1 **ADMITTING CLIENTS**

	S	U	NP	Comments

ROOM PREPARATION

1. Washed hands before preparing room equipment, furniture, and bed.   ___ ___ ___ _____

2. Assembled special equipment.   ___ ___ ___ _____

ASSESSMENT

1. Greeted client and family cordially and introduced self by name and job title.   ___ ___ ___ _____

2. Escorted client and family members to room and introduced roommate.   ___ ___ ___ _____

3. Assessed client's general appearance and condition before beginning admitting procedures (postponed routine procedures when client presented acute physical or psychologic problems).   ___ ___ ___ _____

4. Assessed client's and family members' psychologic response to admitting procedures.   ___ ___ ___ _____

5. Checked physician's admitting orders.   ___ ___ ___ _____

6. Oriented client and family to nursing division policies and procedures; introduced personnel to client; demonstrated use of room equipment, e.g., call light, bed controls.   ___ ___ ___ _____

7. Assessed client's vital signs.   ___ ___ ___ _____

8. Provided for privacy and prepared client for examination.   ___ ___ ___ _____

9. Obtained a complete nursing history. Identified food, drug, and other substance allergies.   ___ ___ ___ _____

10. Conducted physical assessment of appropriate body systems.   ___ ___ ___ _____

NURSING DIAGNOSIS

1. Developed appropriate nursing diagnoses based on assessment data.   ___ ___ ___ _____

PLANNING

1. Developed individualized goals for transfer of client.   ___ ___ ___ _____

2. Informed client of planned procedures or treatment.   ___ ___ ___ _____

3. Identified expected outcomes based on goals of care.   ___ ___ ___ _____

	S	U	NP	Comments

IMPLEMENTATION

1. Informed client of planned procedures or treatments. ___ ___ ___ _____

2. Allowed client opportunity to ask questions about admission procedures or therapies. ___ ___ ___ _____

3. Collected client's valuables and explained policy for ensuring safekeeping. ___ ___ ___ _____

4. Allowed client and family time alone. ___ ___ ___ _____

5. Placed call light within client's reach after assessment; placed bed in low position; raised side rails as needed. ___ ___ ___ _____

6. Washed hands after assessment. ___ ___ ___ _____

EVALUATION

1. Confirmed client's understanding of tests and procedures. ___ ___ ___ _____

2. Observed client for nonverbal signs. ___ ___ ___ _____

3. Monitored client's ability to ambulate independently. ___ ___ ___ _____

4. Checked client's room setup regularly. ___ ___ ___ _____

5. Assessed for unexpected outcomes. ___ ___ ___ _____

RECORDING AND REPORTING

1. Recorded history and assessment findings. ___ ___ ___ _____

2. Notified physician of client's admission; reported unusual assessment findings; secured admission orders. ___ ___ ___ _____

3. Began to develop nursing plan of care. ___ ___ ___ _____

Student _____   Date _____

Instructor _____   Date _____

PERFORMANCE CHECKLIST 1-2 **TRANSFERRING CLIENTS**

	S	U	NP	Comments

ASSESSMENT
1. Assessed reason for client's transfer.

2. Assessed client's physical condition and determined vehicle for transport.

3. Determined client's level of understanding and feelings regarding transfer.

4. Assessed method to transfer client to vehicle.

5. Assessed client's need for analgesic or antiemetic prior to transfer.

6. Assessed if client's family or significant others had been notified of transfer.

NURSING DIAGNOSIS
1. Developed appropriate nursing diagnoses based on assessment data.

PLANNING
1. Developed individualized goals for transfer of client.

2. Identified expected outcomes.

3. Arranged for transport vehicle.

4. Obtained transfer order.

IMPLEMENTATION
1. Explained transfer procedure to client or family.

2. Checked accuracy and completeness of client's record.

3. Obtained signed release from client giving permission to copy necessary part of record.

4. Completed nursing care transfer form.

5. Gathered and secured client's personal items.

6. Attended to any last-minute physical needs of client.

7. Transferred client to stretcher or wheelchair.

8. Performed final assessment of client's physical stability.

	S	U	NP	Comments
9. Accompanied client to transport vehicle.	___	___	___	_____
10. Notified receiving agency of impending transfer and client's status.	___	___	___	_____

EVALUATION

	S	U	NP	Comments
1. Compared final assessment data with previous finding.	___	___	___	_____
2. Inspected client's alignment and positioning in transport vehicle.	___	___	___	_____
3. Confirmed client's understanding of transfer and procedures.	___	___	___	_____
4. Determined if receiving agency had questions regarding client's care.	___	___	___	_____
5. Identified unexpected outcomes.	___	___	___	_____

RECORDING AND REPORTING

	S	U	NP	Comments
1. Verified that admission information was documented by receiving nurse.	___	___	___	_____

Student _____   Date _____

Instructor _____   Date _____

PERFORMANCE CHECKLIST 1-3 **DISCHARGING CLIENTS**

	S	U	NP	Comments
ASSESSMENT				
1. Began assessing client's discharge needs upon admission.	—	—	—	_____
2. Assessed client's and family members' need for health teaching.	—	—	—	_____
3. Assessed existence of environmental barriers in client's home setting.	—	—	—	_____
4. Collaborated with physician and staff in other disciplines about client's need for referral for home health care services or an extended care facility.	—	—	—	_____
5. Assessed client's and family's perceptions of continued health care needs outside the hospital.	—	—	—	_____
6. Assessed client's acceptance of health problems.	—	—	—	_____
7. Consulted other health team members to determine client's discharge needs; made appropriate referrals.	—	—	—	_____
NURSING DIAGNOSIS				
1. Developed appropriate nursing diagnoses based on assessment data.	—	—	—	_____
PLANNING				
1. Developed individualized goals for client's discharge.	—	—	—	_____
2. Identified expected outcomes.	—	—	—	_____
IMPLEMENTATION				
Before Day of Discharge				
1. Suggested ways to change physical arrangement of home environment to meet client's needs.	—	—	—	_____
2. Provided client and family with information about community health care resources.	—	—	—	_____
3. Conducted teaching sessions related to health care needs.	—	—	—	_____
4. Communicated client's response to teaching and proposed discharge plan to other health care team members.	—	—	—	_____
Day of Discharge				
1. Completed any of the following activities prior to discharge, if possible.	—	—	—	_____

	S	U	NP	Comments

2. Allowed client and family opportunity to ask questions and discuss issues related to home health care; considered variations in the home setting for skill performance. ___ ___ ___ _____

3. Checked physician's discharge orders. ___ ___ ___ _____

4. Determined if transportation has been arranged for client. ___ ___ ___ _____

5. Assisted client with dressing and packing personal items. ___ ___ ___ _____

6. Checked all closets and drawers for belongings; obtained copy of valuables list and had valuables delivered to client; accounted for all valuables. ___ ___ ___ _____

7. Gave client prescriptions or medications and reviewed drug information. ___ ___ ___ _____

8. Assisted client in arranging with business office for bill payment. ___ ___ ___ _____

9. Transported client and belongings to source of transportation. ___ ___ ___ _____

10. Assisted client to wheelchair or stretcher using proper body mechanics; escorted client to agency entrance; locked wheelchair wheels; assisted client into transport vehicle with personal belongings. ___ ___ ___ _____

11. Notified admitting or appropriate department of discharge time. ___ ___ ___ _____

EVALUATION

1. Asked client to describe nature of illness, treatment regimens, signs and symptoms to be reported. ___ ___ ___ _____

2. Had client or family member perform treatments to be continued at home. ___ ___ ___ _____

3. Inspected home environment for risks. ___ ___ ___ _____

4. Identified unexpected outcomes. ___ ___ ___ _____

RECORDING AND REPORTING

1. Documented client's discharge. ___ ___ ___ _____

2. Documented status of client's health problems at time of discharge. ___ ___ ___ _____

Student _____   Date _____

Instructor _____   Date _____

PERFORMANCE CHECKLIST 2-1 **ESTABLISHING THERAPEUTIC COMMUNICATION**

	S	U	NP	Comments
ASSESSMENT				
1. Determined client's specific need to communicate.	___	___	___	_____
2. Assessed client's reason for need of health care.	___	___	___	_____
3. Assessed factors about self and client that influence communication.	___	___	___	_____
4. Assessed client's language and ability to speak.	___	___	___	_____
5. Observed client's pattern of communication and verbal and nonverbal behavior.	___	___	___	_____
6. Determined available resources for selection of communication methods.	___	___	___	_____
NURSING DIAGNOSIS				
1. Developed appropriate nursing diagnoses based on assessment data.	___	___	___	_____
PLANNING				
1. Developed individualized client goals for communication based on nursing diagnoses.	___	___	___	_____
2. Identified expected outcomes based on communication goals.	___	___	___	_____
3. Prepared client and physical environment.	___	___	___	_____
IMPLEMENTATION				
1. Created a climate of warmth and acceptance, with consideration of environment and client's status.	___	___	___	_____
2. Addressed client by name and introduced self by name and role.	___	___	___	_____
3. Used appropriate nonverbal behaviors.	___	___	___	_____
4. Observed nonverbal behaviors and actively listened to client.	___	U	___	_____
5. Explained the purpose of the interaction and if the information is to be shared.	___	___	___	_____
6. Encouraged client to seek clarification during the interaction.	___	___	___	_____
7. Used therapeutic communication techniques during the interaction.	___	___	___	_____
8. Avoided barriers to communication.	___	___	___	_____
9. Summarized what was discussed with the client.	___	___	___	_____

	S	U	NP	Comments

EVALUATION

1. Observed client's verbal and nonverbal responses. ___ ___ ___ _____

2. Requested feedback from client on information that was communicated. ___ ___ ___ _____

3. Assessed for unexpected outcomes. ___ ___ ___ _____

RECORDING AND REPORTING

1. Reported pertinent information to health care team members. ___ ___ ___ _____

2. Recorded in nurses' notes communication pertinent to client's status and level of understanding. ___ ___ ___ _____

Student _____   Date _____

Instructor _____   Date _____

PERFORMANCE CHECKLIST 2-2   **COMMUNICATING THROUGHOUT THE PHASES OF THE NURSE-CLIENT RELATIONSHIP**

	S	U	NP	Comments
ASSESSMENT				
1. Determined client's needs, behaviors, and patterns of communication during orientation phase.	___	___	___	_____
2. Assessed own barriers to communication with client.	___	___	___	_____
3. Assessed client's readiness to work toward goal attainment.	___	___	___	_____
4. Considered time frame for client discharge or transfer from the agency.	___	___	___	_____
NURSING DIAGNOSIS				
1. Developed appropriate nursing diagnoses based on assessment data.	___	___	___	_____
PLANNING				
1. Developed individualized client goals for communication based on nursing diagnoses.	___	___	___	_____
2. Prepared for communication during orientation phase by providing warm and accepting environment, establishing trust, and gathering pertinent client data.	___	___	___	_____
3. Prepared for working phase by identifying strategies to achieve desired goals.	___	___	___	_____
4. Prepared for termination phase by identifying methods of summarizing and synthesizing pertinent client information.	___	___	___	_____
IMPLEMENTATION				
Orientation Phase				
1. Introduced self and role to client; provided information and clarified concerns.	___	___	___	_____
2. Identified client's expectations in seeking health care.	___	___	___	_____
Working Phase				
1. Used effective communication skills.	___	___	___	_____
2. Discussed and prioritized problem areas.	___	___	___	_____
3. Provided information to client and helped client express needs and feelings.	___	___	___	_____

	S	U	NP	Comments

Termination Phase

1. Used effective communication skills to discuss discharge/termination issues. ___ ___ ___ _____

2. Summarized goal achievement. ___ ___ ___ _____

EVALUATION

1. Noted client's ability to express self and willingness to share information and concerns during orientation phase. ___ ___ ___ _____

2. Noted nurse's response to client and client's response to nurse; considered alternative techniques, if necessary. ___ ___ ___ _____

3. Determined client's ability to work toward identified goals during working phase. ___ ___ ___ _____

4. Used appropriate communication skills during termination phase; reinforced client's changes and strengths, developed action plan. ___ ___ ___ _____

5. Identified unexpected outcomes. ___ ___ ___ _____

RECORDING AND REPORTING

1. Recorded in nurses' notes communication pertinent to client's health status and response to health care measures. ___ ___ ___ _____

2. Reported observation of behaviors reflecting refusal or acceptance of health care measures. ___ ___ ___ _____

___ ___ ___ _____

Student _____   Date _____

Instructor _____   Date _____

PERFORMANCE CHECKLIST 2-3 **COMMUNICATING WITH THE ANXIOUS CLIENT**

	S	U	NP	Comments
ASSESSMENT				
1. Assessed for physical, behavioral, and verbal cues indicating anxiety.	___	___	___	_____
2. Assessed for possible factors causing client anxiety.	___	___	___	_____
3. Assessed factors influencing communication with client.	___	___	___	_____
4. Assessed own level of anxiety; made conscious effort to remain calm.	___	___	___	_____
NURSING DIAGNOSIS				
1. Developed appropriate nursing diagnoses based on assessment data.	___	___	___	_____
PLANNING				
1. Developed individualized goals for client communication to reduce anxiety.	___	___	___	_____
2. Identified expected outcomes.	___	___	___	_____
3. Recognized and controlled own anxiety.	___	___	___	_____
4. Prepared physical environment to provide quiet, calm area with ample personal space.	___	___	___	_____
IMPLEMENTATION				
1. Provided brief, simple introduction of self and role.	___	___	___	_____
2. Used appropriate nonverbal behaviors and active listening skills.	___	___	___	_____
3. Used clear and concise verbal techniques.	___	___	___	_____
4. Helped client acquire alternate coping strategies (e.g., progressive relaxation, etc.).	___	___	___	_____
5. Minimized noise in physical setting.	___	___	___	_____
6. Provided necessary comfort measures.	___	___	___	_____
EVALUATION				
1. Observed for continuing presence of signs and symptoms and behaviors reflecting anxiety.	___	___	___	_____
2. Had client discuss ways to cope with anxiety in future.	___	___	___	_____

	S	U	NP	Comments
3. Evaluated client's ability to discuss factors causing anxiety.	___	___	___	_____
4. Identified unexpected outcomes.	___	___	___	_____

RECORDING AND REPORTING

	S	U	NP	Comments
1. Recorded in nurses' notes cause of client's anxiety and exhibited signs and symptoms and behaviors.	___	___	___	_____
2. Recorded and reported methods used to relieve anxiety and client's response.	___	___	___	_____

Student _____   Date _____

Instructor _____   Date _____

PERFORMANCE CHECKLIST 2-4 **VERBALLY DEESCALATING THE POTENTIALLY VIOLENT CLIENT**

	S	U	NP	Comments
ASSESSMENT				
1. Observed for behaviors or expressions that indicate client anger.	—	—	—	_____
2. Assessed factors that influence communication of the angry client.	—	—	—	_____
3. Considered available resources to assist in communication with the angry client.	—	—	—	_____
NURSING DIAGNOSIS				
1. Developed appropriate nursing diagnoses based on assessment data.	—	—	—	_____
PLANNING				
1. Developed individualized client goals based on nursing diagnoses.	—	—	—	_____
2. Identified expected outcomes.	—	—	—	_____
3. Prepared self for interaction with the angry client.	—	—	—	_____
4. Prepared environment to deescalate the potentially violent client.	—	—	—	_____
IMPLEMENTATION				
1. Created climate of acceptance for client; maintained nonthreatening communication skills.	—	—	—	_____
2. Responded appropriately to the potentially violent client by using therapeutic silence, answering questions, remaining calm, maintaining personal space and safety, and exploring alternatives to situation.	—	—	—	_____
EVALUATION				
1. Observed for continuing behaviors or expressions of anger.	—	—	—	_____
2. Noted client's ability to answer questions and problem solve.	—	—	—	_____
3. Identified unexpected outcomes.	—	—	—	_____
RECORDING AND REPORTING				
1. Recorded in nurses' notes observations related to anger; reported verbal threats to appropriate agency personnel.	—	—	—	_____
2. Recorded and reported nursing interventions used and client's responses.	—	—	—	_____

Student _____   Date _____

Instructor _____   Date _____

PERFORMANCE CHECKLIST 3-1 **GIVING A CHANGE-OF-SHIFT REPORT**

	S	U	NP	Comments
ASSESSMENT				
1. Gathered pertinent client information from available sources.	—	—	—	_____
PLANNING				
1. Prioritized information.	—	—	—	_____
IMPLEMENTATION				
1. Provided a detailed description of the client's progress, including background information, assessment data, nursing diagnoses, interventions, and evaluation.	—	—	—	_____
a. Described therapy or treatment interventions given, including client's response.	—	—	—	_____
b. Described instructions given and client's progress in discharge plan. Included family information and explanation of current priorities.	—	—	—	_____
2. Clarified report with oncoming shift.	—	—	—	_____

Student _____   Date _____

Instructor _____   Date _____

PERFORMANCE CHECKLIST 3-2 **DOCUMENTING NURSES' PROGRESS NOTES**

	S	U	NP	Comments
ASSESSMENT				
1. Completed assessments and interventions and noted responses.	—	—	—	_____
IMPLEMENTATION				
1. Recorded a summary of nursing care using guidelines for the various recording types, including:				
a. PIE	—	—	—	_____
b. APIE	—	—	—	_____
c. SOAP	—	—	—	_____
d. SOAPE	—	—	—	_____
e. FOCUS	—	—	—	_____
2. Signed progress note with full name and status.	—	—	—	_____

Student _____   Date _____

Instructor _____   Date _____

PERFORMANCE CHECKLIST 3-3 **INCIDENT REPORTING**

	S	U	NP	Comments
ASSESSMENT				
1. Reported accurate, objective, chronological information.	—	—	—	_____
2. Assessed the extent of injury to client or others.	—	—	—	_____
IMPLEMENTATION				
1. Restored individual's safety, if injured.	—	—	—	_____
2. Notified physician if injury occurred.	—	—	—	_____
3. Referred nonclient injury to appropriate setting.	—	—	—	_____
4. Completed incident report correctly and promptly.	—	—	—	_____
5. Documented events of incident in client's chart correctly.	—	—	—	_____
6. Assessed and implemented ordered therapies in case of injured client.	—	—	—	_____

Student _____ Date _____

Instructor _____ Date _____

PERFORMANCE CHECKLIST 4-1 **FALL PREVENTION**

	S	U	NP	Comments
ASSESSMENT				
1. Observed older adult for physiologic changes common to aging process.	—	—	—	_____
2. Assessed risk factors in home and community.	—	—	—	_____
3. Determined potential risk of injury cause by motor-sensory or cognitive changes.	—	—	—	_____
NURSING DIAGNOSIS				
1. Developed appropriate nursing diagnoses based on assessment data.	—	—	—	_____
PLANNING				
1. Developed individualized goals for client.	—	—	—	_____
2. Identified expected outcomes.	—	—	—	_____
IMPLEMENTATION				
Home or Health Care Facility				
1. Provided adequate, non-glare lighting.	—	—	—	_____
2. Removed unnecessary objects from walkways and stairs.	—	—	—	_____
3. Arranged necessary objects in a logical way, in easy to reach locations.	—	—	—	_____
4. Installed grip bars or handrails in hallways and bathrooms, and provided raised toilet seats.	—	—	—	_____
5. Stairs:				
a. Installed appropriately colored and textured treads.				
b. Ensured proper lighting and room for mobility.	—	—	—	_____
c. Kept stairs and walkways in good condition.	—	—	—	_____
6. Secured all carpeting, mats, and tile.	—	—	—	_____
7. Kept floors clean and dry.	—	—	—	_____
In a Health Care Facility				
8. Identified client correctly.	—	—	—	_____
9. Introduced self and role to client.	—	—	—	_____
10. Gathered equipment.	—	—	—	_____
11. Washed hands correctly.	—	—	—	_____

	S	U	NP	Comments

12. Provided privacy. Positioned and draped client as needed. ___ ___ ___ _____

13. Adjusted bed and side rails properly. ___ ___ ___ _____

14. Explained and demonstrated use of call bell/intercom system. Placed call bell within client's reach. ___ ___ ___ _____

15. Side rails:

    a. Explained use to client and family.

    b. Checked agency policy for use. ___ ___ ___ _____

    c. Kept side rails up and bed in lowest position with wheels locked, as indicated. ___ ___ ___ _____

    d. Left one side rail down for oriented, ambulatory client. ___ ___ ___ _____

16. Ambularm monitoring device:

    a. Explained use to client and family.

    b. Measured client for proper size. ___ ___ ___ _____

    c. Tested battery function. ___ ___ ___ _____

    d. Identified contraindications for use. ___ ___ ___ _____

    e. Applied device appropriately. ___ ___ ___ _____

    f. Positioned client for comfort. ___ ___ ___ _____

17. Washed hands. ___ ___ ___ _____

EVALUATION

1. Observed modification of client's environment for safety needs. ___ ___ ___ _____

2. Asked client to identify safety risks. ___ ___ ___ _____

3. Reassessed motor, sensory, and cognitive status. ___ ___ ___ _____

4. Identified unexpected outcomes. ___ ___ ___ _____

RECORDING AND REPORTING

1. Recorded specific interventions to promote safety. ___ ___ ___ _____

2. Reported specific threats to safety and measures taken to reduce threats to all health care providers. ___ ___ ___ _____

Student _____   Date _____

Instructor _____   Date _____

PERFORMANCE CHECKLIST 4-2 **DESIGNING A RESTRAINT-FREE ENVIRONMENT**

	S	U	NP	Comments

ASSESSMENT

1. Assessed client's physical and mental status.   ___ ___ ___ _____

2. Assessed client's knowledge of medical condition and treatment.   ___ ___ ___ _____

NURSING DIAGNOSIS

1. Developed appropriate nursing diagnoses based on assessment data.   ___ ___ ___ _____

PLANNING

1. Developed individualized goals for client.   ___ ___ ___ _____

2. Identified expected outcomes.   ___ ___ ___ _____

IMPLEMENTATION

1. Oriented client and family to surroundings, introduced to staff, and explained all treatments and procedures.   ___ ___ ___ _____

2. Encouraged family and friends to stay with client.   ___ ___ ___ _____

3. Placed client in room close to staff.   ___ ___ ___ _____

4. Provided appropriate visual and auditory stimuli.   ___ ___ ___ _____

5. Met client needs as quickly as possible.   ___ ___ ___ _____

6. Approached client in calm, non-threatening, professional manner.   ___ ___ ___ _____

7. Limited number of care givers interacting with client.   ___ ___ ___ _____

8. Organized treatments to allow for long, uninterrupted periods.   ___ ___ ___ _____

9. Employed stress reduction techniques.   ___ ___ ___ _____

10. Used various disciplines (e.g., physical therapy).   ___ ___ ___ _____

11. Reviewed medications frequently.   ___ ___ ___ _____

EVALUATION

1. Observed client for injuries.   ___ ___ ___ _____

2. Avoided injury to others by client.   ___ ___ ___ _____

3. Identified unexpected outcomes.   ___ ___ ___ _____

	S	U	NP	Comments

RECORDING AND REPORTING

1. Recorded and reported client behaviors and nursing interventions.   __ __ __ _____

Student _____   Date _____

Instructor _____   Date _____

PERFORMANCE CHECKLIST 4-3   **APPLYING RESTRAINTS**

	S	U	NP	Comments
ASSESSMENT				
1. Assessed if client requires restraint.	—	—	—	_____
2. Reviewed agency policy and medical orders.	—	—	—	_____
3. Reviewed manufacturer's instructions for restraint use.	—	—	—	_____
4. Inspected site for restraint placement.	—	—	—	_____
NURSING DIAGNOSIS				
1. Developed appropriate nursing diagnoses based on assessment data.	—	—	—	_____
PLANNING				
1. Developed individualized goals for client.	—	—	—	_____
2. Identified expected outcomes.	—	—	—	_____
IMPLEMENTATION				
1. Identified client.	—	—	—	_____
2. Introduced self and role; explained procedure.	—	—	—	_____
3. Gathered equipment.	—	—	—	_____
4. Washed hands.	—	—	—	_____
5. Provided privacy; draped client.	—	—	—	_____
6. Adjusted bed to working height.	—	—	—	_____
7. Positioned client appropriately.	—	—	—	_____
8. Padded skin and bony prominences beneath restraint.	—	—	—	_____
9. Applied selected restraint correctly:				
a. Jacket restraint.				
b. Belt restraint.	—	—	—	_____
c. Extremity restraint.	—	—	—	_____
d. Clove-hitch restraint, if necessary.	—	—	—	_____
e. Mitten restraint.	—	—	—	_____
10. Attached restraint to bed frame, not side rails.	—	—	—	_____
11. Inserted two fingers under restraint to check for constriction.	—	—	—	_____

	S	U	NP	Comments
12. Checked placement of restraint and status of site/extremity every 30 minutes.	—	—	—	_____
13. Removed restraint for 30 minutes every 2 hours. Obtained assistance, if necessary, for client safety.	—	—	—	_____
14. Secured call bell/intercom within reach.	—	—	—	_____
15. Left bed in lowest position; locked wheels of bed or chair.	—	—	—	_____
16. Washed hands.	—	—	—	_____

EVALUATION

1. Inspected client for injury.	—	—	—	_____
2. Observed IV and urinary catheters for positioning and functioning.	—	—	—	_____
3. Identified unexpected outcomes.	—	—	—	_____

RECORDING AND REPORTING

1. Recorded in nurses' notes client's prior behavior and status; type and specific use of restraint (e.g., where and when applied); nursing interventions to promote client safety; and client's response to restraint.	—	—	—	_____

Student _____   Date _____

Instructor _____   Date _____

PERFORMANCE CHECKLIST 4-4 **SEIZURE PRECAUTIONS**

	S	U	NP	Comments
ASSESSMENT				
1. Assessed client's seizure history.	—	—	—	_____
2. Assessed client for medical and surgical conditions that may lead to or exacerbate existing seizure condition.	—	—	—	_____
3. Assessed client's medication history.	—	—	—	_____
4. Inspected client's environment for potential safety hazards.	—	—	—	_____
NURSING DIAGNOSIS				
1. Developed appropriate nursing diagnoses based on assessment data.	—	—	—	_____
PLANNING				
1. Developed individualized goals for client.	—	—	—	_____
2. Identified expected outcomes.	—	—	—	_____
IMPLEMENTATION				
1. Positioned client safely prior to and during a seizure.	—	—	—	_____
2. Provided privacy.	—	—	—	_____
3. Turned client on side with head flexed slightly forward, if possible.	—	—	—	_____
4. Did not restrain client; loosened clothing.	—	—	—	_____
5. Did not force objects into client's mouth.	—	—	—	_____
6. Remained with client, observing sequence and timing of seizure activity.	—	—	—	_____
7. Explained event and answered client's questions after seizure.	—	—	—	_____
8. Applied clean gloves and inspected oral airway when jaw relaxed for client with status epilepticus; kept own fingers away from client's mouth.	—	—	—	_____
9. Padded side rails and headboard.	—	—	—	_____
10. Assisted client to position of comfort and safety in bed following seizure.	—	—	—	_____
11. Washed hands.	—	—	—	_____

	S	U	NP	Comments

EVALUATION

1. Assessed client for traumatic injury during and after seizure. — — — _____

2. Observed client's color and respiratory status during and after seizure. — — — _____

3. Asked client to verbalize feelings after seizure. — — — _____

4. Identified unexpected outcomes. — — — _____

RECORDING AND REPORTING

1. Recorded the timing of seizure activity and sequence of events, including presence of aura, level of consciousness, and client status following seizure. — — — _____

2. Reported seizure episode to nurse in charge or physician. — — — _____

Student _____   Date _____

Instructor _____   Date _____

PERFORMANCE CHECKLIST 5-1 **REMOVING PAINFUL STIMULI**

	S	U	NP	Comments
ASSESSMENT				
1. Assessed client's level of comfort.	—	—	—	_____
2. Assessed physical and emotional signs and symptoms of acute pain of low to moderate intensity.	—	—	—	_____
3. Assessed physical and emotional signs and symptoms of severe or deep acute pain.	—	—	—	_____
4. Assessed physical and emotional signs and symptoms of chronic pain.	—	—	—	_____
5. Assessed client's behavioral responses to discomfort.	—	—	—	_____
6. Assessed characteristics of pain.	—	—	—	_____
7. Assessed environment for factors contributing to pain.	—	—	—	_____
8. Assessed precipitating factors of pain.	—	—	—	_____
9. Inspected area of pain.	—	—	—	_____
10. Identified current or previous pain management methods.	—	—	—	_____
11. Checked physician's orders for position restrictions.	—	—	—	_____
NURSING DIAGNOSIS				
1. Developed appropriate nursing diagnoses based on assessment data.	—	—	—	_____
PLANNING				
1. Developed individualized goals of comfort measures with client.	—	—	—	_____
2. Identified expected outcomes.	—	—	—	_____
3. Adjusted or controlled environmental factors affecting client's comfort.	—	—	—	_____
4. Closed room curtains or door for privacy.	—	—	—	_____
5. Explained to client that splinting with pillows and positioning can reduce pain.	—	—	—	_____
6. Explained steps to be taken to minimize pain stimuli.	—	—	—	_____

	S	U	NP	Comments

IMPLEMENTATION

1. Washed hands and applied gloves.   — — — _____

2. Removed any painful stimuli: — — — _____

   a. Positioned client so that area of discomfort is accessible.   — — — _____

   b. Kept client draped properly.   — — — _____

   c. Removed soiled dressings.   — — — _____

   d. Smoothed wrinkled bed linen.   — — — _____

   e. Loosened constrictive bandages or devices.   — — — _____

   f. Removed underlying tubes, wires, or equipment.   — — — _____

3. Splinted area of discomfort: — — — _____

   a. Explained purpose of splinting.   — — — _____

   b. Assisted client in placement of hands over painful body part.   — — — _____

   c. Assisted client to splint during coughing, deep breathing, and turning.   — — — _____

4. Positioned client comfortably: — — — _____

   a. Used pillows to support body position.   — — — _____

   b. Avoided positioning on bony prominences.   — — — _____

5. Removed and disposed of gloves and washed hands.   — — — _____

EVALUATION

1. Evaluated client's level of comfort.   — — — _____

2. Identified unexpected outcomes.   — — — _____

RECORDING AND REPORTING

1. Reported changes in character of pain or client status to nurse in charge or physician.   — — — _____

2. Recorded assessment, interventions, and client's response in nurses' notes.   — — — _____

Student _____   Date _____

Instructor _____   Date _____

PERFORMANCE CHECKLIST 5-2   **NONPHARMACOLOGIC AIDS TO PROMOTE COMFORT**

	S	U	NP	Comments
ASSESSMENT				
1. Had client identify level of pain or comfort.	___	___	___	_____
2. Assessed physiologic responses to pain.	___	___	___	_____
3. Assessed intensity and quality of client's pain.	___	___	___	_____
4. Assessed factors related to pain.	___	___	___	_____
5. Assessed factors preceding or aggravating pain experience.	___	___	___	_____
6. Examined site of client's pain.	___	___	___	_____
7. Identified current or past pain management methods.	___	___	___	_____
8. Assessed client's willingness to participate in pain-relief program.	___	___	___	_____
9. Assessed potential types of distraction.	___	___	___	_____
10. Assessed client's language level and identified terms to be used.	___	___	___	_____
NURSING DIAGNOSIS				
1. Developed appropriate nursing diagnoses based on assessment data.	___	___	___	_____
PLANNING				
1. Developed individualized goals for client based on nursing diagnoses.	___	___	___	_____
2. Identified expected outcomes.	___	___	___	_____
3. Explained purpose of technique and expectations of client during procedure. Determined if analgesic was needed prior to initial practice.	___	___	___	_____
4. Planned to explain procedures in advance.	___	U	NP	_____
5. Planned to perform technique before client's rest period.	___	___	___	_____
6. Assisted client to bathroom, if needed.	___	___	___	_____
7. Prepared environment conducive to relaxation.	___	___	___	_____
8. Closed room curtains or door for privacy.	___	___	___	_____
9. Assisted client to comfortable position.	___	___	___	_____

	S	U	NP	Comments

IMPLEMENTATION
Anticipatory Guidance

1. Explained procedure to client. ___ ___ ___ _____

2. Explained time anticipated. ___ ___ ___ _____

3. Described sensory experiences connected with procedural steps. ___ ___ ___ _____

4. Guided client verbally through procedure. ___ ___ ___ _____

5. Assisted client in returning to comfortable position. ___ ___ ___ _____

Massage

1. Washed hands. ___ ___ ___ _____

2. Adjusted bed to high position and lowered side rail. ___ ___ ___ _____

3. Assisted client to comfortable position such as prone or side-lying. ___ ___ ___ _____

4. Exposed only area to be massaged. ___ ___ ___ _____

5. Warmed lotion in hands. ___ ___ ___ _____

6. Used techniques of effleurage, pétrissage, and friction on muscle groups. ___ ___ ___ _____

7. Encouraged patient to deep breathe and relax during massage. ___ ___ ___ _____

8. Massaged client's head and scalp. ___ ___ ___ _____

9. Massaged client's hands and arms. ___ ___ ___ _____

10. Massaged neck. ___ ___ ___ _____

11. Massaged back. ___ ___ ___ _____

12. Massaged feet. ___ ___ ___ _____

13. Told client when massage was completed. ___ ___ ___ _____

14. Completed procedure by having client breathe deeply and slowly assume activity. ___ ___ ___ _____

15. Washed hands. ___ ___ ___ _____

Relaxation

1. Instructed client to breathe slowly and deeply. ___ ___ ___ _____

2. Instructed client to close eyes if desired. ___ ___ ___ _____

3. Provided verbal clues for client to follow during muscle relaxation procedure. ___ ___ ___ _____

4. On completion, instructed client to inhale deeply, exhale, and move slowly initially after a few minutes of rest. ___ ___ ___ _____

Student _____   Date _____

Instructor _____   Date _____

	S	U	NP	Comments

Guided Imagery

1. Directed client through exercise.   ___ ___ ___ _____

2. Directed client imagery with suggestions for sensory experiences.   ___ ___ ___ _____

3. Provided uninterrupted practice time for client.   ___ ___ ___ _____

Distraction

1. Directed client's attention from pain.   ___ ___ ___ _____

2. Asked client to close eyes or focus on a single object.   ___ ___ ___ _____

3. Instructed/guided client in slow rhythmic breathing.   ___ ___ ___ _____

4. Continued skill with method of choice (e.g., music, conversation).   ___ ___ ___ _____

EVALUATION

1. Determined client's physiologic and behavioral response to technique.   ___ ___ ___ _____

2. Identified unexpected outcomes.   ___ ___ ___ _____

REPORTING AND RECORDING

1. Recorded procedure, technique, preparation given to client, and client's response in nurses' notes. Recorded procedure's completion date on Kardex and included technique in Nursing Care Plan.   ___ ___ ___ _____

2. Recorded alterations in client's condition (e.g., vital signs).   ___ ___ ___ _____

3. Reported client's response to technique to nurse in charge.   ___ ___ ___ _____

4. Reported any unusual responses to techniques.   ___ ___ ___ _____

Student _____   Date _____

Instructor _____   Date _____

PERFORMANCE CHECKLIST 5-4 **EPIDURAL ANALGESIA**

	S	U	NP	Comments

ASSESSMENT

1. Assessed client's comfort level and current medical condition.

2. Assessed client's nonverbal response.

3. Assessed characteristics and intensity of pain.

4. Assessed environmental factors.

5. Assessed client's sedation level.

6. Checked client's history of drug allergies.

7. Checked rate, pattern, and depth of respirations.

8. Checked blood pressure.

9. Assessed mobility and motor and sensory function before getting client into or out of bed.

10. Determined if epidural catheter was secured to client's skin.

11. Assessed epidural catheter insertion site for signs of inflammation or infection.

12. Checked physician's order for medication and dosage.

13. If continuous infusion, checked infusion pump for proper calibration and operation.

14. If continuous infusion, checked patency of tubing.

NURSING DIAGNOSIS

1. Developed appropriate nursing diagnoses based on assessment data.

PLANNING

1. Developed individualized goals for client based on nursing diagnoses.

2. Identified expected outcomes.

3. Identified client ID.

4. Explained purpose and function of epidural analgesia and expectations of client during procedure.

5. Attached "epidural line" label for intermittent bolus or continuous infusion.

6. Provided for client's privacy.

	S	U	NP	Comments

IMPLEMENTATION

1. Washed hands and applied gloves.

2. Followed the "five rights" in preparing medication.

3. Followed correct procedure for bolus administration.

4. Followed correct procedure for continuous infusion.

5. Removed and disposed of gloves. Washed hands.

EVALUATION

1. Evaluated comfort level and compared with original assessment data.

2. Observed for signs of adverse reaction to epidurally administered narcotic.

   a. Assessed respiratory status.

   b. Monitored blood pressure and pulse.

   c. Monitored intake and output (I&O).

   d. Observed for pruritus.

   e. Observed for nausea and vomiting.

3. Checked insertion site for clear or bloody drainage. Listened for complaints of headache.

4. Monitored temperature. Observed for signs of inflammation.

5. Evaluated for paresthesias.

6. Identified unexpected outcomes.

RECORDING AND REPORTING

1. Recorded drug, dose, and time given (if injection), or time begun and ended (if infusion). Specified concentration and diluent.

2. Recorded any supplemental analgesic requirements.

3. Recorded medication on narcotic sheet.

4. If continuous infusion, obtained and recorded pump "read out" at required time intervals.

5. Recorded regular periodic assessment of client's status in nurses' notes or appropriate flowsheet.

6. Reported any adverse reactions or complications to physician.

Student _____   Date _____

Instructor _____   Date _____

PERFORMANCE CHECKLIST 6-1   **BATHING A CLIENT**

	S	U	NP	Comments
ASSESSMENT				
1. Determined client's ability to participate in bathing. Identified type of bath to be administered, e.g., complete bed bath, shower, or tub bath.	___	___	___	_____
2. Determined client's preferences for bathing practices.	___	___	___	_____
3. Noted client's awareness of existing skin problems.	___	___	___	_____
4. Identified risks for skin impairment.	___	___	___	_____
5. Assessed client's knowledge of skin hygiene.	___	___	___	_____
6. Checked physician's order for therapeutic bath.	___	___	___	_____
7. Reviewed restrictions affecting client's movement or positioning during bath.	___	___	___	_____
NURSING DIAGNOSIS				
1. Developed appropriate nursing diagnoses based on assessment data.	___	___	___	_____
PLANNING				
1. Developed individualized goals for client based on nursing diagnoses.	___	___	___	_____
2. Identified expected outcomes.	___	___	___	_____
3. Explained procedure to client.	___	___	___	_____
4. Adjusted room temperature and ventilation for client's comfort and provided for client's privacy during bath.	___	___	___	_____
5. Prepared necessary equipment and supplies.	___	___	___	_____
IMPLEMENTATION				
Complete or Partial Bed Bath				
1. Offered bedpan or urinal before bath.	___	___	___	_____
2. Washed hands and applied gloves if needed.	___	___	___	_____
3. Lowered side rail, assisted client in assuming comfortable position, and positioned client to avoid strain on nurse.	___	___	___	_____
4. Used bath blanket properly while removing top linens of bed.	___	___	___	_____
5. Disposed of soiled linen correctly.	___	___	___	_____

	S	U	NP	Comments

6. Removed client's gown correctly.

7. Raised side rail and filled washbasin two-thirds full; checked temperature of bathwater and client's tolerance. Warmed bath lotion, if desired.

8. Removed pillow if allowed and raised head of bed; placed a towel under client's head and a towel over client's chest.

9. Folded washcloth into mitt.

10. Washed and dried client's eyes correctly (without using soap).

11. Washed, rinsed, and dried client's forehead, cheeks, nose, neck, and ears, using or avoiding soap as appropriate.

12. Removed bath blanket from client's far arm and placed bath towel under arm.

13. Bathed client's far arm and axilla.

14. Rinsed and dried arm and axilla thoroughly; provided deodorant (or talcum powder if used by client).

15. Followed procedure for soaking and drying client's hand.

16. Repeated Steps 12-15 for other arm.

17. Checked temperature of bathwater and changed water if necessary.

18. Placed bath towel and blanket correctly for washing client's chest; washed, rinsed, and dried chest correctly.

19. Placed bath towel and blanket correctly for washing client's abdomen.

20. Washed, rinsed, and dried abdomen correctly.

21. Applied clothing if appropriate to maintain client's warmth and comfort.

22. Draped client correctly for washing far leg.

23. Followed procedure for placing towel under client's leg and asked client to hold foot still while positioning basin near foot.

24. Placed foot in basin and allowed it to soak while washing leg.

25. Washed leg from ankle to knee; from knee to thigh. Dried well.

Student _____   Date _____

Instructor _____   Date _____

	S	U	NP	Comments
26. Washed and dried foot correctly. Provided nail care.	___	___	___	_____
27. Repeated Steps 22-26 for other leg and foot.	___	___	___	_____
28. Covered client with bath blanket and changed bathwater.	___	___	___	_____
29. Positioned client correctly for bathing back and buttocks.	___	___	___	_____
30. Kept client properly draped for bathing back and buttocks.	___	___	___	_____
31. Washed, rinsed, and dried client's back from neck to buttocks.	___	___	___	_____
32. Changed bathwater and washcloth. Applied gloves, if not done before.	___	___	___	_____
33. Positioned and draped client in correct position for washing genitalia; washed, rinsed, and dried perineum or allowed client to do so.	___	___	___	_____
34. Disposed of gloves.	___	___	___	_____
35. Applied moisturizing lotion to skin.	___	___	___	_____
36. Assisted client in dressing; combed client's hair.	___	___	___	_____
37. Made client's bed.	___	___	___	_____
38. Disposed of soiled linen properly; cleaned and replaced bathing equipment; replaced call light and personal possessions.	___	___	___	_____
39. Washed hands.	___	___	___	_____

Tub Bath or Shower

	S	U	NP	Comments
1. Considered client's condition and reviewed medical orders.	___	___	___	_____
2. Scheduled use of shower or tub.	___	___	___	_____
3. Cleaned tub or shower according to agency policy; provided rubber bath mat or disposable mat to prevent slipping.	___	___	___	_____
4. Arranged all hygienic aids, toilet items, and linen within reach of client.	___	___	___	_____
5. Assisted client into tub or shower.	___	___	___	_____
6. Instructed client on use of call signal.	___	___	___	_____
7. Placed "occupied" sign on bathroom door.	___	___	___	_____

	S	U	NP	Comments

8. Filled tub halfway, adjusted water temperature, and instructed client on use of faucets. If client took shower, turned shower on and adjusted water temperature before client entered shower stall.   ___ ___ ___ _____

9. Instructed client on use of safety bars and cautioned client against use of bath oil in tub water.   ___ ___ ___ _____

10. Cautioned client against remaining in tub for over 20 minutes and checked on client every 5 minutes.   ___ ___ ___ _____

11. Returned to bathroom when client signaled and knocked before entering.   ___ ___ ___ _____

12. Drained water from tub; placed bath towel over client's shoulders; assisted client in getting out of tub and with drying.   ___ ___ ___ _____

13. Assisted client with dressing.   ___ ___ ___ _____

14. Assisted client in returning to room.   ___ ___ ___ _____

15. Prepared bathroom for next use.   ___ ___ ___ _____

16. Washed hands.   ___ ___ ___ _____

EVALUATION

1. Assessed skin for signs of breakdown or irritation.   ___ ___ ___ _____

2. Assessed extent of range of motion (ROM) during bath.   ___ ___ ___ _____

3. Determined client's comfort and level of fatigue.   ___ ___ ___ _____

4. Assessed vital signs if necessary.   ___ ___ ___ _____

5. Assessed client's knowledge of proper hygiene techniques.   ___ ___ ___ _____

6. Identified unexpected outcomes.   ___ ___ ___ _____

RECORDING AND REPORTING

1. Recorded bath on flowsheet and noted level of assistance required.   ___ ___ ___ _____

2. Recorded condition of skin and significant findings.   ___ ___ ___ _____

3. Reported evidence of alterations in skin integrity to nurse in charge or physician.   ___ ___ ___ _____

Student _____   Date _____

Instructor _____   Date _____

PERFORMANCE CHECKLIST 6-2 **PROVIDING PERINEAL CARE**

	S	U	NP	Comments
ASSESSMENT				
1. Identified client's risk for developing infection of genitalia, urinary tract, or reproductive tract.	___	___	___	_____
2. Assessed client's ability to perform own perineal care.	___	___	___	_____
3. Assessed condition of genitalia.	___	___	___	_____
4. Assessed client's knowledge of importance of perineal hygiene.	___	___	___	_____
NURSING DIAGNOSIS				
1. Developed appropriate nursing diagnoses based on assessment data.	___	___	___	_____
PLANNING				
1. Developed individualized goals for client based on nursing diagnoses.	___	___	___	_____
2. Identified expected outcomes.	___	___	___	_____
3. Explained procedure and its purpose to client.	___	___	___	_____
4. Prepared necessary equipment and supplies.	___	___	___	_____
IMPLEMENTATION				
1. Provided for client's privacy during perineal care; assembled supplies at bedside.	___	___	___	_____
2. Raised client's bed to comfortable working position; lowered side rail and assisted client in assuming proper position.	___	___	___	_____
3. Applied disposable gloves.	___	___	___	_____
4. Removed fecal material, if present. Cleansed, rinsed, and dried buttocks and anus thoroughly.	___	___	___	_____
5. Changed soiled gloves.	___	___	___	_____
6. Folded top bed linen down and raised client's gown.	___	___	___	_____
7. Applied "diamond" drape correctly.	___	___	___	_____
8. Raised side rail. Filled washbasin with water and tested temperature.	___	___	___	_____
9. Placed washbasin and tissue on overbed table. Placed washcloths in basin.	___	___	___	_____

	S	U	NP	Comments

10. Provided perineal care. ___ ___ ___ _____

Female Perineal Care

a. Lowered side rail and positioned client for full exposure of genitalia. ___ ___ ___ _____

b. Uncovered genitalia, washed and dried client's upper thighs. ___ ___ ___ _____

c. Retracted labia and correctly cleansed, rinsed, and dried skinfolds. ___ ___ ___ _____

d. Separated labia to expose urethral meatus and vaginal orifice and correctly cleaned area. ___ ___ ___ _____

e. Poured warm water over perineal area if client was on bedpan and dried perineal area thoroughly. ___ ___ ___ _____

f. Covered client with bath blanket and positioned comfortably. ___ ___ ___ _____

Male Perineal Care

a. Lowered side rail. Noted any mobility restrictions. ___ ___ ___ _____

b. Uncovered perineum. Washed and dried client's upper thighs. ___ ___ ___ _____

c. Positioned towel under penis; gently grasped shaft of penis; retracted foreskin if client uncircumcised. ___ ___ ___ _____

d. Cleansed, rinsed, and dried glans penis correctly. Deferred procedure if client has an erection. ___ ___ ___ _____

e. Returned foreskin to natural position after cleansing. ___ ___ ___ _____

f. Gently washed, rinsed, and dried shaft of penis on all surfaces; rinsed and dried penis thoroughly; instructed client to abduct legs for washing of scrotum. ___ ___ ___ _____

g. Gently washed, rinsed, and dried scrotum, including underlying skinfolds. ___ ___ ___ _____

h. Covered perineum and positioned client on side. ___ ___ ___ _____

11. Applied thin layer of skin barrier over anal and perineal area if client has had bladder or bowel incontinence. ___ ___ ___ _____

12. Removed and disposed of gloves. ___ ___ ___ _____

13. Assisted client to comfortable position and returned covers. ___ ___ ___ _____

Student _____   Date _____

Instructor _____   Date _____

	S	U	NP	Comments

14. Removed bath blanket and disposed of soiled linen. Returned unused equipment.   ___ ___ ___ _____

EVALUATION

1. Inspected surface of external genitalia and surrounding skin after cleansing.   ___ ___ ___ _____

2. Assessed client's level of comfort and cleanliness.   ___ ___ ___ _____

3. Noted presence of any abnormal drainage or discharge from genitalia.   ___ ___ ___ _____

4. Evaluated client's ability to perform hygiene.   ___ ___ ___ _____

5. Identified unexpected outcomes.   ___ ___ ___ _____

RECORDING AND REPORTING

1. Recorded procedure and presence of any abnormal findings in nurses' notes or on flowsheet.   ___ ___ ___ _____

2. Recorded appearance of suture line, if present.   ___ ___ ___ _____

3. Reported any break in suture line or presence of abnormalities to nurse in charge or physician.   ___ ___ ___ _____

Student _____　Date _____

Instructor _____　Date _____

PERFORMANCE CHECKLIST 6-3　**BRUSHING TEETH**

	S	U	NP	Comments
ASSESSMENT				
1. Washed hands. Applied disposable gloves.	—	—	—	_____
2. Made physical assessment of oral cavity (with gloves).	—	—	—	_____
3. Removed gloves and washed hands.	—	—	—	_____
4. Assessed client's risk for oral hygiene problems.	—	—	—	_____
5. Identified presence of common oral problems.	—	—	—	_____
6. Assessed client's oral hygiene practices.	—	—	—	_____
7. Assessed client's ability to grasp and manipulate toothbrush.	—	—	—	_____
NURSING DIAGNOSIS				
1. Developed appropriate nursing diagnoses based on assessment data.	—	—	—	_____
PLANNING				
1. Developed individualized goals for client based on nursing diagnoses.	—	—	—	_____
2. Identified expected outcomes.	—	—	—	_____
3. Prepared equipment at bedside.	—	—	—	_____
4. Explained procedure to client.	—	—	—	_____
IMPLEMENTATION				
1. Arranged equipment on paper towels on bedside table.	—	—	—	_____
2. Raised bed to comfortable working position, lowered side rail, positioned client on side near nurse in semi-Fowler's position to avoid aspiration.	—	—	—	_____
3. Placed towel over client's chest to prevent soiling gown and bed linen.	—	—	—	_____
4. Applied gloves.	—	—	—	_____
5. Applied toothpaste to brush and moistened paste.	—	—	—	_____
6. Held or had client hold toothbrush at 45-degree angle to gum line and used short strokes to brush tooth surfaces from gum to crown; held brush parallel to teeth to clean biting surfaces; brushed sides of teeth, moving bristles back and forth.	—	—	—	_____

	S	U	NP	Comments

7. Held or had client hold brush at 45-degree angle and lightly brushed tongue surface without stimulating gag reflex.   — — — _____

8. Provided water for client to rinse mouth thoroughly.   — — — _____

9. Offered mouthwash for gargling and rinsing.   — — — _____

10. Assisted in wiping client's mouth.   — — — _____

11. Allowed client to floss.   — — — _____

12. Allowed client to rinse mouth thoroughly with tepid water after flossing.   — — — _____

13. Repositioned client comfortably after procedure.   — — — _____

14. Disposed of equipment and soiled linen properly.   — — — _____

15. Washed hands.   — — — _____

EVALUATION

1. Assessed client's comfort level.   — — — _____

2. Applied gloves and inspected condition of oral cavity.   — — — _____

3. Asked client to describe proper hygiene techniques.   — — — _____

4. Observed client brushing.   — — — _____

5. Identified unexpected outcomes.   — — — _____

RECORDING AND REPORTING

1. Recorded procedure on flowsheet. Included condition of oral cavity in nurses' notes.   — — — _____

2. Reported any unusual findings to nurse in charge or physician.   — — — _____

Student _____ Date _____

Instructor _____ Date _____

PERFORMANCE CHECKLIST 6-4   **PERFORMING MOUTH CARE FOR THE UNCONSCIOUS OR DEBILITATED CLIENT**

	S	U	NP	Comments

ASSESSMENT

1. Washed hands. Applied disposable gloves.

2. Tested for presence of gag reflex.

3. Conducted physical assessment of oral cavity.

4. Removed gloves. Washed hands.

5. Assessed client's risk for oral hygiene problems.

NURSING DIAGNOSIS

1. Developed appropriate nursing diagnoses based on assessment data.

PLANNING

1. Developed individualized goals for client based on nursing diagnoses.

2. Identified expected outcomes.

3. Positioned client on side with head turned toward dependent side and head of bed lowered. Raised side rail.

4. Explained procedure to client.

IMPLEMENTATION

1. Washed hands and applied disposable gloves.

2. Properly arranged equipment and turned on suction device.

3. Closed curtain or room door for privacy.

4. Raised bed and lowered side rail to have easy access to client; raised side rail when client was unattended.

5. Positioned client on side of bed near you; kept client positioned on side with head turned toward mattress to prevent aspiration.

6. Placed towel under client's face and positioned emesis basin under client's chin.

7. Separated client's upper and lower teeth correctly with tongue blade.

	S	U	NP	Comments
8. Cleaned teeth and mucosa using brush or padded tongue blade moistened in water and peroxide; thoroughly swabbed areas of accumulated crusts or secretions; suctioned oral cavity as secretions accumulated (may have second nurse assist); thoroughly rinsed oral cavity.	___	___	___	_____
9. Applied water-soluble jelly to lips.	___	___	___	_____
10. Informed client that procedure was completed.	___	___	___	_____
11. Removed gloves and disposed in proper receptacle.	___	___	___	_____
12. Repositioned client safely and comfortably after procedure.	___	___	___	_____
13. Disposed of equipment and soiled linen properly.	___	___	___	_____
14. Washed hands.	___	___	___	_____

EVALUATION

	S	U	NP	Comments
1. Applied gloves and inspected oral cavity.	___	___	___	_____
2. Assessed client's level of comfort.	___	___	___	_____
3. Assessed client's respirations on an ongoing basis.	___	___	___	_____
4. Identified unexpected outcomes.	___	___	___	_____

RECORDING AND REPORTING

	S	U	NP	Comments
1. Recorded procedure including description of the condition of the oral cavity.	___	___	___	_____
2. Reported any unusual findings to nurse in charge or physician.	___	___	___	_____

Student _____   Date _____

Instructor _____   Date _____

PERFORMANCE CHECKLIST 6-5 **CLEANING DENTURES**

	S	U	NP	Comments

ASSESSMENT

1. Assessed condition of gums and mucosa and surfaces of dentures.   ___ ___ ___ _____

2. Determined if dentures are loose fitting.   ___ ___ ___ _____

3. Assessed type of denture cleaner client uses.   ___ ___ ___ _____

4. Assessed home routines for denture care.   ___ ___ ___ _____

NURSING DIAGNOSIS

1. Developed appropriate nursing diagnoses based on assessment data.   ___ ___ ___ _____

PLANNING

1. Developed individualized goals for client based on nursing diagnoses.   ___ ___ ___ _____

2. Identified expected outcomes.   ___ ___ ___ _____

3. Explained procedure to client.   ___ ___ ___ _____

IMPLEMENTATION

1. Washed hands.   ___ ___ ___ _____

2. Arranged supplies on bedside table or near sink.   ___ ___ ___ _____

3. Added tepid water to emesis basin or sink lined with washcloth.   ___ ___ ___ _____

4. Applied disposable gloves.   ___ ___ ___ _____

5. Asked client to remove dentures. If client unable to remove dentures, removed dentures by grasping upper denture at front with thumb and index finger wrapped in gauze and pulling downward; lifted lower denture and rotated one side downward; placed dentures in emesis basin or sink.   ___ ___ ___ _____

6. Thoroughly brushed all denture surfaces with denture or regular toothbrush and dentifrice.   ___ ___ ___ _____

7. Thoroughly rinsed dentures with tepid water.   ___ ___ ___ _____

8. Stored dentures securely in denture cup containing tepid water.   ___ ___ ___ _____

9. Emptied emesis basin and added fresh water; used soft toothbrush to brush client's gums, palate, and tongue.   ___ ___ ___ _____

	S	U	NP	Comments
10. Had client rinse mouth thoroughly.	——	——	——	_____
11. Reinserted dentures according to client's preferences (moistened denture before reinsertion); checked to see if dentures were sealed in place.	——	——	——	_____
12. Disposed of gloves. Cleaned and stored supplies after procedure. Washed hands.	——	——	——	_____

EVALUATION

1. Questioned client regarding comfort of dentures.	——	——	——	_____
2. Inspected condition of oral cavity.	——	——	——	_____
3. Asked client to explain steps in denture care.	——	——	——	_____
4. Identified unexpected outcomes.	——	——	——	_____

RECORDING AND REPORTING

1. Correctly recorded procedure on flowsheets or nurses' notes. Noted any abnormalities.	——	——	——	_____

Student _____   Date _____

Instructor _____   Date _____

PERFORMANCE CHECKLIST 6-6   **SHAMPOOING THE HAIR OF A BEDRIDDEN CLIENT**

	S	U	NP	Comments

ASSESSMENT

1. Identified any factors that contraindicated shampooing.   ___ ___ ___ _____

2. Assessed positioning restrictions.   ___ ___ ___ _____

3. Determined if medicated soap was ordered.   ___ ___ ___ _____

4. Determined client's routine for hair care practices.   ___ ___ ___ _____

5. Assessed client's hair and scalp.   ___ ___ ___ _____

NURSING DIAGNOSIS

1. Developed appropriate nursing diagnoses based on assessment data.   ___ ___ ___ _____

PLANNING

1. Developed individualized goals for client based on nursing diagnoses.   ___ ___ ___ _____

2. Identified expected outcomes.   ___ ___ ___ _____

3. Explained procedure to client.   ___ ___ ___ _____

IMPLEMENTATION

1. Washed hands.   ___ ___ ___ _____

2. Arranged equipment within easy reach and lowered side rail.   ___ ___ ___ _____

3. Protected bed linen with waterproof pad; properly positioned client supine with shampoo trough under head and washbasin at end of trough.   ___ ___ ___ _____

4. Placed rolled towel under client's neck; draped client's shoulders with towel.   ___ ___ ___ _____

5. Brushed and combed client's hair before shampooing.   ___ ___ ___ _____

6. Checked water temperature.   ___ ___ ___ _____

7. Provided client with towel to cover eyes during shampooing.   ___ ___ ___ _____

8. Rinsed hair thoroughly before shampooing.   ___ ___ ___ _____

9. Lathered hair thoroughly; worked from hairline toward back of neck to sides of head; used fingertips to massage scalp.   ___ ___ ___ _____

	S	U	NP	Comments
10. Rinsed hair thoroughly.	___	___	___	_____
11. Repeated Steps 8-10 if needed.	___	___	___	_____
12. Applied conditioner or cream rinse as client desired.	___	___	___	_____
13. Used bath towel to wrap client's head and dried moisture from around eyes, face, and neck.	___	___	___	_____
14. Dried hair thoroughly.	___	___	___	_____
15. Combed hair gently to remove tangles and completed drying with dryer if desired.	___	___	___	_____
16. Applied oil or conditioner if desired.	___	___	___	_____
17. Brushed and styled hair with client in comfortable position.	___	___	___	_____
18. Returned equipment to its proper place, disposed of soiled linen, and washed hands.	___	___	___	_____

EVALUATION

	S	U	NP	Comments
1. Asked client how hair felt after shampooing.	___	___	___	_____
2. Inspected condition of hair.	___	___	___	_____
3. Identified unexpected outcomes.	___	___	___	_____

RECORDING AND REPORTING

	S	U	NP	Comments
1. Recorded pertinent findings related to condition of hair or scalp.	___	___	___	_____

Student _____   Date _____

Instructor _____   Date _____

PERFORMANCE CHECKLIST 6-7 **SHAVING A CLIENT**

	S	U	NP	Comments
ASSESSMENT				
1. Determined if client has bleeding tendency.	—	—	—	_____
2. Assessed client's ability to manipulate razor.	—	—	—	_____
3. Assessed client's preferences for hygiene products to use to shave.	—	—	—	_____
NURSING DIAGNOSIS				
1. Developed appropriate nursing diagnoses based on assessment data.	—	—	—	_____
PLANNING				
1. Developed individualized goals for client based on nursing diagnoses.	—	—	—	_____
2. Identified expected outcomes.	—	—	—	_____
3. Prepared client by instructing him to indicate if shave became uncomfortable and asked if there were special steps to follow while shaving.	—	—	—	_____
IMPLEMENTATION				
Disposable Razor				
1. Arranged supplies at bedside table and adjusted lighting.	—	—	—	_____
2. Assisted client to sitting or supine position with head of bed elevated.	—	—	—	_____
3. Placed towel over client's chest and around shoulders.	—	—	—	_____
4. Adjusted water temperature to comfortable level or as client preferred.	—	—	—	_____
5. Applied warm, damp cloth to client's face to soften beard.	—	—	—	_____
6. Applied shaving cream or soap to client's face. Applied gloves, if indicated.	—	—	—	_____
7. Shaved one side of face at a time, using nondominant hand to pull skin taut; used short strokes in same direction as hair grows.	—	—	—	_____
8. Removed cream from blade by dipping razor in water.	—	—	—	_____
9. Rinsed client's face with warm, moist washcloth.	—	—	—	_____

	S	U	NP	Comments

10. Dried face and applied aftershave if client desired.

11. Assisted client to comfortable position.

12. Returned supplies to proper place, discarded soiled linen properly, (removed gloves, if worn) washed hands.

Electric Razor

1. Performed Steps 1-3 for disposable razor procedure.

2. Applied skin conditioner or pre-shave lotion.

3. Shaved one side of face at a time, holding skin taut and using gentle downward strokes.

4. Applied aftershave if client requested.

5. Performed Steps 11 and 12 for disposable razor procedure.

Mustache and Beard Care

1. Performed Steps 1-3 for disposable razor.

2. Gently combed mustache or beard if necessary.

3. Allowed client to use mirror to direct areas to trim with scissors.

EVALUATION

1. Inspected condition of shaved area and skin underneath beard or mustache.

2. Assessed client's level of comfort and satisfaction with degree of participation.

3. Identified unexpected outcomes.

Student _____ Date _____

Instructor _____ Date _____

PERFORMANCE CHECKLIST 6-8 **PERFORMING NAIL AND FOOT CARE**

	S	U	NP	Comments
ASSESSMENT				
1. Inspected all surfaces of feet and nails.	—	—	—	_____
2. Assessed circulatory status of toes, feet, and fingers.	—	—	—	_____
3. Observed client's gait and determined relationship to local foot or nail problems.	—	—	—	_____
4. Assessed female client's use of nail polish or polish removal.	—	—	—	_____
5. Assessed type of footwear worn by client.	—	—	—	_____
6. Identified client's risk for foot or nail problems.	—	—	—	_____
7. Assessed client's use of home remedies for foot problems.	—	—	—	_____
8. Assessed client's ability to perform foot and nail care.	—	—	—	_____
9. Assessed client's knowledge of foot and nail care practices.	—	—	—	_____
NURSING DIAGNOSIS				
1. Developed appropriate nursing diagnoses based on assessment data.	—	—	—	_____
PLANNING				
1. Developed individualized goals for client based on nursing diagnoses.	—	—	—	_____
2. Identified expected outcomes.	—	—	—	_____
3. Explained procedure to client.	—	—	—	_____
4. Obtained physician's order to cut nails.	—	—	—	_____
IMPLEMENTATION				
1. Washed hands and arranged supplies on overbed table.	—	—	—	_____
2. Closed room door or curtain for privacy.	—	—	—	_____
3. Assisted client to chair (when possible); placed bath mat under client's feet.	—	—	—	_____
4. Prepared washbasin with water; tested water temperature.	—	—	—	_____
5. Placed washbasin on bath mat on floor and helped client place feet in basin; put call light within reach.	—	—	—	_____

S   U   NP   Comments

6. Adjusted overbed table to low position and placed it over client's lap.
___ ___ ___ _____

7. Filled emesis basin with water and tested temperature; placed emesis basin on overbed table.
___ ___ ___ _____

8. Instructed client to position fingertips in basin, with arms in comfortable position.
___ ___ ___ _____

9. Had client soak fingers and feet for approximately 10-20 minutes and rewarmed water as needed during soaking.
___ ___ ___ _____

10. Used orange stick gently to clean debris from under fingernails while fingers were immersed; removed emesis basin and dried fingers thoroughly.
___ ___ ___ _____

11. Clipped fingernails straight across and shaped with file or emery board; avoided cutting nails at nail bed. Filed nails of client with circulatory problems.
___ ___ ___ _____

12. Used orange stick to gently push back cuticles.
___ ___ ___ _____

13. Moved overbed table away from client.
___ ___ ___ _____

14. Applied disposable gloves before giving foot care; scrubbed calluses of feet with washcloth.
___ ___ ___ _____

15. Cleaned under toenails gently with orange stick; dried feet thoroughly.
___ ___ ___ _____

16. Trimmed toenails using procedures in Steps 11 and 12, avoided filing corners of toenails.
___ ___ ___ _____

17. Applied lotion to feet and hands and assisted client back to bed and into comfortable position.
___ ___ ___ _____

18. Properly disposed of gloves and soiled linen, cleaned and returned equipment and supplies to proper place, washed hands.
___ ___ ___ _____

EVALUATION

1. Inspected nails and skin surfaces after soaking.
___ ___ ___ _____

2. Asked client to explain or demonstrate nail care.
___ ___ ___ _____

3. Assessed client's walk after nail care.
___ ___ ___ _____

4. Identified unexpected outcomes.
___ ___ ___ _____

RECORDING AND REPORTING

1. Recorded procedure and observations related to condition of nails and feet.
___ ___ ___ _____

2. Reported presence of foot ulcers or other breaks in skin to nurse in charge or physician.
___ ___ ___ _____

Student _____   Date _____

Instructor _____   Date _____

PERFORMANCE CHECKLIST 7-1 **MAKING AN UNOCCUPIED BED**

	S	U	NP	Comments

ASSESSMENT

1. Verified client's activity orders and assessed client's ability to get out of bed.

2. Assessed potential for client incontinence or excess drainage on linen.

3. Determined if client should assume any position precautions while out of bed.

NURSING DIAGNOSIS

1. Developed appropriate nursing diagnoses.

PLANNING

1. Developed individualized goals for client based on assessment data.

2. Identified expected outcomes.

3. Determined best time to change linens. Explained procedure to client; assisted client to chair if needed.

IMPLEMENTATION

1. Washed hands and donned gloves.

2. Assembled all necessary equipment with linen stacked in order of use (top to bottom). Removed furniture and equipment from around bed before making.

3. Lowered side rails and removed call light from bed; adjusted bed to a comfortable working height position.

4. Loosened all soiled linen from under mattress.

5. Removed bedspread and blanket separately and discarded properly; did not shake or allow linen to come in contact with uniform.

6. When reusing blanket or spread, folded each correctly into square.

7. Removed soiled pillowcases correctly by slipping each pillow out from case.

8. Folded each piece of soiled linen separately before discarding.

	S	U	NP	Comments

9. Repositioned mattress toward head of bed; cleaned any moisture off mattress with appropriate disinfectant.

10. Stood at side of bed where linen is placed, and spread mattress pad over mattress; smoothed out all wrinkles on pad.

11. Applied bottom sheet correctly to bed, one side at a time, keeping seam edge down.

12. Made mitered corner in top corner of bottom sheet.

13. Tucked bottom sheet tightly under mattress; applied drawsheet to bed correctly; tucked excess edge of drawsheet under mattress, keeping palms down.

14. Moved to opposite side of bed.

15. Spread fanfolded bottom sheet smoothly over bed.

16. Mitered top corner of bottom sheet.

17. Used good body mechanics by keeping back straight while tucking linen tightly under mattress. Frequently observed client for tolerance to sitting in chair.

18. Smoothed folded drawsheet over bottom sheet and tucked tightly.

19. Applied waterproof pads according to client's need.

20. Moved to side of bed where linen was placed and applied all top linen to one side of bed at a time.

21. Correctly made horizontal toe pleat in top sheet.

22. Tucked in remaining portion of top sheet under foot of mattress (optional).

23. Placed blanket correctly on bed.

24. Placed bedspread over bed according to Step 8.

25. Made cuff out of top edge of sheet, blanket, and bedspread.

26. Correctly tucked bottom linen together under mattress at foot of bed.

27. Made a modified mitered corner at bottom edge of mattress.

28. Moved to opposite side of bed to complete application of top linen.

Student _____   Date _____

Instructor _____   Date _____

	S	U	NP	Comments
29. Correctly applied a clean pillowcase over pillow.	___	___	___	_____
30. Placed pillow at center of head of bed; placed call light within client's reach. Returned bed to low comfortable height.	___	___	___	_____
31. Folded back top linen to side or fanfolded linen down to bottom third of bed.	___	___	___	_____
32. Rearranged furniture around bedside and placed client's personal items within easy reach.	___	___	___	_____
33. Discarded dirty linen properly. Removed gloves and washed hands.	___	___	___	_____

EVALUATION

	S	U	NP	Comments
1. Assessed client's tolerance to sitting in chair.	___	___	___	_____
2. Assessed client's level of comfort and condition of skin upon return to bed.	___	___	___	_____
3. Identified unexpected outcomes.	___	___	___	_____

RECORDING AND REPORTING

	S	U	NP	Comments
1. Documentation not required. Record only changes in client status.	___	___	___	_____

Student _____   Date _____

Instructor _____   Date _____

PERFORMANCE CHECKLIST 7-2 **MAKING AN OCCUPIED BED**

	S	U	NP	Comments
ASSESSMENT				
1. Determined need to apply waterproof pads.	—	—	—	_____
2. Assessed restrictions affecting client's positioning and movement during bed making.	—	—	—	_____
NURSING DIAGNOSIS				
1. Developed appropriate nursing diagnoses.	—	—	—	_____
PLANNING				
1. Developed individualized goals for client based on assessment data.	—	—	—	_____
2. Identified expected outcomes.	—	—	—	_____
3. Explained procedure to client.	—	—	—	_____
IMPLEMENTATION				
1. Washed hands and donned gloves.	—	—	—	_____
2. Assembled equipment with linen stacked in order of use (top to bottom). Removed unnecessary equipment.	—	—	—	_____
3. Closed curtain or room door for client's privacy.	—	—	—	_____
4. Adjusted bed to comfortable working height; lowered side rail on working side and removed call light.	—	—	—	_____
5. Loosened top linen sheet at foot of bed.	—	—	—	_____
6. Removed bedspread and blanket separately by folding and discarding into linen bag. Did not allow soiled linen to come in contact with uniform.	—	—	—	_____
7. When reusing blanket or spread, folded each correctly into a square.	—	—	—	_____
8. Covered client with bath blanket and removed top sheet without exposing body parts.	—	—	—	_____
9. Repositioned mattress toward head of bed with assistance from another nurse.	—	—	—	_____
10. Assisted client to side-lying position. Elevated side rail.	—	—	—	_____
11. Loosened bottom linen from head to foot of bed.	—	—	—	_____

	S	U	NP	Comments

12. Fanfolded soiled bottom and drawsheet and tucked them under client's shoulders, back, and buttocks.

13. Cleaned soiled mattress with appropriate disinfectant.

14. Applied clean bottom linen to one side of bed at a time.

15. Correctly made mitered corner in top corner of bottom sheet.

16. Tucked bottom sheet tightly under mattress.

17. Put drawsheet in place correctly.

18. Placed waterproof pad on bed.

19. Raised side rail on working side and moved to other side of bed.

20. Lowered side rail and assisted client in rolling over folds of linen; loosened edges of soiled linen from underneath mattress.

21. Discarded linen correctly in linen bag. Cleaned mattress, if necessary.

22. Spread clean, fanfolded linen smoothly over edge of mattress from head to foot of bed.

23. Positioned client supine on bottom linen.

24. Mitered top corner of bottom sheet.

25. Tucked all bottom linen under mattress.

26. Smoothed fanfolded drawsheet and tucked under mattress.

27. Placed top sheet over client and unfolded from head to foot.

28. Removed bath blanket and discarded it into linen bag.

29. Placed blanket correctly on bed.

30. Placed bedspread correctly on bed.

31. Made cuff out of top edge of sheet, blanket, and bedspread.

32. Tucked top sheet, blanket, and spread under mattress.

33. Made modified mitered corner with top sheet, blanket, and spread.

34. Raised side rail. Made other side of bed.

Student _____   Date _____

Instructor _____   Date _____

	S	U	NP	Comments

35. Removed and discarded soiled pillow case. Correctly applied clean pillow case over pillow.   ___ ___ ___ _____

36. Repositioned pillow under client's head.   ___ ___ ___ _____

37. Placed call light within client's reach and returned bed to comfortable position.   ___ ___ ___ _____

38. Opened room curtains. Rearranged furniture around bedside and placed client's personal items within easy reach. Returned bed to comfortable height.   ___ ___ ___ _____

39. Discarded linen bag properly. Removed gloves and washed hands.   ___ ___ ___ _____

EVALUATION

1. Assessed client's level of comfort.   ___ ___ ___ _____

2. Inspected skin for irritated areas.   ___ ___ ___ _____

3. Observed for signs of fatigue, dyspnea, pain, or discomfort.   ___ ___ ___ _____

4. Identified unexpected outcomes.   ___ ___ ___ _____

RECORDING AND REPORTING

1. Documentation not required.   ___ ___ ___ _____

Student _____   Date _____

Instructor _____   Date _____

PERFORMANCE CHECKLIST 8-1 **RISK ASSESSMENT AND PREVENTION STRATEGIES**

	S	U	NP	Comments

ASSESSMENT

1. Identified client's risk for pressure ulcer formation.

2. Selected risk assessment tool.

3. Obtained client's "Risk Score."

4. Assessed condition of client's skin, particularly over potential pressure sites.

5. Assessed client for additional areas of potential pressure.

6. Observed client for preferred positions when in bed or chair.

7. Assessed client's ability to initiate and assist with position changes.

8. Assessed client's and support person's understanding of risks of pressure ulcers.

NURSING DIAGNOSIS

1. Developed appropriate nursing diagnoses based on assessment data.

PLANNING

1. Developed individualized goals for client based on nursing diagnoses.

2. Identified expected outcomes.

3. Explained procedure(s) and purpose to client and family.

4. Washed hands and prepared needed equipment and supplies.

IMPLEMENTATION

1. Provided for client's privacy.

2. Applied disposable gloves.

3. Positioned client comfortably so that ulcer was easily accessible.

4. Assessed for redness in area that was under pressure. Palpated areas of discoloration or mottling.

5. Monitored length of time area of redness persisted.

	S	U	NP	Comments

6. Implemented Pressure Ulcer Prevention Points. ___ ___ ___ _____

7. Removed gloves, disposed of properly. Washed hands. ___ ___ ___ _____

EVALUATION

1. Assessed condition of skin areas at risk for change in color, texture. ___ ___ ___ _____

2. Assessed client's tolerance of position changes. ___ ___ ___ _____

3. Compared subsequent risk assessment scores. ___ ___ ___ _____

4. Identified unexpected outcomes. ___ ___ ___ _____

RECORDING AND REPORTING

1. Recorded client's "Risk Score." ___ ___ ___ _____

2. Recorded appearance of skin area under pressure. ___ ___ ___ _____

3. Recorded positions, turning intervals, and other preventive measures. ___ ___ ___ _____

4. Reported need for additional consultations for the high-risk client. ___ ___ ___ _____

Student _____   Date _____

Instructor _____   Date _____

PERFORMANCE CHECKLIST 8-2   **TREATMENT OF PRESSURE ULCERS**

	S	U	NP	Comments
ASSESSMENT				
1. Assessed client's level of comfort and need for pain medication.	—	—	—	_____
2. Determined presence of allergies to topical agents.	—	—	—	_____
3. Reviewed physician's order for topical agent or dressing.	—	—	—	_____
4. Washed hands and applied clean gloves; closed room door or bedside curtains.	—	—	—	_____
5. Positioned client to allow dressing removal.	—	—	—	_____
6. Assessed pressure ulcer and surrounding skin to determine stage and color of pressure ulcer.	—	—	—	_____
7. Removed gloves, disposed of properly. Washed hands.	—	—	—	_____
8. Completed an entire assessment of client, including nutritional status.	—	—	—	_____
9. Assessed client's and support persons' understanding of pressure ulcer characteristics and purpose of treatment.	—	—	—	_____
NURSING DIAGNOSIS				
1. Developed appropriate nursing diagnoses based on assessment data.	—	—	—	_____
PLANNING				
1. Developed individualized goals for client based on nursing diagnoses.	—	—	—	_____
2. Identified expected outcomes.	—	—	—	_____
3. Explained procedure and its purpose to client and family.	—	—	—	_____
4. Prepared necessary equipment and supplies.	—	—	—	_____
IMPLEMENTATION				
1. Assembled needed supplies at bedside. Washed hands, donned gloves. Opened sterile packages and topical solution containers.	—	—	—	_____
2. Removed client's bed linen and gown to expose ulcer and surrounding skin; kept remaining body parts draped.	—	—	—	_____

S   U   NP   Comments

3. Gently washed skin surrounding ulcer with warm water and soap.

4. Rinsed area thoroughly with water.

5. Gently dried skin by patting with towel.

6. Changed gloves.

7. Cleansed ulcer thoroughly with normal saline or prescribed cleansing agent. Utilized whirlpool treatments for debridement, as indicated.

8. Applied topical agents if prescribed:

    a. Applied enzymes if prescribed.

    b. Applied dextranomer beads correctly.

    c. Applied hydrocolloid beads or paste correctly.

    d. Applied hydrogel agent correctly.

    e. Applied calcium alginates correctly.

9. Repositioned client comfortably off pressure ulcer.

10. Removed gloves. Disposed of soiled supplies. Washed hands.

EVALUATION

1. Inspected condition of skin surrounding pressure ulcer.

2. Inspected ulcer and dressing.

3. Compared subsequent ulcer measurements.

4. Avoided use of pressure ulcer staging system to measure healing.

5. Identified unexpected outcomes.

RECORDING AND REPORTING

1. Recorded appearance of ulcer in nurses' notes.

2. Described type of topical agent and dressing applied, including client's response.

3. Reported worsening of ulcer to nurse in charge or physician.

Student _____   Date _____

Instructor _____   Date _____

PERFORMANCE CHECKLIST 9-1   **TAKING CARE OF CONTACT LENSES**

	S	U	NP	Comments
ASSESSMENT				
1. Placed towel below client's face.	__	__	__	_____
2. Determined if contact lenses were in place.	__	__	__	_____
3. Assessed for eye discomfort and determined length of time client usually wears lenses.	__	__	__	_____
4. Assessed client's ability to manipulate and hold lenses.	__	__	__	_____
5. Assessed for any unusual visual symptoms.	__	__	__	_____
6. Assessed type of medications client receives.	__	__	__	_____
7. Inspected condition of cornea after removal of lenses.	__	__	__	_____
NURSING DIAGNOSIS				
1. Developed appropriate nursing diagnoses based on assessment data.	__	__	__	_____
PLANNING				
1. Developed individualized goals for client based on nursing diagnoses.	__	__	__	_____
2. Identified expected outcomes.	__	__	__	_____
3. Discussed procedure with client.	__	__	__	_____
4. Positioned client in sitting or supine position. Side-lying position used, if indicated.	__	__	__	_____
5. Assembled supplies at bedside.	__	__	__	_____
IMPLEMENTATION				
Removing Soft Lenses				
1. Washed hands. Applied disposable gloves if needed.	__	__	__	_____
2. Placed towel just below client's face.	__	__	__	_____
3. Added saline drops to client's eye.	__	__	__	_____
4. Told client to look straight ahead.	__	__	__	_____
5. Retracted lower eyelid.	__	__	__	_____
6. Slid lens off cornea onto white of eye with pad of index finger.	__	__	__	_____
7. Compressed lens correctly between thumb and index finger.	__	__	__	_____

	S	U	NP	Comments

8. Removed lens from eye. ___ ___ ___ _____

9. Soaked lens in sterile saline to return lens to normal shape if needed. ___ ___ ___ _____

10. Placed lens in correct cup of storage case after cleansing and rinsing. ___ ___ ___ _____

11. Repeated Steps 3-10 for other lens. ___ ___ ___ _____

12. Disposed of towel, removed gloves, and washed hands. ___ ___ ___ _____

Removing Rigid Lenses

1. Washed hands. Applied gloves, if needed. ___ ___ ___ _____

2. Placed towel just below client's face. ___ ___ ___ _____

3. Determined position of lens before removal. ___ ___ ___ _____

4. Retracted outer corner of eye toward client's ear. ___ ___ ___ _____

5. Instructed client to blink. ___ ___ ___ _____

6. Depressed lower eyelid against edge of lens correctly if lens failed to pop out. ___ ___ ___ _____

7. Removed lens from eye. Held lens in cupped hand. Lens suction cup used for confused or unconscious clients. ___ ___ ___ _____

8. Placed lens in correct cup of storage case after cleansing and rinsing. ___ ___ ___ _____

9. Repeated Steps 3-8 for other lens. Secured cover over storage case. ___ ___ ___ _____

10. Disposed of towel, removed gloves, and washed hands. ___ ___ ___ _____

Cleansing and Disinfecting Contact Lenses

1. Washed hands and applied gloves if needed. ___ ___ ___ _____

2. Assembled supplies at bedside. Placed towel over work area. Checked expiration date of all solutions. ___ ___ ___ _____

3. Opened lens storage case carefully. ___ ___ ___ _____

4. Removed lens from storage case and applied 1-2 drops of cleaner on lens in palm of hand. ___ ___ ___ _____

5. Used fingertips to distribute cleansing solution over lens surfaces for 20-30 seconds. ___ ___ ___ _____

6. Rinsed lens thoroughly in recommended rinsing solution (soft lenses) or cold tap water (rigid lenses). ___ ___ ___ _____

7. Placed lenses in storage case with recommended solution. ___ ___ ___ _____

8. Repeated Steps 3-7 for other lens. ___ ___ ___ _____

Student _____   Date _____

Instructor _____   Date _____

	S	U	NP	Comments

Inserting Soft Lenses

1. Washed hands with mild soap, rinsed well, and dried with lint-free or paper towel.   ___ ___ ___ _____

2. Placed towel over client's chest.   ___ ___ ___ _____

3. Removed right lens from storage case and rinsed with recommended solution.   ___ ___ ___ _____

4. Checked that lens was not inverted or damaged.   ___ ___ ___ _____

5. Retracted upper lid using proper technique.   ___ ___ ___ _____

6. Pulled down lower lid using proper finger.   ___ ___ ___ _____

7. Instructed client to look straight ahead and gently placed lens on cornea.   ___ ___ ___ _____

8. Correctly positioned lens over cornea if it was on sclera.   ___ ___ ___ _____

9. Instructed client to blink a few times.   ___ ___ ___ _____

10. Determined if lens was centered properly.   ___ ___ ___ _____

11. Repositioned lens if client's vision was blurred after insertion.   ___ ___ ___ _____

12. Repeated Steps 3-10 for other eye.   ___ ___ ___ _____

13. Assisted client to comfortable position.   ___ ___ ___ _____

14. Discarded soiled supplies, rinsed storage case and allowed to air dry, washed hands.   ___ ___ ___ _____

Inserting Rigid Lenses

1. Washed hands with mild soap, rinsed well, and dried with lint-free or paper towel.   ___ ___ ___ _____

2. Placed towel over client's chest.   ___ ___ ___ _____

3. Removed right lens from storage case.   ___ ___ ___ _____

4. Rinsed lens with cold tap water.   ___ ___ ___ _____

5. Wet both sides of lens with prescribed wetting solution.   ___ ___ ___ _____

6. Placed right lens concave side up on tip of index finger of dominant hand.   ___ ___ ___ _____

7. Instructed client to look straight ahead; retracted eyelids and placed lens over center of cornea.   ___ ___ ___ _____

8. Instructed client to close eyes.   ___ ___ ___ _____

9. Determined if lens was centered. Repositioned lens, if vision blurred and lens not centered.   ___ ___ ___ _____

	S	U	NP	Comments
10. Repeated Steps 3-9 for left eye.	___	___	___	_____
11. Assisted client to comfortable position.	___	___	___	_____
12. Discarded soiled supplies, rinsed storage case and allowed to air dry, washed hands.	___	___	___	_____

EVALUATION

1. Determined if lens fit correctly.	___	___	___	_____
2. Inspected eye for signs of infection or injury.	___	___	___	_____
3. Assessed client's visual acuity.	___	___	___	_____
4. Evaluated client's understanding and performance of lens care.	___	___	___	_____
5. Identified unexpected outcomes.	___	___	___	_____

RECORDING AND REPORTING

1. Recorded and reported signs or symptoms of visual alterations noted during procedure.	___	___	___	_____
2. Recorded on nursing care plan or Kardex times of lens insertion and removal.	___	___	___	_____

Student _____   Date _____

Instructor _____   Date _____

PERFORMANCE CHECKLIST 9-2   **TAKING CARE OF AN ARTIFICIAL EYE**

	S	U	NP	Comments
ASSESSMENT				
1. Determined which eye is artificial.	—	—	—	_____
2. Inspected condition of eyelids and eye socket.	—	—	—	_____
3. Assessed client's routines for prosthesis care.	—	—	—	_____
4. Assessed client's ability to remove, clean, and replace prosthesis.	—	—	—	_____
NURSING DIAGNOSIS				
1. Developed appropriate nursing diagnoses based on assessment data.	—	—	—	_____
PLANNING				
1. Developed individualized goals for client based on nursing diagnoses.	—	—	—	_____
2. Identified expected outcomes.	—	—	—	_____
3. Discussed procedure with client.	—	—	—	_____
4. Assisted client to supine position with head elevated.	—	—	—	_____
IMPLEMENTATION				
1. Washed hands. Applied disposable gloves.	—	—	—	_____
2. Retracted lower eyelid against lower orbital ridge. Exerted slight pressure below eyelid to loosen prosthesis.	—	—	—	_____
3. Used bulb syringe or medicine dropper bulb to apply direct suction to prosthesis.	—	—	—	_____
4. Removed prosthesis and placed in palm of hand.	—	—	—	_____
5. Washed prosthesis with saline or mild soap and water using thumb and index finger; rinsed and dried prosthesis thoroughly.	—	—	—	_____
6. Stored prosthesis in labeled container when not used.	—	—	—	_____
7. Retracted upper and lower eyelids and washed socket with warm water or saline; dried socket thoroughly; washed lid margin by cleansing from inner to outer canthus; dried eyelids.	—	—	—	_____
8. Dampened prosthesis in water before insertion.	—	—	—	_____
9. Retracted upper eyelid.	—	—	—	_____

	S	U	NP	Comments

10. Inserted prosthesis with notched edge toward nose. ___ ___ ___ _____

11. Slid prosthesis with notched edge toward nose and pushed down lower lid to allow prosthesis to slip into place. ___ ___ ___ _____

12. Wiped prosthesis from outer to inner canthus if necessary. ___ ___ ___ _____

13. Helped client assume comfortable position. ___ ___ ___ _____

14. Disposed of soiled supplies, removed gloves, and washed hands. ___ ___ ___ _____

EVALUATION

1. Asked client feelings regarding prosthesis removal. ___ ___ ___ _____

2. Observed position of prosthesis. ___ ___ ___ _____

3. Asked client if prosthesis fits comfortably. ___ ___ ___ _____

4. Inspected condition of eyelids and socket. ___ ___ ___ _____

5. Asked client to explain or demonstrate procedure. ___ ___ ___ _____

6. Identified unexpected outcomes. ___ ___ ___ _____

RECORDING AND REPORTING

1. Documented removal of prosthesis for client going to surgery. ___ ___ ___ _____

2. Recorded and reported any alterations in integrity of tissues surrounding eye. ___ ___ ___ _____

Student _____   Date _____

Instructor _____   Date _____

PERFORMANCE CHECKLIST 9-3 **TAKING CARE OF AN IN-THE-EAR HEARING AID**

	S	U	NP	Comments
ASSESSMENT				
1. Assessed client's knowledge of and routines for hearing aid care.	___	___	___	_____
2. Assessed client's hearing with aid in place.	___	___	___	_____
3. Assessed function of aid through battery check.	___	___	___	_____
4. Checked that earmold was intact.	___	___	___	_____
5. Inspected for cerumen around earmold and external ear canal.	___	___	___	_____
NURSING DIAGNOSIS				
1. Developed appropriate nursing diagnoses based on assessment data.	___	___	___	_____
PLANNING				
1. Developed individualized goals for client based on nursing diagnoses.	___	___	___	_____
2. Identified expected outcomes.	___	___	___	_____
3. Asked client for additional suggestions on techniques and explained procedure to be performed.	___	___	___	_____
IMPLEMENTATION				
Cleaning Hearing Aid				
1. Washed hands. Applied disposable gloves.	___	___	___	_____
2. Assembled supplies at bedside table or sink area.	___	___	___	_____
3. Removed cerumen from holes in the aid.	___	___	___	_____
4. Washed, rinsed, and dried ear canal.	___	___	___	_____
5. Placed in storage case if indicated. Kept device dry.	___	___	___	_____
6. Opened battery door to air dry.	___	___	___	_____
7. Labeled client's storage case.	___	___	___	_____
Inserting Hearing Aid				
1. Checked battery function before insertion of hearing aid.	___	___	___	_____
2. Turned aid off and volume control down.	___	___	___	_____
3. Held aid correctly to prepare for insertion in ear.	___	___	___	_____
4. Inserted aid into ear canal correctly.	___	___	___	_____

	S	U	NP	Comments

5. Adjusted volume to comfortable level.   ___ ___ ___ _____

6. Disposed of soiled equipment properly and washed hands.   ___ ___ ___ _____

EVALUATION

1. Determined client's ability to hear with aid in place.   ___ ___ ___ _____

2. Asked client to explain or perform insertion and cleaning.   ___ ___ ___ _____

3. Observed client's response to environmental sounds.   ___ ___ ___ _____

4. Determined client's level of comfort.   ___ ___ ___ _____

5. Identified unexpected outcomes.   ___ ___ ___ _____

RECORDING AND REPORTING

1. Documented removal and storage of aid when client went to surgery or for special procedure.   ___ ___ ___ _____

2. Reported client's communication problems to nursing staff.   ___ ___ ___ _____

Student _____   Date _____

Instructor _____   Date _____

PERFORMANCE CHECKLIST 10-1 **MEASURING BODY TEMPERATURE**

	S	U	NP	Comments

ASSESSMENT

1. Determined need to measure client's temperature.   ___ ___ ___ _____

2. Assessed for signs and symptoms of temperature alterations.   ___ ___ ___ _____

3. Assessed for factors that normally influence temperature.   ___ ___ ___ _____

4. Assessed site for most appropriate temperature measurement.   ___ ___ ___ _____

5. Determined client's baseline temperature from client's record.   ___ ___ ___ _____

NURSING DIAGNOSIS

1. Developed appropriate nursing diagnoses based on assessment.   ___ ___ ___ _____

PLANNING

1. Developed individualized goals for assessing client's body temperature.   ___ ___ ___ _____

2. Identified expected outcomes.   ___ ___ ___ _____

3. Explained procedure to client.   ___ ___ ___ _____

4. Waited 30 minutes before measuring oral temperature if client smoked or ingested hot or cold liquids or foods.   ___ ___ ___ _____

IMPLEMENTATION
Oral Temperature—Glass Thermometer

1. Washed hands.   ___ ___ ___ _____

2. Positioned client comfortably.   ___ ___ ___ _____

3. Applied disposable gloves.   ___ ___ ___ _____

4. Held color-coded end of glass thermometer with fingertips.   ___ ___ ___ _____

5. Read mercury level while gently rotating thermometer at eye level.   ___ ___ ___ _____

6. Shook thermometer down briskly to proper level (Below 35.5° C, 96° F).   ___ ___ ___ _____

7. Inserted thermometer into plastic sleeve cover.   ___ ___ ___ _____

8. Placed thermometer under tongue in posterior sublingual pocket.   ___ ___ ___ _____

	S	U	NP	Comments

9. Asked client to hold thermometer with closed lips; cautioned client against biting down on thermometer.

10. Left thermometer in place for 3 minutes or according to agency policy.

11. Removed thermometer and disposed of plastic sleeve cover. Correctly held thermometer at eye level while reading temperature.

12. Informed client of temperature reading.

13. Removed secretions from thermometer by wiping from fingers toward bulb in rotating fashion. Discarded tissue properly.

14. Cleaned thermometer in lukewarm soapy water, rinsed, dried, and returned to container.

15. Removed and disposed of gloves and washed hands.

Oral Temperature—Electronic Thermometer

1. Washed hands and applied disposable gloves.

2. Positioned client comfortably.

3. Correctly attached oral probe to unit.

4. Placed disposable plastic cover over probe.

5. Inserted thermometer under tongue in posterior sublingual pocket.

6. Asked client to hold thermometer with closed lips.

7. Left probe in place until audible signal occurred, read temperature on digital display, and informed client of temperature reading.

8. Correctly discarded plastic probe cover.

9. Returned probe to storage well.

10. Removed and disposed of gloves and washed hands.

11. Returned thermometer to charger.

Rectal Temperature—Glass Thermometer

1. Washed hands and applied disposable gloves.

2. Provided for client's privacy and positioned client correctly.

3. Prepared thermometer following Steps 4-7 of Oral Temperature Measurement with Glass Thermometer.

4. Applied lubricant to thermometer bulb.

Student _____ Date _____

Instructor _____ Date _____

	S	U	NP	Comments

5. Correctly exposed client's anus and instructed client to breathe slowly and relax. ___ ___ ___ _____

6. Gently inserted thermometer correct distance into anus. ___ ___ ___ _____

7. Withdrew thermometer if resistance was felt. ___ ___ ___ _____

8. Held thermometer in place for 2 minutes or according to agency policy. ___ ___ ___ _____

9. Carefully removed thermometer, disposed of plastic sleeve cover, and wiped off secretions with tissue. Wiped in rotating fashion from fingers toward bulb. Discarded tissue. ___ ___ ___ _____

10. Read thermometer while gently rotating thermometer at eye level. ___ ___ ___ _____

11. Informed client of temperature reading. ___ ___ ___ _____

12. Wiped client's anal area, disposed of tissue, and helped client return to comfortable position. ___ ___ ___ _____

13. Washed thermometer in lukewarm soapy water, rinsed, dried, and replaced in storage container. ___ ___ ___ _____

14. Removed and disposed of gloves and washed hands. ___ ___ ___ _____

Rectal Temperature—Electronic Thermometer

1. Washed hands and applied disposable gloves. ___ ___ ___ _____

2. Provided for client's privacy. ___ ___ ___ _____

3. Positioned client correctly. ___ ___ ___ _____

4. Correctly attached rectal probe to unit. ___ ___ ___ _____

5. Placed disposable plastic cover over probe. Applied lubricant. ___ ___ ___ _____

6. Correctly exposed client's anus and asked client to breathe slowly and relax. ___ ___ ___ _____

7. Gently inserted thermometer correct distance into anus. ___ ___ ___ _____

8. Held probe in place until audible signal occurred and read temperature on digital display. ___ ___ ___ _____

9. Carefully removed probe from rectum and informed client of temperature reading. ___ ___ ___ _____

10. Correctly discarded plastic probe cover and returned probe to storage well. ___ ___ ___ _____

S   U   NP   Comments

11. Wiped client's anal area and removed and disposed of gloves.

12. Helped client return to comfortable position.

13. Washed hands.

14. Returned thermometer to charger.

Axillary Temperature—Glass Thermometer

1. Washed hands.

2. Provided for client's privacy.

3. Positioned client correctly.

4. Moved clothing or gown away from client's shoulder and arm.

5. Prepared glass thermometer following Steps 4-7 of Oral Temperature Measurement with Glass Thermometer.

6. Inserted thermometer in center of axilla, lowered client's arm over thermometer, and placed arm across client's chest.

7. Held thermometer in place for 3 minutes or according to agency policy.

8. Removed thermometer, disposed of plastic sleeve cover, and wiped off secretions with tissue. Wiped in rotating fashion from fingers toward bulb. Discarded tissue.

9. Read while gently rotating thermometer at eye level.

10. Informed client of temperature reading.

11. Washed thermometer in lukewarm soapy water, rinsed, dried, and replaced in storage container.

12. Assisted client in replacing clothing or gown.

13. Washed hands.

Axillary Temperature—Electronic Thermometer

1. Washed hands.

2. Provided for client's privacy.

3. Positioned client correctly.

4. Moved clothing or gown away from client's shoulder and arm.

5. Prepared thermometer following Steps 3 and 4 for Oral Temperature Measurement with Electronic Thermometer.

Student _____   Date _____

Instructor _____   Date _____

	S	U	NP	Comments

6. Inserted probe in center of axilla, lowered client's arm over thermometer, and placed arm across client's chest.

7. Held electronic probe in place until audible signal occurred and read temperature on digital display.

8. Removed probe from axilla and informed client of temperature reading.

9. Correctly discarded plastic probe cover and returned probe to storage well.

10. Assisted client in replacing clothing or gown.

11. Washed hands.

12. Returned thermometer to charger.

Tympanic Membrane Temperature—Electronic Thermometer

1. Washed hands.

2. Assisted client to comfortable position, with head turned to side, away from nurse.

3. Removed thermometer from charging base without applying pressure to ejection button.

4. Slid disposable speculum cover over tip until locked in place.

5. Inserted speculum into ear canal per manufacturer's instructions and client's age.

6. Depressed scan button on unit. Left thermometer in place until audible signal heard and temperature read.

7. Removed speculum from ear canal, and informed client of temperature reading.

8. Correctly discarded plastic probe cover.

9. Returned unit to charging base.

10. Assisted client to comfortable position.

11. Washed hands.

EVALUATION

1. Established client's temperature as a baseline if within normal range.

	S	U	NP	Comments

2. Compared client's temperature with client's baseline and normal temperature range.   ___ ___ ___ _____

3. Identified unexpected outcomes.   ___ ___ ___ _____

REPORTING AND RECORDING

1. Recorded and reported temperature correctly on vital signs flowsheet and/or nurses' notes.   ___ ___ ___ _____

2. Reported abnormal findings to nurse in charge or physician.   ___ ___ ___ _____

Student _____   Date _____

Instructor _____   Date _____

PERFORMANCE CHECKLIST 10-2   **ASSESSING A CLIENT'S APICAL PULSE**

	S	U	NP	Comments

ASSESSMENT

1. Determined need to assess client's pulse: noted conditions or alterations increasing client's risk for pulse alterations and assessed for signs and symptoms of cardiovascular alterations.

2. Identified factors that normally may influence client's pulse.

3. Identified client's baseline heart rate from client's records.

NURSING DIAGNOSIS

1. Developed appropriate nursing diagnoses based on assessment data.

PLANNING

1. Identified individualized goals for assessing pulse.

2. Identified expected outcomes.

3. Explained assessment procedure to client and the need to wait 5-10 minutes to assess pulse after client has been active.

4. Positioned client supine or sitting. Child may sit in parent's lap.

IMPLEMENTATION
Apical Pulse

1. Washed hands.

2. Provided privacy.

3. Exposed client's sternum and left side of chest for auscultation.

4. Used palpation correctly. Located apex of heart at point of maximal impulse.

5. Warmed diaphragm of stethoscope between hands.

6. Placed diaphragm over point of maximal impulse (PMI) and auscultated for S_1 and S_2 heart sounds.

7. Was able to determine rate of S_1 and S_2 sounds accurately.

	S	U	NP	Comments
8. With regular heart rate, counted for 30 seconds and correctly converted to minute rate.	___	___	___	_____
9. With irregular heart rate, counted for 1 minute.	___	___	___	_____
10. Assessed regularity of any existing dysrhythmia.	___	___	___	_____
11. Replaced client's gown. Assisted client in returning to comfortable position.	___	___	___	_____
12. Discussed findings with client.	___	___	___	_____
13. Washed hands.	___	___	___	_____
14. Cleaned stethoscope earpieces and diaphragm with alcohol swab.	___	___	___	_____

EVALUATION

	S	U	NP	Comments
1. Established client's baseline pulse.	___	___	___	_____
2. Compared client's pulse rate and character with baseline and/or normal range for age-group.	___	___	___	_____
3. If pulse character was abnormal, asked another nurse to assess pulse.	___	___	___	_____
4. Identified unexpected outcomes.	___	___	___	_____

RECORDING AND REPORTING

	S	U	NP	Comments
1. Recorded findings in vital signs flowsheet and/or nurses' notes.	___	___	___	_____
2. Reported abnormal findings to nurse in charge or physician.	___	___	___	_____

Student _____ Date _____

Instructor _____ Date _____

PERFORMANCE CHECKLIST 10-3 ASSESSING A CLIENT'S RADIAL PULSE

	S	U	NP	Comments
ASSESSMENT				
1. Determined need to assess client's pulse: noted conditions or alterations increasing client's risk for pulse alterations and assessed for signs and symptoms of cardiovascular alterations.	___	___	___	_____
2. Identified factors that normally may influence client's pulse.	___	___	___	_____
3. Identified client's baseline heart rate from client's records.	___	___	___	_____
NURSING DIAGNOSIS				
1. Developed appropriate nursing diagnoses based on assessment data.	___	___	___	_____
PLANNING				
1. Identified individualized goals for assessing pulse.	___	___	___	_____
2. Identified expected outcomes.	___	___	___	_____
3. Explained assessment procedure to client and the need to wait 5-10 minutes to assess pulse after client has been active.	___	___	___	_____
4. Positioned client supine or sitting. Child may sit in parent's lap.	___	___	___	_____
IMPLEMENTATION				
Radial Pulse				
1. Washed hands. Provided privacy, if necessary.	___	___	___	_____
2. If supine, placed client's forearm across lower chest with wrist extended and palm down. If sitting, bent client's elbow 90 degrees and supported lower arm on chair or on nurse's arm. Slightly extended wrist with palm down.	___	___	___	_____
3. Placed fingertips of first two fingers over radial pulse.	___	___	___	_____
4. Was able to palpate client's radial pulse and determine strength of pulse.	___	___	___	_____
5. Began to count rate when pulse was felt regularly.	___	___	___	_____
6. With regular rate, counted pulse rate for 30 seconds and converted to minute rate.	___	___	___	_____

	S	U	NP	Comments

7. With irregular rate, counted pulse rate for full minute. ___ ___ ___ _____

8. Assessed regularity frequency of any dysrhythmia. Assessed for pulse deficit, if indicated. ___ ___ ___ _____

9. Determined strength and character of pulse. ___ ___ ___ _____

10. Assisted client in returning to comfortable position. ___ ___ ___ _____

11. Discussed findings with client. ___ ___ ___ _____

12. Washed hands. ___ ___ ___ _____

EVALUATION

1. Established client's baseline pulse. ___ ___ ___ _____

2. Compared client's pulse rate and character with baseline and/or normal range for age-group. ___ ___ ___ _____

3. Identified unexpected outcomes. ___ ___ ___ _____

RECORDING AND REPORTING

1. Recorded findings in vital signs flowsheet and/or nurses' notes, including site assessed and signs and symptoms of pulse alterations. ___ ___ ___ _____

2. Reported abnormal findings to nurse in charge or physician. ___ ___ ___ _____

Student _____   Date _____

Instructor _____   Date _____

PERFORMANCE CHECKLIST 10-4 **ASSESSING ARTERIAL BLOOD PRESSURE**

	S	U	NP	Comments

ASSESSMENT

1. Determined need to assess client's blood pressure: identified conditions or alterations increasing client's risk for blood pressure alterations, identified common signs and symptoms of blood pressure alterations, and determined client's age.

2. Assessed for factors that normally influence blood pressure.

3. Determined best site for blood pressure assessment.

4. Determined client's previous baseline blood pressure from client's record.

NURSING DIAGNOSIS

1. Developed appropriate nursing diagnoses based on assessment data.

PLANNING

1. Developed individualized goals for assessing client's blood pressure.

2. Identified expected outcomes.

3. Postponed assessment for 30 minutes if client had recently exercised or smoked.

4. Assisted client in assuming proper sitting or lying position.

5. Explained procedure to client and had client rest at least 5 minutes before procedure.

IMPLEMENTATION
Auscultation Method—Upper Extremities

1. Washed hands.

2. Positioned client's forearm at heart level with palm of hand turned up.

3. Removed constricting clothing from around upper arm.

4. Palpated brachial artery, positioned cuff properly above brachial artery, and wrapped deflated cuff evenly and snugly around upper arm.

5. Positioned manometer correctly for viewing.

	S	U	NP	Comments

6. Identified approximate systolic pressure by palpating brachial or radial pulse during cuff inflation. ___ ___ ___ _____

7. Waited 30 seconds after deflating cuff before auscultation. ___ ___ ___ _____

8. Checked stethoscope amplification of sound. ___ ___ ___ _____

9. Applied stethoscope correctly over brachial artery. ___ ___ ___ _____

10. Tightened valve of pressure bulb. ___ ___ ___ _____

11. Correctly inflated cuff to 30 mm Hg above that of palpated systolic pressure. ___ ___ ___ _____

12. Allowed mercury to fall evenly at rate of 2-3 mm Hg/sec during auscultation. ___ ___ ___ _____

13. Noted point on manometer when first clear sound was heard. ___ ___ ___ _____

14. Continued to deflate cuff gradually, noting point at which muffled or dampened sound appeared in children, and point at which sound disappeared in adults. ___ ___ ___ _____

15. Rapidly deflated cuff completely and removed from client's arm. ___ ___ ___ _____

16. If first assessment, repeated procedure on other arm. ___ ___ ___ _____

17. Assisted client in returning to comfortable position. ___ ___ ___ _____

18. Informed client of blood pressure reading. ___ ___ ___ _____

19. Washed hands. ___ ___ ___ _____

20. Cleaned earpieces and diaphragm of stethoscope with alcohol swab (optional). ___ ___ ___ _____

Auscultation Method—Lower Extremities

1. Washed hands. ___ ___ ___ _____

2. Assisted client in assuming prone position (supine optional). ___ ___ ___ _____

3. Removed constricting clothing from around leg. ___ ___ ___ _____

4. Palpated popliteal artery. ___ ___ ___ _____

5. Applied leg cuff to posterior aspect of middle thigh. ___ ___ ___ _____

6. Followed Steps 5-16 of Auscultation Method for Upper Extremities using popliteal artery. ___ ___ ___ _____

7. Identified systolic and diastolic pressures. ___ ___ ___ _____

Student _____ Date _____

Instructor _____ Date _____

	S	U	NP	Comments

8. Assisted client in returning to comfortable position.

9. Informed client of blood pressure reading.

10. Washed hands.

Palpation Method

1. Began palpation by following Steps 1-5 of auscultation method.

2. Identified approximate systolic pressure by palpating brachial or radial pulse during cuff inflation.

3. Allowed mercury to fall evenly at rate of 2-3 mm Hg/sec.

4. Noted manometer reading when pulse was again palpable.

5. Rapidly deflated cuff completely and removed from client's arm.

6. Assisted client in returning to comfortable position.

7. Informed client of reading.

8. Washed hands.

EVALUATION

1. When blood pressure was inaudible or difficult to obtain, repeated measurement after waiting 1-2 minutes.

2. Established blood pressure as baseline, if assessed for first time and found within normal range.

3. Compared client's blood pressure reading with previous baseline and/or normal average blood pressure for client's age.

4. Identified unexpected outcomes.

RECORDING AND REPORTING

1. Recorded blood pressure in nurses' notes and/or flowsheet.

2. Reported abnormal findings to nurse in charge or physician.

Student _____   Date _____

Instructor _____   Date _____

PERFORMANCE CHECKLIST 10-5   **ASSESSING A CLIENT'S RESPIRATIONS**

	S	U	NP	Comments
ASSESSMENT				
1. Determined need to assess client's respirations: described conditions that increase client's risk for respiratory alterations and identified common signs and symptoms of respiratory alterations.	___	___	___	_____
2. Assessed factors that normally influence client's respirations.	___	___	___	_____
3. Assessed results of pertinent laboratory valves.	___	___	___	_____
4. Determined client's baseline respiratory rate from client's record.	___	___	___	_____
NURSING DIAGNOSIS				
1. Developed appropriate nursing diagnoses based on assessment data.	___	___	___	_____
PLANNING				
1. Developed individualized goals for assessing respirations.	___	___	___	_____
2. Identified expected outcomes.	___	___	___	_____
3. Waited 5-10 minutes before assessing respirations if client had been active.	___	___	___	_____
4. Assessed respirations as first vital sign in infant or child.	___	___	___	_____
5. Assessed respirations after pulse measurement in adult.	___	___	___	_____
6. Assisted client in assuming comfortable position.	___	___	___	_____
IMPLEMENTATION				
1. Washed hands. Provided privacy.	___	___	___	_____
2. Positioned client and self properly to ensure view of chest wall movement.	___	___	___	_____
3. Was able to observe complete respiratory cycle.	___	___	___	_____
4. Correctly began count of respiration rate.	___	___	___	_____
5. Correctly counted respirations for 30 seconds in normal adult and multiplied by 2; counted rate for full minute in child. If respirations were irregular in adult, counted rate for full minute.	___	___	___	_____
6. Assessed respiratory depth.	___	___	___	_____

	S	U	NP	Comments
7. Assessed respiratory rhythm.	——	——	——	_____
8. Replaced client's gown and covered client with bed linen.	——	——	——	_____
9. Washed hands.	——	——	——	_____
10. Discussed findings with client.	——	——	——	_____

EVALUATION

1. Determined client's baseline respirations.	——	——	——	_____
2. Compared characteristics of client's respirations with previous baseline data and/or normal range for client's age.	——	——	——	_____
3. Identified unexpected outcomes.	——	——	——	_____

RECORDING AND REPORTING

1. Recorded respiratory rate, rhythm, and depth on vital signs flowsheet and/or nurse's notes.	——	——	——	_____
2. Reported abnormal findings to nurse in charge or physician.	——	——	——	_____
3. Correlated findings with data obtained from other measurements (e.g., arterial blood gases).	——	——	——	_____

Student _____ Date _____

Instructor _____ Date _____

PERFORMANCE CHECKLIST 10-6   MEASURING OXYGEN SATURATION (PULSE OXIMETRY)

	S	U	NP	Comments
ASSESSMENT				
1. Assessed clinical status of clients who would benefit from pulse oximetry.	—	—	—	_____
2. Assessed client's respiratory status.	—	—	—	_____
3. Reviewed client's medical record for physician's order.	—	—	—	_____
4. Assessed site for sensor probe placement.	—	—	—	_____
5. Determined previous baseline SaO_2, if available.	—	—	—	_____
NURSING DIAGNOSIS				
1. Developed appropriate nursing diagnoses based on assessment data.	—	—	—	_____
PLANNING				
1. Developed individualized goals for client based on nursing diagnoses.	—	—	—	_____
2. Identified expected outcomes.	—	—	—	_____
3. Obtained equipment and placed at bedside.	—	—	—	_____
4. Explained purpose of procedure to client and family.	—	—	—	_____
IMPLEMENTATION				
1. Washed hands.	—	—	—	_____
2. Positioned client correctly.	—	—	—	_____
3. Instructed client to breathe normally.	—	—	—	_____
4. Removed fingernail polish if using finger site.	—	—	—	_____
5. Attached sensor probe to selected site.	—	—	—	_____
6. Watched pulse bar for pulse sensing.	—	—	—	_____
7. Correlated oximeter with radial pulse rate and read saturation.	—	—	—	_____
8. Discussed findings with client.	—	—	—	_____
9. Removed probe and turned oximeter off (intermittent readings).	—	—	—	_____
10. Assisted client to comfortable position.	—	—	—	_____
11. Washed hands.	—	—	—	_____

	S	U	NP	Comments

EVALUATION

1. Established SaO_2 as baseline, if assessed for first time and within normal limits.   ___ ___ ___ _____

2. Compared SaO_2 with previous baseline and normals. Noted use of oxygen therapy.   ___ ___ ___ _____

3. Identified unexpected outcomes.   ___ ___ ___ _____

RECORDING AND REPORTING

1. Recorded SaO_2 in nurses' notes and/or flow sheet; identified use of continuous or intermittent pulse oximetry.   ___ ___ ___ _____

2. Reported abnormal findings to nurse in charge or physician.   ___ ___ ___ _____

3. Correlated findings with arterial blood gas measurements, if available.   ___ ___ ___ _____

4. Reported SaO_2 and response to change in therapy to oncoming shift.   ___ ___ ___ _____

Student _____   Date _____

Instructor _____   Date _____

PERFORMANCE CHECKLIST 11-1   **PERFORMING A GENERAL SURVEY**

	S	U	NP	Comments
ASSESSMENT				
1. Noted if client is experiencing any acute distress.	___	___	___	_____
2. Determined client's primary language.	___	___	___	_____
3. Reconfirmed client's primary reason for seeking health care.	___	___	___	_____
4. Asked if client knows personal normal pulse rate and blood pressure at rest.	___	___	___	_____
5. Assessed factors or conditions that may alter vital sign reading.	___	___	___	_____
6. Asked what client's normal height and weight are.	___	___	___	_____
7. Determined whether client had a history of sudden weight change.	___	___	___	_____
8. Reviewed client's past intake and output records.	___	___	___	_____
9. Assessed for history of dieting or exercise.	___	___	___	_____
10. Determined type of diet client needs.	___	___	___	_____
11. Determined client's perceptions about personal health.	___	___	___	_____
PLANNING				
1. Developed individualized goals for assessment.	___	___	___	_____
2. Identified expected outcomes or normal findings.	___	___	___	_____
3. Prepared client for examination.	___	___	___	_____
IMPLEMENTATION				
1. Measured vital signs correctly.	___	___	___	_____
2. Calibrated scale.	___	___	___	_____
3. Correctly measured weight of weight-bearing client.	___	___	___	_____
4. Correctly measured height of weight-bearing client.	___	___	___	_____
5. Correctly measured weight of non–weight-bearing client.	___	___	___	_____
6. Correctly measured height of non–weight-bearing client.	___	___	___	_____

	S	U	NP	Comments

7. Correctly weighed and measured height of infant or toddler.   — — — _____

8. Measured skinfold thickness with calipers.   — — — _____

9. Observed pertinent verbal and nonverbal behaviors.   — — — _____

10. Observed client's behavior and appearance.   — — — _____

11. Noted possible indications of abuse.   — — — _____

EVALUATION

1. Asked client if expectations for visit and examination were met.   — — — _____

2. Compared vital signs with client's baseline or normal range for client's age.   — — — _____

3. Compared client's height and weight with normal standards.   — — — _____

4. Compared client's skinfold thickness with 50th percentile.   — — — _____

5. Compared client's appearance and behaviors with those typified as normal.   — — — _____

6. Compared client's appearance and behaviors with those characteristic of an abusive relationship.   — — — _____

7. Identified unexpected outcomes.   — — — _____

NURSING DIAGNOSIS

1. Developed appropriate nursing diagnoses based on assessment data.   — — — _____

RECORDING AND REPORTING

1. Recorded vital signs on flowsheet.   — — — _____

2. Recorded client's height and weight in nurses' notes or flowsheet.   — — — _____

3. Recorded description of client's general appearance and skinfold thickness.   — — — _____

4. Described client's behavior using objective terms.   — — — _____

5. Reported abnormalities in vital signs to nurse in charge or physician.   — — — _____

Student _____ Date _____

Instructor _____ Date _____

PERFORMANCE CHECKLIST 11-2 **ASSESSING THE SKIN**

	S	U	NP	Comments
ASSESSMENT				
1. Asked client if changes in skin have been noted.	___	___	___	_____
2. Determined whether client spends time outside exposed to sun and if sunscreen used.	___	___	___	_____
3. Determined history of occupational exposure.	___	___	___	_____
4. Assessed client's bathing practices.	___	___	___	_____
5. Determined whether client experienced recent skin trauma.	___	___	___	_____
6. Determined whether client has a history of allergies.	___	___	___	_____
7. Determined whether client uses topical medications or home remedies.	___	___	___	_____
8. Determined whether client uses sunlamps, tanning pills, or tanning salons.	___	___	___	_____
9. Determined whether client has family history of serious skin disorders.	___	___	___	_____
PLANNING				
1. Developed individualized goals for skin assessment.	___	___	___	_____
2. Identified expected outcomes.	___	___	___	_____
3. Prepared equipment.	___	___	___	_____
4. Prepared client for skin examination by positioning and draping client and explaining procedure.	___	___	___	_____
IMPLEMENTATION				
1. Washed hands; applied gloves if open or moist lesions present.	___	___	___	_____
2. Conducted overall visual sweep of body.	___	___	___	_____
3. Inspected color of skin surfaces, comparing color of symmetric body parts. Assessed sun-exposed areas.	___	___	___	_____
4. Inspected color of face, oral mucosa, nail beds, lips, palms of hands, sclerae, and conjunctivae.	___	___	___	_____
5. Assessed condition of skin.	___	___	___	_____
6. Palpated skin to detect level of hydration.	___	___	___	_____

	S	U	NP	Comments
8. Palpated skin to assess skin temperature.	—	—	—	_____
9. Determined skin texture.	—	—	—	_____
10. Palpated localized areas of hardness. Inspected character of any secretions.	—	—	—	_____
11. Inspected skin lesions for color, location, size, type, grouping, and distribution.	—	—	—	_____
12. Palpated skin lesions for mobility, contour, and consistency.	—	—	—	_____
13. Noted client's complaint of any tenderness during palpation.	—	—	—	_____
14. Inspected skin for presence of edema.	—	—	—	_____
15. Palpated areas of edema for mobility, consistency, and tenderness.	—	—	—	_____
16. Assessed areas of edema for pitting.	—	—	—	_____
17. Removed and disposed of gloves. Washed hands.	—	—	—	_____

EVALUATION

1. Compared findings with previous observations and normal skin characteristics.	—	—	—	_____
2. Asked client to describe warning signals for cancerous skin lesions.	—	—	—	_____
3. Identified unexpected outcomes.	—	—	—	_____

NURSING DIAGNOSIS

1. Developed appropriate nursing diagnoses based on assessment data.	—	—	—	_____

RECORDING AND REPORTING

1. Recorded condition of client's skin in nurses' notes.	—	—	—	_____
2. Reported skin abnormalities to nurse in charge or physician.	—	—	—	_____

Student _____   Date _____

Instructor _____   Date _____

PERFORMANCE CHECKLIST 11-3   **ASSESSING THE HAIR AND SCALP**

	S	U	NP	Comments
ASSESSMENT				
1. Asked if client is wearing wig or hairpiece.	___	___	___	_____
2. Assessed if client noted recent change in growth or loss of hair.	___	___	___	_____
3. Assessed shampoo and hair care products used.	___	___	___	_____
4. Determined if there has been recent trauma to scalp.	___	___	___	_____
5. Asked if client takes chemotherapy medications.	___	___	___	_____
6. Determined risk for potential tick exposure.	___	___	___	_____
7. Reviewed diet history.	___	___	___	_____
PLANNING				
1. Developed individualized goals for hair assessment.	___	___	___	_____
2. Identified expected outcomes.	___	___	___	_____
3. Prepared client.	___	___	___	_____
4. Explained procedure for inspecting hair to client.	___	___	___	_____
IMPLEMENTATION				
1. Washed hands and applied gloves if lice or lesions expected.	___	___	___	_____
2. Inspected distribution and condition of hair.	___	___	___	_____
3. Inspected areas of baldness or thinning of hair.	___	___	___	_____
4. Inspected scalp for cleanliness and presence of lesions.	___	___	___	_____
5. Inspected scalp contour and palpated masses or prominences.	___	___	___	_____
6. Inspected hair follicles for lice.	___	___	___	_____
7. Inspected scalp for bites or pustular eruptions. Assessed for ticks.	___	___	___	_____
8. Inspected hair over perineal area for crab lice.	___	___	___	_____
9. Properly disposed of soiled gloves and washed hands.	___	___	___	_____
10. Inspected hair distribution over lower extremities.	___	___	___	_____

	S	U	NP	Comments

EVALUATION

1. Compared findings with previous observations and normal characteristics of hair.   — — — _____

2. Identified unexpected outcomes.   — — — _____

NURSING DIAGNOSIS

1. Developed appropriate nursing diagnoses based on assessment data.   — — — _____

RECORDING AND REPORTING

1. Recorded condition of hair and scalp in nurses' notes.   — — — _____

Student _____   Date _____

Instructor _____   Date _____

PERFORMANCE CHECKLIST 11-4 **ASSESSING THE NAILS**

	S	U	NP	Comments

ASSESSMENT

1. Asked if client has had recent trauma to nails.

2. Assessed client's nail care practices.

3. Determined if client noted changes in nail growth or appearance.

4. Determined risks for nail or foot problems.

PLANNING

1. Developed individualized goals for nail assessment.

2. Identified expected outcomes.

3. Prepared client for examination by positioning client comfortably and explaining procedure.

4. Asked client to remove nail polish or artificial nails when necessary.

IMPLEMENTATION

1. Inspected condition of each nail's entire surface.

2. Palpated nail bed for firmness.

3. Palpated nail bed to assess capillary return.

EVALUATION

1. Compared condition of nails with normal nail characteristics.

2. Asked client to describe nail care practices.

3. Identified unexpected outcomes.

NURSING DIAGNOSIS

1. Developed appropriate nursing diagnoses based on assessment data.

RECORDING AND REPORTING

1. Recorded condition of nails in nurses' notes.

Student _____   Date _____

Instructor _____   Date _____

PERFORMANCE CHECKLIST 11-5 **ASSESSING THE EYES**

	S	U	NP	Comments

ASSESSMENT

1. Determined whether client has history of eye disease, diabetes, or hypertension.   ___ ___ ___ _____

2. Assessed for presence of signs and symptoms indicating eye disease.   ___ ___ ___ _____

3. Assessed client's occupational history.   ___ ___ ___ _____

4. Determined whether client has visited an eye doctor recently.   ___ ___ ___ _____

5. Determined whether client has family history of eye disorders.   ___ ___ ___ _____

6. Determined if client normally wears glasses or contact lenses.   ___ ___ ___ _____

7. Assessed medications client is currently taking, including eye drops.   ___ ___ ___ _____

PLANNING

1. Developed individualized goals for assessment.   ___ ___ ___ _____

2. Identified expected outcomes.   ___ ___ ___ _____

3. Prepared client correctly.   ___ ___ ___ _____

IMPLEMENTATION

1. Assessed visual acuity: ___ ___ ___ _____

   a. Had client read print.   ___ ___ ___ _____

   b. Assessed client with reduced acuity by measuring each eye separately.   ___ ___ ___ _____

   c. Performed Snellen test correctly for more accurate assessment.   ___ ___ ___ _____

   d. Had client with severe visual impairment count upraised fingers, or tested for light perception when client unable to see objects.   ___ ___ ___ _____

2. Assessed visual fields correctly.   ___ ___ ___ _____

3. Assessed extraocular movements correctly.   ___ ___ ___ _____

4. Assessed eye alignment correctly.   ___ ___ ___ _____

5. Assessed external eye structures: ___ ___ ___ _____

   a. Had client remove contact lenses.   ___ ___ ___ _____

   b. Positioned client correctly.   ___ ___ ___ _____

   c. Applied disposable gloves.   ___ ___ ___ _____

	S	U	NP	Comments

d. Inspected position and alignment of eyes. ___ ___ ___ _____

e. Measured distance between pupils of client with abnormal eye placement. ___ ___ ___ _____

f. Observed eyebrows for symmetry, hair growth, and movement. Asked client to raise and lower brows. ___ ___ ___ _____

g. Inspected for flaking of skin around eyebrows. ___ ___ ___ _____

h. Inspected eyelid position with eyes open normally. ___ ___ ___ _____

i. Noted position of conjunctivae. ___ ___ ___ _____

j. Inspected eyelid position when client closed eyes. ___ ___ ___ _____

k. Inspected upper eyelids for color, edema, and presence of lesions. ___ ___ ___ _____

l. Inspected lower eyelids. ___ ___ ___ _____

m. Inspected condition of eyelashes. ___ ___ ___ _____

n. Inspected lacrimal apparatus. ___ ___ ___ _____

o. Inspected for excess tearing. ___ ___ ___ _____

p. Palpated lower eyelid correctly if tearing noted. ___ ___ ___ _____

q. Correctly assessed conjunctiva by retracting upper and lower eyelids. ___ ___ ___ _____

r. Inspected cornea for opacities. ___ ___ ___ _____

s. Inspected character of pupils. ___ ___ ___ _____

t. Inspected iris. ___ ___ ___ _____

u. Correctly tested pupillary reflex to light. ___ ___ ___ _____

v. Assessed pupillary accommodation reflex. ___ ___ ___ _____

6. Performed ophthalmoscopic examination correctly. ___ ___ ___ _____

EVALUATION

1. Compared assessment findings with normal characteristics of eye. ___ ___ ___ _____

2. Asked client to identify common symptoms of eye problems. ___ ___ ___ _____

3. Identified unexpected outcomes. ___ ___ ___ _____

NURSING DIAGNOSIS

1. Identified appropriate nursing diagnoses based on assessment data. ___ ___ ___ _____

RECORDING AND REPORTING

1. Recorded findings of Snellen test correctly. ___ ___ ___ _____

2. Recorded observations made of eye structures and results of functional assessments. ___ ___ ___ _____

3. Reported serious abnormalities to nurse in charge or physician. ___ ___ ___ _____

Student _____   Date _____

Instructor _____   Date _____

PERFORMANCE CHECKLIST 11-6 **ASSESSING THE EARS**

	S	U	NP	Comments
ASSESSMENT				
1. Assessed for signs and symptoms indicative of ear infection or hearing loss.	___	___	___	_____
2. Determined risk factors for hearing loss.	___	___	___	_____
3. Assessed for hearing loss hazards in client's work setting.	___	___	___	_____
4. Observed for behaviors indicative of hearing loss.	___	___	___	_____
5. Assessed for use of antibiotics and aspirin.	___	___	___	_____
6. Determined whether client uses a hearing aid.	___	___	___	_____
7. Determined whether client has had a recent hearing problem.	___	___	___	_____
8. Assessed for repeated history of cerumen buildup.	___	___	___	_____
PLANNING				
1. Developed individualized goals for assessment.	___	___	___	_____
2. Identified expected outcomes.	___	___	___	_____
3. Prepared equipment.	___	___	___	_____
4. Explained procedure and positioned client for examination.	___	___	___	_____
IMPLEMENTATION				
External Ear				
1. Washed hands and applied gloves, if indicated.	___	___	___	_____
2. Inspected placement, size, and symmetry of auricle.	___	___	___	_____
3. Noted color of auricles.	___	___	___	_____
4. Palpated auricle for texture, tenderness, and presence of lesions; in presence of pain, palpated external ear to locate source of discomfort.	___	___	___	_____
5. Inspected skin of auricle and ear canal.	___	___	___	_____
6. Observed ear canal for signs of infection or inflammation.	___	___	___	_____
7. Inspected canal for cerumen.	___	___	___	_____
Otoscopic Examination				
1. Checked for foreign objects in canal.	___	___	___	_____
2. Positioned client for otoscopic examination.	___	___	___	_____

	S	U	NP	Comments

3. Inserted speculum of otoscope into client's ear canal.

4. Braced otoscope while examining ear structures.

5. Inspected inner canal for proper color and any disorder.

6. Inspected structures in eardrum.

7. Disposed of gloves and washed hands.

Hearing Acuity

1. Asked client to remove hearing aid, if used.

2. Assessed client's ability to hear spoken words.

3. Repeated in conversational or loud tones if needed. Tested both ears to compare results.

4. Performed Weber's and Rinne's tests with tuning fork if hearing loss suspected.

EVALUATION

1. Compared findings with normal assessment characteristics of ears.

2. Asked client to describe risks for hearing loss.

3. Identified unexpected outcomes.

NURSING DIAGNOSIS

1. Identified appropriate nursing diagnoses based on assessment data.

RECORDING AND REPORTING

1. Recorded observations made during assessment in nurses' notes.

2. Recorded results of hearing acuity tests.

3. Reported hearing loss to charge nurse or physician.

Student _____   Date _____

Instructor _____   Date _____

PERFORMANCE CHECKLIST 11-7 **ASSESSING THE NOSE AND SINUSES**

	S	U	NP	Comments

ASSESSMENT

1. Determined if client has experienced trauma to nose.

2. Assessed if client has history of allergies, nasal discharge, epistaxis, or postnasal drip.

3. Assessed character of nasal discharge, if present, and associated symptoms.

4. Assessed for history of nosebleeds.

5. Asked if client uses nasal spray or drops.

6. Asked if client snores at night or has difficulty breathing.

PLANNING

1. Developed individualized goals for assessment.

2. Identified expected outcomes.

3. Prepared client for examination by explaining procedure and positioning client properly.

IMPLEMENTATION

1. Washed hands and applied gloves, if necessary.

2. Inspected external nose for shape, color, alignment, and any deformities.

3. Palpated gently if swelling or deformities exist, noting tenderness, masses, and any underlying deviations.

4. Occluded one naris at a time to check client's breathing through nose with mouth closed.

5. Illuminated anterior nares and inspected nasal mucosa, noting color, presence of lesions, swelling, discharge, or bleeding.

6. Inspected nares for excoriation, inflammation, or sloughing for clients with nasogastric, nasotracheal tubes.

7. Asked client to tip head back slightly and inspected septum.

8. Inserted nasal speculum into nares properly (optional).

	S	U	NP	Comments
9. Palpated frontal sinus with gentle pressure.	___	___	___	_____
10. Palpated maxillary sinuses with gentle upward pressure.	___	___	___	_____
11. Transilluminated sinuses, if tenderness present or infection suspected.	___	___	___	_____
12. Removed gloves, washed hands, and disposed of supplies.	___	___	___	_____

EVALUATION

	S	U	NP	Comments
1. Compared findings with normal characteristics of nose and sinuses.	___	___	___	_____
2. Had client report on use of nasal spray.	___	___	___	_____
3. Identified unexpected outcomes.	___	___	___	_____

NURSING DIAGNOSIS

	S	U	NP	Comments
1. Developed appropriate nursing diagnoses based on assessment data.	___	___	___	_____

RECORDING AND REPORTING

	S	U	NP	Comments
1. Recorded observations in nurses' notes.	___	___	___	_____
2. Reported abnormalities to nurse in charge or physician.	___	___	___	_____

Student _____   Date _____

Instructor _____   Date _____

PERFORMANCE CHECKLIST 11-8   **ASSESSING THE MOUTH AND PHARYNX**

	S	U	NP	Comments

ASSESSMENT

1. Determined whether client wears dentures and inquired about fit.

2. Assessed for change in appetite or weight.

3. Assessed if client has pain from chewing, swallowing, or moving jaw; checked for lesions.

4. Assessed client's dental hygiene practices.

5. Determined whether client smokes or chews tobacco.

6. Reviewed client's history for alcohol consumption.

PLANNING

1. Developed individualized goals for assessment.

2. Identified expected outcomes.

3. Positioned client and explained need to open mouth fully.

IMPLEMENTATION

1. Washed hands and applied gloves.

2. Had client close mouth normally and inspected lips.

3. Asked client to clench teeth and smile; checked for position of upper teeth in relation to lower teeth.

4. Asked client to remove dental appliances.

5. Inspected and counted teeth, noting position, wear, presence of caries, and alignment.

6. Inspected mucosa and gums.

7. Palpated any lesions for tenderness, size, and consistency.

8. Asked client to open mouth to check all aspects of buccal mucosa.

9. Palpated cheek.

10. Palpated gums gently.

11. Inspected all sides of tongue and floor of mouth.

	S	U	NP	Comments

12. Asked client to raise and move tongue to check for symmetry. ___ ___ ___ _____

13. Grasped tip of tongue with gauze square and gently palpated length of tongue. ___ ___ ___ _____

14. Inspected hard and soft palates with client extending head backward and holding mouth open. ___ ___ ___ _____

15. Asked client to say "ah" in order to view movement of uvula and soft palate. ___ ___ ___ _____

16. Used penlight to view posterior pharynx. ___ ___ ___ _____

17. Noted throughout procedure if client has halitosis. ___ ___ ___ _____

18. Removed gloves, washed hands, and disposed of supplies. ___ ___ ___ _____

EVALUATION

1. Compared findings with assessment characteristics of mouth and pharynx. ___ ___ ___ _____

2. Had client describe oral care practices. ___ ___ ___ _____

3. Had client describe warning signs and risk factors of oral cancer. ___ ___ ___ _____

4. Identified unexpected outcomes. ___ ___ ___ _____

NURSING DIAGNOSIS

1. Identified appropriate nursing diagnoses based on assessment data. ___ ___ ___ _____

RECORDING AND REPORTING

1. Recorded condition of oral cavity in nurses' notes. ___ ___ ___ _____

2. Reported any abnormalities to nurse in charge or physician. ___ ___ ___ _____

Student _____   Date _____

Instructor _____   Date _____

PERFORMANCE CHECKLIST 11-9 **ASSESSING THE STRUCTURES OF THE NECK**

	S	U	NP	Comments

ASSESSMENT

1. Determined whether client has had recent infection or cold.   ___ ___ ___ _____

2. Determined whether client has a history of thyroid problems or takes thyroid medications.   ___ ___ ___ _____

3. Asked client, if has enlarged lymph node, about recent infections.   ___ ___ ___ _____

4. Determined whether client experiences changes associated with thyroid dysfunction.   ___ ___ ___ _____

PLANNING

1. Developed individualized goals for assessment.   ___ ___ ___ _____

2. Identified expected outcomes.   ___ ___ ___ _____

3. Assisted client to sitting position and explained procedure.   ___ ___ ___ _____

IMPLEMENTATION

1. Assessed client's neck muscle function.   ___ ___ ___ _____

2. Inspected client's neck with chin hyperextended.   ___ ___ ___ _____

3. Palpated any apparent masses.   ___ ___ ___ _____

4. Inspected neck bilaterally for lymph node enlargement.   ___ ___ ___ _____

5. Systematically and carefully palpated each lymphatic chain.   ___ ___ ___ _____

6. Palpated supraclavicular nodes.   ___ ___ ___ _____

7. Inspected area of neck overlying thyroid gland.   ___ ___ ___ _____

8. Instructed client to extend neck and swallow.   ___ ___ ___ _____

9. Palpated thyroid gland using either posterior or anterior approach.   ___ ___ ___ _____

10. Auscultated thyroid when gland is enlarged.   ___ ___ ___ _____

11. Palpated trachea.   ___ ___ ___ _____

EVALUATION

1. Compared findings with normal assessment characteristics of neck structures.   ___ ___ ___ _____

2. Identified unexpected outcomes.   ___ ___ ___ _____

	S	U	NP	Comments

NURSING DIAGNOSIS

1. Developed appropriate nursing diagnoses based on assessment data. ___ ___ ___ _____

RECORDING AND REPORTING

1. Recorded observations in nurses' notes. ___ ___ ___ _____

2. Reported abnormalities to physician immediately. ___ ___ ___ _____

Student _____   Date _____

Instructor _____   Date _____

PERFORMANCE CHECKLIST 11-10   **ASSESSING THE THORAX AND LUNGS**

	S	U	NP	Comments
ASSESSMENT				
1. Assessed client's smoking history.	—	—	—	_____
2. Assessed for symptoms of respiratory alterations.	—	—	—	_____
3. Determined whether client exposed to environmental pollutants.	—	—	—	_____
4. Reviewed client history for risk factors associated with tuberculosis and infection with human immunodeficiency virus (HIV).	—	—	—	_____
5. Assessed for history of allergies.	—	—	—	_____
6. Reviewed family history for risk factors.	—	—	—	_____
PLANNING				
1. Developed individualized goals for assessment.	—	—	—	_____
2. Identified expected outcomes.	—	—	—	_____
3. Assisted client to assume correct positions throughout procedure; exposed chest wall for assessment; explained steps of procedure.	—	—	—	_____
IMPLEMENTATION				
Posterior Thorax				
1. Inspected appearance of thorax.	—	—	—	_____
2. Determined rate and rhythm of breathing.	—	—	—	_____
3. Palpated posterior chest wall and costal and intercostal spaces.	—	—	—	_____
4. Palpated chest excursion.	—	—	—	_____
5. Noted chest symmetry.	—	—	—	_____
6. Palpated for fremitus over chest wall.	—	—	—	_____
7. Percussed intercostal spaces over chest wall.	—	—	—	_____
8. Auscultated breath sounds.	—	—	—	_____
9. If abnormality detected, assessed intercostal spaces using voice sounds.	—	—	—	_____
10. Auscultated lobes with client whispering.	—	—	—	_____
Lateral Thorax				
1. Inspected lateral chest wall with client's arms raised.	—	—	—	_____
2. Extended assessment to lateral sides of chest.	—	—	—	_____

	S	U	NP	Comments

Anterior Thorax

1. Inspected accessory muscles.

2. Inspected angle of costal margins and tip of sternum.

3. Measured client's respiratory character.

4. Palpated for swelling or tenderness.

5. Palpated anterior chest excursion.

6. Palpated for fremitus over chest wall.

7. Percussed thorax between intercostal spaces.

8. Auscultated breath sounds in anterior thorax.

EVALUATION

1. Compared findings with normal assessment characteristics of thorax and lungs.

2. Had client identify factors leading to lung disease.

3. Identified unexpected outcomes.

NURSING DIAGNOSIS

1. Developed appropriate nursing diagnoses based on assessment data.

RECORDING AND REPORTING

1. Recorded observations and findings in nurses' notes or flowsheet.

2. Recorded respiratory rate and character in vital signs flowsheet.

3. Reported abnormalities to nurse in charge or physician.

Student _____   Date _____

Instructor _____   Date _____

PERFORMANCE CHECKLIST 11-11   **ASSESSING THE HEART AND VASCULAR SYSTEM**

	S	U	NP	Comments
ASSESSMENT				
1. Assessed for risk factors for heart and vascular disease.	—	—	—	_____
2. Determined client's medication history.	—	—	—	_____
3. Assessed for symptoms of heart disease.	—	—	—	_____
4. Determined whether client has a stressful lifestyle.	—	—	—	_____
5. Assessed client and family history for heart disease.	—	—	—	_____
6. Assessed client for history of heart problems.	—	—	—	_____
7. Determined whether client has preexisting diabetes, lung disease, or obesity.	—	—	—	_____
8. Assessed client's caffeine intake.	—	—	—	_____
9. Assessed client for symptoms of peripheral vascular disease.	—	—	—	_____
10. Determined whether client has pain in lower extremities and its relation to activity if present.	—	—	—	_____
11. Determined whether female client wears constrictive clothing.	—	—	—	_____
12. Reassessed client's medical history for vascular disorders.	—	—	—	_____
PLANNING				
1. Developed individualized goals for assessment.	—	—	—	_____
2. Identified expected outcomes.	—	—	—	_____
3. Assisted client to proper position and explained procedure.	—	—	—	_____
IMPLEMENTATION				
Heart				
1. Located anatomic sites to assess heart function.	—	—	—	_____
2. Used inspection and palpation over anatomic landmarks to detect pulsations.	—	—	—	_____
3. Timed any pulsations in relation to heart sounds.	—	—	—	_____
4. Located PMI by palpation.	—	—	—	_____

	S	U	NP	Comments

5. Turned client to left side when unable to locate PMI. ___ ___ ___ _____

6. Inspected epigastric area and palpated abdominal aorta. ___ ___ ___ _____

7. Auscultated heart sounds, repositioning client when indicated. ___ ___ ___ _____

8. Auscultated heart sounds using diaphragm and bell of stethoscope.

   a. Auscultated S_1 sound at various anatomic landmarks. ___ ___ ___ _____

   b. Listened for S_2 sound at each site. ___ ___ ___ _____

   c. Determined apical pulse rate. ___ ___ ___ _____

   d. Assessed heart rhythm. ___ ___ ___ _____

   e. Assessed for a pulse deficit if heart rate irregular. ___ ___ ___ _____

9. Auscultated for extra heart sounds. ___ ___ ___ _____

10. Characterized any murmurs present. ___ ___ ___ _____

Vascular

1. Auscultated brachial blood pressure in standing, sitting, supine positions. ___ ___ ___ _____

2. Assessed carotid arteries using inspection, palpation, and auscultation. ___ ___ ___ _____

3. Assessed jugular veins separately, measuring from appropriate landmarks. ___ ___ ___ _____

4. Assessed skin condition, color, venous tenderness, temperature, edema, hair distribution, etc. on face and upper and lower extremities. ___ ___ ___ _____

5. Assessed each peripheral artery for vessel elasticity, pulse rate and rhythm, strength, and type and equality of pulse. ___ ___ ___ _____

6. Palpated radial pulse. ___ ___ ___ _____

7. Palpated ulnar pulse. ___ ___ ___ _____

8. Palpated brachial pulse. ___ ___ ___ _____

9. Palpated femoral pulse. ___ ___ ___ _____

10. Palpated popliteal pulse. ___ ___ ___ _____

11. Palpated dorsalis pedis pulse. ___ ___ ___ _____

12. Palpated posterior tibial pulse. ___ ___ ___ _____

Student _____   Date _____

Instructor _____   Date _____

	S	U	NP	Comments

13. Correctly used ultrasound stethoscope to assess nonpalpable pulse. ___ ___ ___ _____

14. Correctly assessed inguinal lymphatics. ___ ___ ___ _____

EVALUATION

1. Compared findings with normal assessment characteristics for heart and vascular system. ___ ___ ___ _____

2. If pulses were not palpable, had another nurse assess for pulses. ___ ___ ___ _____

3. Asked client to describe behaviors that increase the risk of cardiovascular disease. ___ ___ ___ _____

4. Identified unexpected outcomes. ___ ___ ___ _____

NURSING DIAGNOSIS

1. Formulated appropriate nursing diagnoses based on assessment data. ___ ___ ___ _____

RECORDING AND REPORTING

1. Recorded all findings for heart and vascular assessment in nurses' notes. ___ ___ ___ _____

2. Recorded instruction given to client and client's response. ___ ___ ___ _____

3. Reported abnormalities to nurse in charge or physician. ___ ___ ___ _____

Student _____   Date _____

Instructor _____   Date _____

PERFORMANCE CHECKLIST 11-12 **ASSESSING THE BREASTS**

	S	U	NP	Comments

ASSESSMENT

1. Assessed for high risk factors for occurrence of breast cancer.

2. Determined whether client has had signs or symptoms of breast cancer.

3. Determined whether female client performs monthly self-examination of breasts.

4. Determined what medications client is taking (including oral contraceptives and hormones).

5. Determined history of fibrocystic disease.

PLANNING

1. Developed individualized goals for assessment.

2. Identified expected outcomes.

3. Prepared equipment correctly.

4. Prepared client for examination by correctly draping and positioning client, providing mirror for client to observe examination, explaining steps of procedure, and encouraging client's questions.

IMPLEMENTATION

Female Client

1. Used anatomic landmarks to describe findings.

2. Inspected appearance of each breast.

3. Checked for retraction using appropriate maneuver.

4. Inspected skin color and venous patterns.

5. Inspected appearance of areola and nipples.

6. Correctly palpated lymph nodes.

   a. Had client sit in proper position for axillary node palpation.

   b. Correctly palpated axillary lymph nodes.

   c. Correctly palpated supraclavicular and infraclavicular lymph nodes.

   d. Noted consistency, mobility, and any tenderness of palpable nodes.

S   U   NP   Comments

7. Had client lie supine with right arm abducted and hand under head.

8. Reviewed steps of BSE with client.

9. If client complained of lump or mass, began examination with opposite breast.

10. Examined breast using proper technique.

11. Noted consistency of tissue during breast palpation.

12. Palpated any mass for seven characteristics.

13. Palpated areola and nipples.

14. Repeated procedure for other breast.

15. Had client demonstrate self-examination.

Male Client
1. Inspected appearance of areola and nipples and palpated breast tissue in same systematic pattern as for females.

EVALUATION
1. Compared findings with normal assessment characteristics.

2. Had female client perform self-examination.

3. Asked female client to describe findings of self-examination.

4. Identified unexpected outcomes.

NURSING DIAGNOSIS
1. Formulated appropriate nursing diagnoses based on assessment data.

RECORDING AND REPORTING
1. Recorded findings and client education in nurses' notes.

2. Reported abnormalities to nurse in charge or physician.

Student _____ Date _____

Instructor _____ Date _____

PERFORMANCE CHECKLIST 11-13 **ASSESSING THE ABDOMEN**

	S	U	NP	Comments
ASSESSMENT				
1. Assessed for character of existing abdominal or low back pain.	___	___	___	_____
2. Observed for signs of pain associated with positioning.	___	___	___	_____
3. Assessed client's bowel habits.	___	___	___	_____
4. Assessed for history of abdominal surgery or trauma.	___	___	___	_____
5. Assessed for weight change or diet intolerance.	___	___	___	_____
6. Assessed for signs and symptoms of abdominal alterations.	___	___	___	_____
7. Asked whether client taking antiinflammatory medications or antibiotics.	___	___	___	_____
8. Inquired about family history of cancer, kidney disease, alcoholism, hypertension, or heart disease.	___	___	___	_____
9. Determined if female client is pregnant.	___	___	___	_____
10. Assessed client's usual intake of alcohol.	___	___	___	_____
11. Reviewed client's history for risk factors of HBV exposure.	___	___	___	_____
PLANNING				
1. Developed individual goals for assessment.	___	___	___	_____
2. Identified expected outcomes.	___	___	___	_____
3. Prepared client by allowing voiding of bladder before assessment, correctly draping and positioning client, and explaining steps of procedure.	___	___	___	_____
IMPLEMENTATION				
1. Described findings in relation to anatomic landmarks.	___	___	___	_____
2. Stood, then sat, to inspect abdomen's surface.	___	___	___	_____
3. Inspected skin of abdomen. Questioned client if bruising present.	___	___	___	_____
4. Inspected condition of umbilicus.	___	___	___	_____
5. Noted contour and symmetry of abdomen.	___	___	___	_____
6. Had client roll onto side if distention present.	___	___	___	_____
7. Asked client if abdomen felt unusually tight.	___	___	___	_____
8. Measured abdominal girth if distention suspected.	___	___	___	_____
9. Observed for abdominal contour while client took deep breath and held it.	___	___	___	_____

	S	U	NP	Comments
10. Assessed for any bulges while client raised head.				
11. Observed for movement across abdominal surface.				
12. Prepared for auscultation by asking client not to talk or turning nasogastric suction off if applicable.				
13. Auscultated bowel sounds systematically with diaphragm of stethoscope.				
14. Used bell of stethoscope to auscultate vascular sounds and notified physician if aortic bruit auscultated.				
15. Had client roll to side and placed bell of stethoscope over CVA.				
16. Had client return to supine position and percussed four abdominal quadrants.				
17. Percussed abdomen systematically.				
18. Located liver borders by percussion.				
19. Percussed for presence of kidney inflammation.				
20. Performed light palpation of abdomen.				
21. Palpated bladder area.				
22. Noted characteristics of any masses present.				
23. Assessed for rebound tenderness if area was tender on palpation.				
24. Palpated for lower liver border and spleen.				
25. Assessed aortic pulsation.				

EVALUATION

1. Compared findings with normal assessment characteristics of the abdomen.				
2. Asked client to describe signs and symptoms of colon cancer.				
3. Identified unexpected outcomes.				

NURSING DIAGNOSIS

1. Formulated appropriate nursing diagnoses based on assessment data.				

RECORDING AND REPORTING

1. Recorded results of assessment in nurses' notes or flowsheet.				
2. Recorded client instruction.				
3. Reported abnormalities to nurse in charge or physician.				

Student _____ Date _____

Instructor _____ Date _____

PERFORMANCE CHECKLIST 11-14 **ASSESSING THE FEMALE GENITALIA**

	S	U	NP	Comments

ASSESSMENT

1. Assessed for history of illness or surgery affecting reproductive organs.

2. Reviewed client's menstrual history.

3. Assessed for warning signs of cervical cancer.

4. Assessed client's obstetric history.

5. Reviewed client's contraceptive practices. Determined use of safe sex practices. Discussed risks of human immunodeficiency virus (HIV) and sexually transmitted diseases.

6. Assessed for history of genitourinary problems.

7. Assessed client's sexual history.

8. Assessed for signs and symptoms of sexually transmitted disease.

9. Assessed for warning signs of colorectal cancer or other gastrointestinal alterations.

PLANNING

1. Developed individualized goals for assessment.

2. Identified expected outcomes.

3. Prepared client for examination by asking her to void before procedure, assisting her to lithotomy position, draping her correctly, and explaining steps of procedure.

4. Asked colleague to be present.

IMPLEMENTATION
External Genitalia

1. Washed hands and applied disposable gloves.

2. Inspected outer perineum.

3. Touched client's thigh before touching perineum to avoid startling client.

4. Retracted labia correctly and inspected external genitalia systematically.

5. Inspected labia minora.

6. Inspected clitoris for size, color, signs of infection.

S   U   NP   Comments

7. Inspected vaginal opening.   ___ ___ ___   _____

8. Palpated Bartholin's gland if inflammation or edema present.   ___ ___ ___   _____

9. Observed urethral orifice for inflammation, discharge, mass.   ___ ___ ___   _____

10. Palpated Skene's gland. Changed gloves if drainage present.   ___ ___ ___   _____

11. Assessed muscular wall support of vaginal opening while asking client to bear down.   ___ ___ ___   _____

12. Assessed anal area if desired to do so at this time (Skill 11-16).   ___ ___ ___   _____

13. Offered perineal hygiene if examination completed. Removed gloves and washed hands.   ___ ___ ___   _____

Internal Genitalia

1. Assisted examiner in selecting correct size speculum.   ___ ___ ___   _____

2. Placed speculum blades under warm running water.   ___ ___ ___   _____

3. Adjusted light for proper visualization of genitalia.   ___ ___ ___   _____

4. Talked with client or explained procedure as examiner inserts and positions speculum.   ___ ___ ___   _____

5. Explained sensations client should expect while cervix is inspected.   ___ ___ ___   _____

6. Remained at examiner's side as cervix inspected.   ___ ___ ___   _____

7. Assisted examiner in obtaining Pap smear.   ___ ___ ___   _____

8. Remained at examiner's side and informed client that speculum was being removed.   ___ ___ ___   _____

9. Assisted client to more comfortable position after examination.   ___ ___ ___   _____

10. Offered perineal hygiene.   ___ ___ ___   _____

11. Disposed of gloves and washed hands.   ___ ___ ___   _____

EVALUATION

1. Compared findings with normal assessment characteristics for genitalia.   ___ ___ ___   _____

2. Evaluated client's emotional status following examinations.   ___ ___ ___   _____

3. Discussed importance of routine vaginal examinations with client.   ___ ___ ___   _____

4. Identified unexpected outcomes.   ___ ___ ___   _____

Student _____   Date _____

Instructor _____   Date _____

	S	U	NP	Comments

NURSING DIAGNOSIS

1. Formulated appropriate nursing diagnoses based on assessment data.   ___ ___ ___ _____

RECORDING AND REPORTING

1. Recorded all assessment findings and described client's reaction to examination.   ___ ___ ___ _____

2. Recorded instruction provided and client response.   ___ ___ ___ _____

3. Recorded time and date specimens were collected and sent to laboratory.   ___ ___ ___ _____

4. Recorded speculum size.   ___ ___ ___ _____

5. Reported abnormalities to nurse in charge or physician.   ___ ___ ___ _____

Student _____   Date _____

Instructor _____   Date _____

PERFORMANCE CHECKLIST 11-15   **ASSESSING THE MALE GENITALIA**

	S	U	NP	Comments
ASSESSMENT				
1. Assessed client's urinary elimination pattern.	__	__	__	_____
2. Assessed client's sexual history and use of safe sex practices.	__	__	__	_____
3. Assessed history of surgery or illness of urinary or reproductive systems.	__	__	__	_____
4. Assessed for signs and symptoms commonly associated with sexually transmitted diseases.	__	__	__	_____
5. Assessed for inguinal enlargement, if present, associated with pain, straining, lifting, or coughing.	__	__	__	_____
6. Assessed for signs and symptoms of testicular cancer.	__	__	__	_____
PLANNING				
1. Developed individualized goals for assessment.	__	__	__	_____
2. Identified expected outcomes.	__	__	__	_____
3. Prepared client by explaining procedure, asking client to empty bladder, positioning and draping client correctly.	__	__	__	_____
IMPLEMENTATION				
1. Washed hands and applied disposable gloves.	__	__	__	_____
2. Observed size and shape of penis and testes, color of scrotal skin, and pubic hair.	__	__	__	_____
3. Inspected skin covering genitalia.	__	__	__	_____
4. Inspected structures of penis; retracted foreskin of uncircumcised males; inspected urethra, glans, and shaft; milked penis if discharge present; palpated any existing lesions; returned foreskin to normal position.	__	__	__	_____
5. Inspected condition of scrotum.	__	__	__	_____
6. Lifted scrotal sac to view posterior surface.	__	__	__	_____
7. Palpated testes and epididymis.	__	__	__	_____
8. Instructed client on method for testicular self-examination.	__	__	__	_____
9. Inspected condition of inguinal rings before and after client held breath and bore down.	__	__	__	_____

	S	U	NP	Comments

10. Palpated inguinal ring and canal correctly.   ___ ___ ___ _____

11. Palpated lymph nodes in the inguinal area.   ___ ___ ___ _____

12. Removed gloves and washed hands.   ___ ___ ___ _____

EVALUATION

1. Compared findings with normal assessment characteristics for genitalia and rectum.   ___ ___ ___ _____

2. Evaluated client's anxiety level after examination.   ___ ___ ___ _____

3. Determined if client could perform testicular examination correctly.   ___ ___ ___ _____

4. Had client explain symptoms and STD and testicular cancer.   ___ ___ ___ _____

5. Identified unexpected outcomes.   ___ ___ ___ _____

NURSING DIAGNOSIS

1. Formulated appropriate nursing diagnoses based on assessment data.   ___ ___ ___ _____

RECORDING AND REPORTING

1. Recorded assessment findings and client's response to examination in nurses' notes.   ___ ___ ___ _____

2. Recorded instruction provided and client response.   ___ ___ ___ _____

3. Reported abnormalities to nurse in charge or physician.   ___ ___ ___ _____

4. Reported and recorded date and time cultures were sent to laboratory.   ___ ___ ___ _____

Student _____   Date _____

Instructor _____   Date _____

PERFORMANCE CHECKLIST 11-16   **ASSESSING THE RECTUM AND ANUS**

	S	U	NP	Comments

ASSESSMENT

1. Assessed for warning signs of colorectal cancer or other gastrointestinal alterations. ___ ___ ___ _____

2. Determined whether client has personal or family history of risk factors for colorectal cancer. Noted if client over age 40. ___ ___ ___ _____

3. Assessed dietary habits for high-fat or insufficient fiber intake. ___ ___ ___ _____

4. Determined whether client has undergone screening for colorectal cancer. ___ ___ ___ _____

5. Assessed medication history for laxatives or cathartic medications. ___ ___ ___ _____

6. Assessed for use of codeine or iron preparations. ___ ___ ___ _____

7. Assessed male for warning signs of prostate cancer. ___ ___ ___ _____

PLANNING

1. Developed individualized goals for assessment. ___ ___ ___ _____

2. Identified expected outcomes. ___ ___ ___ _____

3. Prepared and positioned client. ___ ___ ___ _____

IMPLEMENTATION

1. Washed hands and donned disposable gloves. ___ ___ ___ _____

2. Assessed symmetry of child's gluteal folds. ___ ___ ___ _____

3. For child, scratched skin around anus and noted response. ___ ___ ___ _____

4. Gently retracted buttocks of adult with nondominant hand. ___ ___ ___ _____

5. Inspected condition of perianal tissues. ___ ___ ___ _____

6. Had client bear down. ___ ___ ___ _____

7. Applied lubricant to gloved index finger of dominant hand. ___ ___ ___ _____

8. Had client bear down gently. ___ ___ ___ _____

9. Instructed client on sensations to be felt during assessment. ___ ___ ___ _____

10. Inserted fingertip into anus as sphincter relaxed. ___ ___ ___ _____

11. Noted tone of anal sphincter. ___ ___ ___ _____

	S	U	NP	Comments

12. Palpated along each side of rectal wall systematically; checked for contour, irregularities, tenderness.

13. Asked client to bear down when finger was at full extent of rectum.

14. Palpated prostate gland in male client.

15. Assessed for tone of sphincter by asking client to tighten muscles.

16. Tested any stool collected on gloves for evidence of blood.

17. Cleaned perineal/rectal area, assisted client to sitting position, and draped lower torso.

18. Disposed of gloves properly and washed hands.

EVALUATION

1. Compared findings with normal assessment characteristics for rectum.

2. Determined if client had pain during examination.

3. Asked client to describe risks for and signs of colorectal or prostate cancer.

4. Identified unexpected outcomes.

NURSING DIAGNOSIS

1. Formulated appropriate nursing diagnoses based on assessment data.

RECORDING AND REPORTING

1. Recorded all assessment findings and described client's reaction to examination.

2. Recorded instruction provided and client response.

3. Reported abnormalities to nurse in charge or physician.

4. Reported and recorded date and time specimens were collected and sent to laboratory.

Student _____   Date _____

Instructor _____   Date _____

PERFORMANCE CHECKLIST 11-17 **ASSESSING THE MUSCULOSKELETAL SYSTEM**

	S	U	NP	Comments
ASSESSMENT				
1. Reviewed history of trauma, injury, or disease involving musculoskeletal structures.	___	___	___	_____
2. Reviewed client's history for risk factors of osteoporosis.	___	___	___	_____
3. Determined risk factors for sports injury.	___	___	___	_____
4. Assessed nature and extent of client's pain.	___	___	___	_____
5. Determined client's perceptions of alterations in activities of daily living and social functions.	___	___	___	_____
6. Assessed height loss of female client over age 50.	___	___	___	_____
NURSING DIAGNOSIS				
1. Developed appropriate nursing diagnoses based on assessment data.	___	___	___	_____
PLANNING				
1. Developed individualized goals for assessment.	___	___	___	_____
2. Identified expected outcomes.	___	___	___	_____
3. Prepared client by integrating assessment into other portions of examination when appropriate, providing rest periods during assessment, assisting client properly in positioning, explaining steps of procedure.	___	___	___	_____
IMPLEMENTATION				
1. Observed client's gait.	___	___	___	_____
2. Observed for postural deformities.	___	___	___	_____
3. Observed client's gait and balance while walking straight line.	___	___	___	_____
4. Made a general observation of symmetry of joints, muscles, and extremity length.	___	___	___	_____
5. Palpated all bones, joints, and surrounding muscles gently.	___	___	___	_____
6. Measured joint ROM for all major joints.	___	___	___	_____
7. Used goniometer to measure precise degree of joint motion.	___	___	___	_____
8. Palpated for joint instability while measuring ROM.	___	___	___	_____

	S	U	NP	Comments
9. Assessed for muscular resistance.	——	——	——	_____
10. Assessed strength of each major muscle group.	——	——	——	_____
11. In presence of muscle weakness measured size of muscle and compared with opposite side of body.	——	——	——	_____

EVALUATION

	S	U	NP	Comments
1. Compared findings with normal assessment characteristics of musculoskeletal structures.	——	——	——	_____
2. Determined level of client's discomfort throughout examination.	——	——	——	_____
3. Identified unexpected outcomes.	——	——	——	_____

NURSING DIAGNOSIS

	S	U	NP	Comments
1. Formulated appropriate nursing diagnoses based on assessment data.	——	——	——	_____

RECORDING AND REPORTING

	S	U	NP	Comments
1. Recorded findings in nurses' notes.	——	——	——	_____
2. Reported abnormalities to nurse in charge or physician.	——	——	——	_____

Student _____   Date _____

Instructor _____   Date _____

PERFORMANCE CHECKLIST 11-18 **ASSESSING THE NEUROLOGIC SYSTEM**

	S	U	NP	Comments

ASSESSMENT

1. Determined whether client was taking medications that alter level of consciousness or behavior. ___ ___ ___ _____

2. Assessed for symptoms of central and peripheral nervous system alterations. ___ ___ ___ _____

3. Discussed with family members/friends changes in client's behavior. ___ ___ ___ _____

4. Assessed client for a history of changes in senses. ___ ___ ___ _____

PLANNING

1. Developed individualized goals for assessment. ___ ___ ___ _____

2. Identified expected outcomes. ___ ___ ___ _____

3. Prepared client by explaining procedures, integrating assessment into other portions of examination, positioning client correctly, screening client's neurologic function. ___ ___ ___ _____

IMPLEMENTATION
Mental and Emotional Status

1. Conducted mental status examination, if appropriate. ___ ___ ___ _____

2. Assessed client's level of consciousness. ___ ___ ___ _____

3. Rephrased questions that client seemed unable to understand. ___ ___ ___ _____

4. Asked questions about person, place, and time if client's initial answers were inappropriate. ___ ___ ___ _____

5. Tested ability to follow commands if client was disoriented. ___ ___ ___ _____

6. Assessed response to pain when appropriate. ___ ___ ___ _____

Behavior and Appearance

1. Made pertinent observations of client's behavior/mood throughout assessment. ___ ___ ___ _____

2. Observed manner of client's speech. ___ ___ ___ _____

3. Observed client's appearance. ___ ___ ___ _____

Language Function

1. Assessed ability of client to understand spoken or written words and to express self. ___ ___ ___ _____

	S	U	NP	Comments

Intellectual Function

1. Assessed client's immediate recall.   ___ ___ ___ _____

2. Assessed client's recent memory.   ___ ___ ___ _____

3. Assessed client's past memory.   ___ ___ ___ _____

4. Assessed client's knowledge of illness or hospitalization.   ___ ___ ___ _____

5. Tested client's ability to explain meaning of stated proverb.   ___ ___ ___ _____

6. Asked client to identify similarities or associations between simple terms or concepts.   ___ ___ ___ _____

7. Asked client why health care was sought and what would be done in response to sudden illness.   ___ ___ ___ _____

Cranial Nerve Function

1. Correctly assessed function of each of twelve cranial nerves.   ___ ___ ___ _____

Sensory Function

1. Tested sensory function with client's eyes closed.   ___ ___ ___ _____

2. Assessed client's sensory response to pain, temperature, light touch, vibration, position, two-point discrimination.   ___ ___ ___ _____

3. Measured sensation by applying stimuli in random, unpredictable order.   ___ ___ ___ _____

4. Compared sensation in symmetric body parts.   ___ ___ ___ _____

5. Asked client to say when particular stimulus perceived.   ___ ___ ___ _____

6. Placed familiar object in client's hand and asked client to identify object.   ___ ___ ___ _____

Motor Function

1. Assessed gait, stance, muscle strength, and tone.   ___ ___ ___ _____

2. Assessed client's ability to perform rapid repeating movements of upper extremity.   ___ ___ ___ _____

3. Assessed client's ability to perform skilled motor act.   ___ ___ ___ _____

4. Assessed client's upper extremity coordination.   ___ ___ ___ _____

5. Measured client's ability to perform rapid, repeated movement of lower extremities.   ___ ___ ___ _____

6. Assessed client's ability to perform heel-shin test.   ___ ___ ___ _____

7. Performed Romberg test.   ___ ___ ___ _____

8. Asked client to close eyes, stand on one foot, then the other.   ___ ___ ___ _____

Student _____   Date _____

Instructor _____   Date _____

	S	U	NP	Comments

Reflexes

1. Assessed deep tendon reflexes correctly and graded according to scale.   ___ ___ ___ _____

EVALUATION

1. Compared findings with normal assessment characteristics.   ___ ___ ___ _____

2. Identified unexpected outcomes.   ___ ___ ___ _____

NURSING DIAGNOSIS

1. Formulated appropriate nursing diagnoses based on assessment data.   ___ ___ ___ _____

RECORDING AND REPORTING

1. Recorded assessment findings in nurses' notes.   ___ ___ ___ _____

2. Reported abnormalities to nurse in charge or physician.   ___ ___ ___ _____

Student _____   Date _____

Instructor _____   Date _____

PERFORMANCE CHECKLIST 12-1   **APPLYING A NASAL CANNULA OR OXYGEN MASK**

	S	U	NP	Comments

ASSESSMENT

1. Observed for signs and symptoms associated with hypoxia.

2. Observed for patent airway and removed airway secretions.

3. Obtained results of client's most recent arterial blood gases (ABGs) study.

4. Reviewed client's medical record for medical order for oxygen therapy; noted method, flow rate, and duration of oxygen therapy.

5. Completed total respiratory system assessment.

NURSING DIAGNOSIS

1. Developed appropriate nursing diagnoses based on assessment data.

PLANNING

1. Developed individualized goals for client based on nursing diagnoses.

2. Identified expected outcomes.

3. Explained procedure and its purpose to client and family.

4. Correctly placed "Oxygen in use" signs.

IMPLEMENTATION

1. Washed hands.

2. Attached nasal cannula or oxygen mask to oxygen tubing and to humidified oxygen source (for flow rates more than 4L/min).

3. Adjusted oxygen flow rate to prescribed dosage.

4. Applied oxygen delivery device and adjusted to client's comfort. Allowed sufficient slack on oxygen tubing and secured to client's clothing.

5. Observed proper function of oxygen delivery device.

6. Followed up with physician if ABGs were necessary.

7. Washed hands.

	S	U	NP	Comments

EVALUATION

1. Reassessed client to determine response to oxygen administration. ___ ___ ___ _____

2. Observed client's mucous membrane and face for skin breakdown. ___ ___ ___ _____

3. Monitored ABGs or pulse oximetry. ___ ___ ___ _____

4. Assessed adequacy of oxygen flow each shift. ___ ___ ___ _____

5. Identified unexpected outcomes. ___ ___ ___ _____

RECORDING AND REPORTING

1. Recorded in nurses' notes respiratory assessment findings before and during oxygen therapy; method of oxygen delivery, flow rate, patency, client's response; any adverse reactions or side effects; change in physician's orders. ___ ___ ___ _____

Student _____   Date _____

Instructor _____   Date _____

PERFORMANCE CHECKLIST 12-2   **ADMINISTERING OXYGEN THERAPY TO A CLIENT WITH AN ARTIFICIAL AIRWAY**

	S	U	NP	Comments

ASSESSMENT

1. Observed for signs and symptoms associated with hypoxia.

2. Observed for patent airway and removed airway secretions.

3. Noted client's most recent ABG results.

4. Reviewed client's medical order for oxygen therapy.

5. Completed assessment of respiratory system.

NURSING DIAGNOSIS

1. Developed appropriate nursing diagnoses based on assessment data.

PLANNING

1. Developed individualized goals for client based on nursing diagnoses.

2. Identified expected outcomes.

3. Explained purpose of T-tube or tracheostomy collar to client and family.

4. Correctly placed "oxygen in use" signs.

IMPLEMENTATION

1. Washed hands. Applied gloves and goggles.

2. Attached T-tube or tracheostomy collar to large-bore oxygen tubing and to humidified oxygen source.

3. Adjusted oxygen flow rate at 10 L/min or as ordered and adjusted nebulizer to proper FiO_2 setting. Attached T-tube or tracheostomy collar to endotracheal or tracheostomy tube.

4. Monitored changes in flow rate with pulse oximetry.

5. Obtained ABGs 10-15 minutes after initiating T-tube.

6. Observed for T-tube pulling on endotracheal or tracheostomy tube. Suctioned secretions in T-tube or tracheostomy collar if necessary.

	S	U	NP	Comments

7. Observed oxygen tubing frequently for accumulation of fluid, and drained tubing correctly.   ___ ___ ___ _____

8. Set up suction equipment at client's bedside.   ___ ___ ___ _____

9. Removed gloves and goggles; washed hands.   ___ ___ ___ _____

EVALUATION

1. Assessed client's response to procedure, including respiratory status, LOC, etc.   ___ ___ ___ _____

2. Determined that oxygen delivery device was not pulling on artificial airway.   ___ ___ ___ _____

3. Monitored arterial blood gas levels or pulse oximetry.   ___ ___ ___ _____

4. Identified unexpected outcomes.   ___ ___ ___ _____

RECORDING AND REPORTING

1. Recorded in nurses' notes and included in report respiratory assessment findings before and during oxygen therapy; method of oxygen delivery, flow rate, client's response; any adverse reactions or side effects; change in physician's orders.   ___ ___ ___ _____

Student _____   Date _____

Instructor _____   Date _____

PERFORMANCE CHECKLIST 12-3   **USING INCENTIVE SPIROMETRY**

	S	U	NP	Comments
ASSESSMENT				
1. Identified clients who would benefit from incentive spirometry.	—	—	—	_____
2. Observed client's respiratory status.	—	—	—	_____
3. Reviewed physician's order for incentive spirometry.	—	—	—	_____
NURSING DIAGNOSIS				
1. Developed appropriate nursing diagnoses based on assessment data.	—	—	—	_____
PLANNING				
1. Developed individualized goals for client based on nursing diagnoses.	—	—	—	_____
2. Explained to client and family purpose and reason for using incentive spirometry.	—	—	—	_____
3. Identified expected outcomes.	—	—	—	_____
IMPLEMENTATION				
1. Washed hands.	—	—	—	_____
2. Instructed client to assume proper position.	—	—	—	_____
3. Demonstrated how to place mouthpiece.	—	—	—	_____
4. Instructed client to inhale slowly and maintain a constant flow through the unit, then hold breath for 2-3 seconds and exhale slowly. Instructed client to breathe normally for short period.	—	—	—	_____
5. Had client repeat maneuver.	—	—	—	_____
6. Washed hands.	—	—	—	_____
EVALUATION				
1. Reassessed client to determine response and ability to use incentive spirometry.	—	—	—	_____
2. Identified unexpected outcomes.	—	—	—	_____
RECORDING AND REPORTING				
1. Recorded in nurses' notes respiratory assessment before and after incentive spirometry, frequency of use, volumes achieved, and any adverse effects.	—	—	—	_____

Student _____   Date _____

Instructor _____   Date _____

PERFORMANCE CHECKLIST 12-4 **ADMINISTERING MECHANICAL VENTILATION**

	S	U	NP	Comments

ASSESSMENT

1. Observed for signs and symptoms associated with hypoxia.

2. Observed for patent airway and removed airway secretions.

3. Noted client's most recent ABG results if available.

4. Reviewed medical order for mechanical ventilation and ventilation settings.

5. Completed assessment of respiratory system.

NURSING DIAGNOSIS

1. Developed appropriate nursing diagnoses based on assessment data.

PLANNING

1. Developed individualized goals for client based on nursing diagnoses.

2. Identified expected outcomes.

3. Explained purpose of mechanical ventilation to client and others.

IMPLEMENTATION

1. Washed hands and applied gloves and goggles.

2. Attached mechanical ventilator to endotracheal or tracheostomy tube. Observed for proper functioning of mechanical ventilator.

3. Assessed for client anxiety and respiration in synchronization with mechanical ventilation. Monitored vital signs.

4. Secured ventilator tubing to prevent dislodging of artificial airway.

5. Set up suction equipment.

6. Followed up with physician frequently about client status and response to therapy.

7. Removed gloves and goggles; washed hands.

EVALUATION

1. Evaluated client's response to mechanical ventilation.

	S	U	NP	Comments
2. Assessed integrity of client's ventilator system.	___	___	___	_____
3. Identified unexpected outcomes.	___	___	___	_____

RECORDING AND REPORTING

1. Recorded in nurses' notes method of oxygen delivery, flow rate, client's response, any adverse effects, change in physician's orders.

    ___ ___ ___ _____

Student _____   Date _____

Instructor _____   Date _____

PERFORMANCE CHECKLIST 12-5   **MEASURING PEAK EXPIRATORY FLOW RATES (PEFR)**

	S	U	NP	Comments

ASSESSMENT

1. Observed for signs and symptoms of airway obstruction.

2. Observed for patent airway and need for removal of secretions.

3. Completed total respiratory assessment.

4. Reviewed client's medical record for order to measure PEFR and expected rate client is to achieve.

NURSING DIAGNOSES

1. Formulated appropriate nursing diagnoses based on assessment data.

PLANNING

1. Developed individualized client goals based on nursing diagnoses.

2. Identified expected outcomes.

3. Explained procedure to client and family.

IMPLEMENTATION

1. Placed indicator at the bottom of the numbered scale.

2. Had client stand up and sit on edge of bed or in high Fowler's position.

3. Had client take deep breath.

4. Had client place meter in mouth and close lips around mouthpiece.

5. Had client blow out as hard and as fast as possible.

6. Had client repeat Steps 1-5 two more times, noting highest number achieved.

EVALUATION

1. Determined client's PEFR and compared with the client's personal best.

2. Reassessed client for improvement in symptoms if bronchodilator therapy has been initiated.

3. Observed client performing PEFR.

4. Identified unexpected outcomes.

S   U   NP   Comments

RECORDING AND REPORTING

1. Recorded in nurses' notes and included in report PEFR measurement, client's ability to use peak flowmeter, any symptoms client had, and any therapy client may have received as result of PEFR measurement.

___ ___ ___ _____

Student _____   Date _____

Instructor _____   Date _____

PERFORMANCE CHECKLIST 13-1   **PERFORMING POSTURAL DRAINAGE**

	S	U	NP	Comments
ASSESSMENT				
1. Assessed for impairment in airway clearance.	—	—	—	_____
2. Identified signs and symptoms that indicated need to perform postural drainage.	—	—	—	_____
3. Identified, through appropriate measures, which bronchial segments needed to be drained.	—	—	—	_____
4. Determined client's understanding of and ability to perform home postural drainage.	—	—	—	_____
NURSING DIAGNOSIS				
1. Developed appropriate nursing diagnoses based on assessment data.	—	—	—	_____
PLANNING				
1. Developed individualized goals for client based on nursing diagnoses.	—	—	—	_____
2. Identified expected outcomes.	—	—	—	_____
3. Correctly prepared client for procedure and instructed client to remove any tight or restrictive clothing.	—	—	—	_____
IMPLEMENTATION				
1. Washed hands.	—	—	—	_____
2. Selected areas to be drained.	—	—	—	_____
3. Correctly positioned client.	—	—	—	_____
4. Had client maintain posture for 10-15 minutes.	—	—	—	_____
5. Performed percussion, vibration, or rib shaking with hands in correct position.	—	—	—	_____
6. After drainage in first position, had client sit up and cough, and saved expectorated secretions.	—	—	—	_____
7. Allowed client to rest.	—	—	—	_____
8. Had client sip water.	—	—	—	_____
9. Repeated Steps 3-8 for all congested areas in accepted time frame.	—	—	—	_____
10. Washed hands.	—	—	—	_____
EVALUATION				
1. Evaluated changes in chest assessment after drainage.	—	—	—	_____

	S	U	NP	Comments
2. Assessed character of sputum.	—	—	—	_____
3. Reviewed diagnostic reports on client's pulmonary function.	—	—	—	_____
4. Evaluated client's understanding of procedure.	—	—	—	_____
5. Identified unexpected outcomes.	—	—	—	_____

RECORDING AND REPORTING

1. Recorded procedure in nurses' notes.	—	—	—	_____
2. Recorded client education for home care and referrals.	—	—	—	_____

Student _____ Date _____

Instructor _____ Date _____

PERFORMANCE CHECKLIST 13-2 **PERFORMING PERCUSSION, VIBRATION, AND RIB SHAKING**

	S	U	NP	Comments
ASSESSMENT				
1. Assessed client's breathing patterns.	—	—	—	_____
2. Identified signs and symptoms and conditions that indicated need to perform skills.	—	—	—	_____
3. Assessed rib cage and bronchial segment being drained.	—	—	—	_____
4. Assessed client's understanding and ability to perform procedure at home.	—	—	—	_____
NURSING DIAGNOSIS				
1. Developed appropriate nursing diagnoses based on assessment data.	—	—	—	_____
PLANNING				
1. Developed individualized goals for client based on nursing diagnoses.	—	—	—	_____
2. Identified expected outcomes.	—	—	—	_____
3. Prepared client for procedure.	—	—	—	_____
IMPLEMENTATION				
1. With client in correct position, assessed and identified chest wall area to be percussed and vibrated.	—	—	—	_____
2. Instructed client in relaxation and breathing techniques.	—	—	—	_____
3. Used good body mechanics.	—	—	—	_____
4. Performed chest wall percussion.	—	—	—	_____
5. Performed chest wall vibration.	—	—	—	_____
6. Assessed client's tolerance of vibration.	—	—	—	_____
7. Performed rib shaking as needed.	—	—	—	_____
8. Completed vibration and rib shaking in each posture.	—	—	—	_____
9. Taught client and family techniques for percussion, vibration, and rib shaking.	—	—	—	_____
EVALUATION				
1. Evaluated changes in chest wall after procedure.	—	—	—	_____
2. Assessed character of mucus.	—	—	—	_____

	S	U	NP	Comments

3. Reviewed diagnostic test results for pulmonary function.

4. Observed care giver perform percussion, vibration, and rib shaking.

5. Identified unexpected outcomes.

RECORDING AND REPORTING

1. Correctly recorded treatment given and client response.

2. Recorded home teaching given to client and family.

Student _____   Date _____

Instructor _____   Date _____

PERFORMANCE CHECKLIST 14-1 **PERFORMING ORAL PHARYNGEAL (YANKAUER) SUCTIONING**

	S	U	NP	Comments

ASSESSMENT

1. Observed for signs and symptoms of airway obstruction requiring oral pharyngeal suctioning. — — — _____

2. Assessed client's knowledge of catheter use. — — — _____

3. Assessed for risk factors. — — — _____

NURSING DIAGNOSIS

1. Developed appropriate nursing diagnoses based on assessment data. — — — _____

PLANNING

1. Developed individualized goals for client based on nursing diagnoses. — — — _____

2. Identified expected outcomes. — — — _____

3. Explained procedure to client. — — — _____

4. Positioned client correctly; placed towel across client's chest. — — — _____

IMPLEMENTATION

1. Washed hands and applied gloves. Applied mask or face shield if indicated. — — — _____

2. Filled cup or basin with approximately 100 ml of water. — — — _____

3. Turned suction device to appropriate pressure. — — — _____

4. Connected tubing properly, filled cup with water, and checked that apparatus was functioning properly. — — — _____

5. Removed oxygen mask if present. — — — _____

6. Inserted catheter into mouth and suctioned correctly. Replaced oxygen mask. — — — _____

7. Rinsed catheter. Turned off suction. — — — _____

8. Assessed client's respiratory status. Repeated procedure, if indicated. — — — _____

9. Disposed of towel properly and repositioned client. — — — _____

10. Discarded water and cup, washed and dried basin, placed catheter in clean, dry area. — — — _____

	S	U	NP	Comments

11. Removed and disposed of gloves, mask, and face shield. Washed hands. ___ ___ ___ _____

EVALUATION

1. Compared assessments before and after procedure. ___ ___ ___ _____

2. Auscultated chest and airways for adventitious sounds. ___ ___ ___ _____

3. Observed client or care giver perform procedure. ___ ___ ___ _____

4. Identified unexpected outcomes. ___ ___ ___ _____

RECORDING AND REPORTING

1. Recorded procedure, client's respiratory status, and education provided in nurses' notes. ___ ___ ___ _____

Student _____   Date _____

Instructor _____   Date _____

PERFORMANCE CHECKLIST 14-2   **PERFORMING NASAL PHARYNGEAL AND NASAL TRACHEAL SUCTIONING**

	S	U	NP	Comments

ASSESSMENT

1. Identified signs and symptoms of upper and lower airway obstruction requiring nasal and oral tracheal suctioning.   ___ ___ ___ _____

2. Determined factors that normally influence lower airway functioning.   ___ ___ ___ _____

3. Assessed client's understanding of procedure.   ___ ___ ___ _____

4. Obtained physician's order if required.   ___ ___ ___ _____

NURSING DIAGNOSIS

1. Developed appropriate nursing diagnoses based on assessment data.   ___ ___ ___ _____

PLANNING

1. Developed individualized goals for client based on nursing diagnosis.   ___ ___ ___ _____

2. Identified expected outcomes.   ___ ___ ___ _____

3. Explained procedure and importance of coughing to client.   ___ ___ ___ _____

4. Positioned client.   ___ ___ ___ _____

5. Placed towel across client's chest.   ___ ___ ___ _____

IMPLEMENTATION

1. Washed hands and applied face shield.   ___ ___ ___ _____

2. Connected tubing to suction machine, turned suction device on, and set vacuum regulator to appropriate pressure.   ___ ___ ___ _____

3. Increased supplemental oxygen as indicated or ordered by physician. Encouraged deep breathing.   ___ ___ ___ _____

4. Prepared suction catheter correctly.   ___ ___ ___ _____

5. Applied sterile gloves properly.   ___ ___ ___ _____

6. Connected catheter to tubing properly.   ___ ___ ___ _____

7. Checked that equipment was functioning correctly.   ___ ___ ___ _____

8. Coated distal end of catheter with water-soluble lubricant.   ___ ___ ___ _____

	S	U	NP	Comments

9. Removed oxygen delivery device, if present. Inserted catheter gently into naris on inhalation.

10. Applied intermittent suction, encouraging client to cough as appropriate. (Performed tracheal suctioning first.) Replaced oxygen device, if applicable.

11. Rinsed catheter and connecting tubing with saline.

12. Reassessed need to repeat suctioning. Allowed time between suction passes for oxygenation. Asked client to deep breathe and cough.

13. Performed oral pharyngeal suctioning after trachea and pharynx were cleared of secretions.

14. Discarded catheter correctly. Removed and discarded gloves correctly.

15. Discarded towel and repositioned client.

16. Readjusted oxygen to original level if indicated.

17. Discarded saline and basin (washed and stored reusable basin).

18. Removed and disposed of face shield. Washed hands.

19. Placed unopened suction kit at head of bed.

EVALUATION

1. Compared assessments before and after suctioning.

2. Asked client if breathing is easier.

3. Identified unexpected outcomes.

RECORDING AND REPORTING

1. Recorded procedure and client assessments in nurses' notes.

Student _____   Date _____

Instructor _____   Date _____

PERFORMANCE CHECKLIST 14-3 **PERFORMING ENDOTRACHEAL OR TRACHEOSTOMY TUBE SUCTIONING**

	S	U	NP	Comments

ASSESSMENT

1. Observed for signs and symptoms indicating need for endotracheal or tracheostomy tube suctioning.

2. Determined factors that influence normal airway functioning.

3. Examined sputum laboratory data.

4. Assessed client's understanding of procedure and when suctioning is necessary.

NURSING DIAGNOSIS

1. Developed appropriate nursing diagnoses based on assessment data.

PLANNING

1. Developed individualized goals for client based on nursing diagnoses.

2. Identified expected outcomes.

3. Explained procedure to client.

4. Positioned client.

5. Placed towel across client's chest.

IMPLEMENTATION

1. Washed hands and applied face shield.

2. Connected tubing to suction machine, turned suction device on, and set vacuum regulator to appropriate pressure.

3. Prepared suction catheter correctly.

4. Applied lubricant to sterile catheter package if indicated.

5. Applied gloves properly.

6. Connected catheter to tubing properly.

7. Checked that equipment was functioning correctly.

8. Coated distal end of catheter with water-soluble lubricant if indicated.

9. Oxygenated client.

S   U   NP   Comments

10. Opened swivel adapter or removed oxygen or humidity device with nondominant hand.   ___ ___ ___   _____

11. Inserted catheter gently and pulled catheter back 1 cm when resistance was met.   ___ ___ ___   _____

12. Applied intermittent suction, encouraging client to cough as appropriate. Observed for respiratory distress.   ___ ___ ___   _____

13. Closed swivel adapter or replaced oxygen delivery device. Encouraged client to deep breathe.   ___ ___ ___   _____

14. Rinsed catheter and connecting tubing with normal saline.   ___ ___ ___   _____

15. Assessed client's cardiopulmonary status. Repeated Steps 1-15 if needed.   ___ ___ ___   _____

16. Performed nasal and oral pharyngeal suctioning when tracheobronchial tree was clear.   ___ ___ ___   _____

17. Disconnected catheter. Discarded gloves and catheter correctly.   ___ ___ ___   _____

18. Discarded towel.   ___ ___ ___   _____

19. Repositioned client.   ___ ___ ___   _____

20. Discarded saline and basin (washed and stored reusable basin).   ___ ___ ___   _____

21. Removed and discarded face shield. Washed hands.   ___ ___ ___   _____

22. Placed unopened suction kit at head of bed.   ___ ___ ___   _____

EVALUATION

1. Compared assessments before and after procedure.   ___ ___ ___   _____

2. Asked client if breathing easier.   ___ ___ ___   _____

3. Observed airway secretions.   ___ ___ ___   _____

4. Identified unexpected outcomes.   ___ ___ ___   _____

RECORDING AND REPORTING

1. Recorded procedure and client assessments in nurses' notes.   ___ ___ ___   _____

Student _____   Date _____

Instructor _____   Date _____

PERFORMANCE CHECKLIST 14-4 **PERFORMING ENDOTRACHEAL OR TRACHEOSTOMY TUBE SUCTIONING USING A CLOSED SYSTEM (IN-LINE) CATHETER**

	S	U	NP	Comments

ASSESSMENT

1. Observed for signs and symptoms of lower airway obstruction requiring ET or tracheostomy tube suctioning.

2. Determined factors that influence normal airway function.

3. Examined sputum microbiology data.

4. Assessed client's understanding of procedure and feeling need to be suctioned.

NURSING DIAGNOSIS

1. Formulated appropriate nursing diagnoses based on assessment data.

PLANNING

1. Developed individualized client goals based on nursing diagnoses.

2. Identified expected outcomes.

3. Explained procedure to client.

4. Positioned client comfortably.

5. Placed towel across client's chest.

IMPLEMENTATION

1. Washed hands. Optional: applied gloves.

2. Attached suction according to agency policy and prepared suction apparatus correctly.

3. Hyperinflated and/or hyperoxygenated client according to institutional protocol and clinical status.

4. Unlocked suction control mechanism if required. Opened saline port and attached saline.

5. Picked up enclosed suction catheter with dominant hand. Advanced catheter and administered saline correctly if indicated.

6. Inserted catheter correctly after saline dispension.

7. Applied suction correctly and withdrew catheter.

	S	U	NP	Comments

8. Assessed need for repeated suctioning and performed suctioning if needed. Reassessed cardiopulmonary status. ___ ___ ___ _____

9. Withdrew catheter completely and rinsed properly. ___ ___ ___ _____

10. Performed oral or nasal suctioning if indicated. ___ ___ ___ _____

11. Repositioned client. ___ ___ ___ _____

12. Removed and disposed of gloves. Washed hands. ___ ___ ___ _____

13. Turned off suction device. ___ ___ ___ _____

EVALUATION

1. Compared client's respiratory assessments before and after suctioning. ___ ___ ___ _____

2. Observed airway secretions. ___ ___ ___ _____

3. Asked client if breathing is easier. ___ ___ ___ _____

4. Identified unexpected outcomes. ___ ___ ___ _____

RECORDING AND REPORTING

1. Charted in nurses' notes: respiratory assessments before and after suctioning; size of suction catheter used; amount of negative suction pressure used; duration of suctioning period; route(s) used to suction; secretions obtained and odor, amount, color, consistency; frequency of suctioning; client's tolerance of procedure. ___ ___ ___ _____

Student _____   Date _____

Instructor _____   Date _____

PERFORMANCE CHECKLIST 14-5   **PERFORMING ENDOTRACHEAL TUBE CARE**

	S	U	NP	Comments

ASSESSMENT

1. Observed for signs and symptoms of need to perform ET tube care.

2. Identified factors placing client at greater risk.

3. Assessed client's knowledge of procedure.

NURSING DIAGNOSIS

1. Developed appropriate nursing diagnoses based on assessment data.

PLANNING

1. Developed individualized goals for client based on nursing diagnoses.

2. Identified expected outcomes.

3. Asked another nurse to assist with procedure.

4. Positioned client.

5. Placed towel across chest.

IMPLEMENTATION

1. Washed hands. Applied face shield if indicated.

2. Administered endotracheal nasal and oral pharyngeal suction.

3. Left suction catheter connected to suction source.

4. Prepared adhesive tape correctly.

5. Applied gloves and instructed assistant to apply gloves and hold ET tube firmly.

6. Removed tape carefully from tube and client's face and discarded tape properly.

7. Cleared excess adhesive from client's face.

8. Removed oral airway or bite block and placed on towel.

9. Cleaned mouth, gums, and teeth opposite ET tube.

10. For oral ET tube only, moved ET tube to opposite side of mouth with assistant's help.

11. Repeated oral cleaning as in Step 9 for second side of mouth.

	S	U	NP	Comments

12. Cleaned and dried face and neck. Shaved male client as necessary.

13. Applied small amount of skin protectant to face.

14. Positioned tape carefully under head and neck.

15. Secured tape from ear to naris and secured tape across upper lip if oral ET tube or across top of nose if nasal ET tube.

16. Secured tape to remaining side of face and secured tape to tube correctly.

17. Cleaned and rinsed oral airway.

18. Reinserted oral airway. Secured with tape, if indicated.

19. Discarded soiled items.

20. Repositioned client.

21. Nurse and assistant removed gloves and washed hands. Removed face shield.

EVALUATION

1. Compared assessments before and after procedure.

2. Observed depth and position of ET tube.

3. Assessed security of tape.

4. Assessed skin around mouth and oral mucous membranes.

5. Identified unexpected outcomes.

RECORDING AND REPORTING

1. Charted in Kardex appropriate depth of ET tube and frequency of care.

2. Recorded procedure and client assessments in nurses' notes.

Student _____   Date _____

Instructor _____   Date _____

PERFORMANCE CHECKLIST 14-6 **PERFORMING TRACHEOSTOMY CARE**

	S	U	NP	Comments

ASSESSMENT

1. Observed for signs and symptoms of need to perform tracheostomy care.

2. Observed for factors influencing tracheostomy airway function.

3. Assessed client's understanding of and ability to perform own tracheostomy care.

4. Checked when tracheostomy care was last done.

NURSING DIAGNOSIS

1. Developed appropriate nursing diagnoses based on assessment data.

PLANNING

1. Developed individualized goals for client based on nursing diagnoses.

2. Identified expected outcomes.

3. Asked another nurse or family member to assist with procedure.

4. Explained procedure to client.

5. Positioned client comfortably.

6. Placed towel across client's chest.

IMPLEMENTATION

1. Washed hands and donned gloves. Applied face shield if indicated.

2. Suctioned tracheostomy.

3. Prepared equipment at bedside table.

4. Applied gloves. Kept dominant hand sterile throughout procedure.

*5. Removed oxygen source and inner cannula. Dropped inner cannula into hydrogen peroxide basin.

6. Placed tracheostomy collar oxygen source over outer cannula. Placed T-tube and ventilator oxygen sources near outer cannula.

*For tracheostomy tube with inner cannula, nurse completed Steps 5-17. For tracheostomy tube with no inner cannula or Kistner button, nurse completed Steps 9-17.

	S	U	NP	Comments

7. Removed secretions inside and outside inner cannula.

8. Rinsed inner cannula correctly.

9. Replaced inner cannula and secured locking mechanism.

10. Cleaned outer cannula surfaces and stoma under faceplate.

11. Rinsed outer cannula and stoma under faceplate.

12. Patted skin and outer cannula lightly with gauze.

13. Cut new ties properly with assistant's help as needed.

14. Inserted fresh tracheostomy dressing under clean ties and faceplate.

15. Positioned client comfortably and assessed respiratory status.

16. Removed and discarded gloves, face shield, and soiled ties correctly.

17. Stored supplies correctly.

18. Washed hands.

EVALUATION

1. Compared assessments before and after procedure.

2. Assessed comfort of new tracheostomy ties.

3. Observed inner and outer cannula for secretions.

4. Assessed stoma for signs of infection or skin breakdown.

5. Identified unexpected outcomes

RECORDING AND REPORTING

1. Charted in Kardex: type and size of tracheostomy tube and frequency of care.

2. Recorded procedure and client assessment in nurses' notes.

Student _____   Date _____

Instructor _____   Date _____

PERFORMANCE CHECKLIST 14-7 **INFLATING THE CUFF ON AN ENDOTRACHEAL OR TRACHEOSTOMY TUBE**

	S	U	NP	Comments

ASSESSMENT

1. Observed for signs and symptoms indicating need to perform cuff care. ___ ___ ___ _____

2. Determined caregiver's understanding of procedure if client discharged with a cuffed tracheostomy tube. ___ ___ ___ _____

NURSING DIAGNOSIS

1. Developed appropriate nursing diagnoses based on assessment data. ___ ___ ___ _____

PLANNING

1. Developed individualized goals for client based on nursing diagnoses. ___ ___ ___ _____

2. Identified expected outcomes. ___ ___ ___ _____

3. Explained procedure to client. ___ ___ ___ _____

4. Positioned client comfortably. ___ ___ ___ _____

IMPLEMENTATION

1. Washed hands, applied gloves and face shield if indicated. ___ ___ ___ _____

2. Suctioned client. ___ ___ ___ _____

3. Connected syringe to pilot balloon. ___ ___ ___ _____

4. Assessed proper cuff inflation with stethoscope. ___ ___ ___ _____

5. Removed all air from cuff if no air leak heard. ___ ___ ___ _____

6. Correctly inflated cuff and assessed for minimal leak with stethoscope. ___ ___ ___ _____

7. Slowly reinflated cuff if excessive air was heard. ___ ___ ___ _____

8. Cleansed stethoscope with alcohol wipe after removal. ___ ___ ___ _____

9. Removed syringe and discarded in appropriate receptacle. ___ ___ ___ _____

10. Repositioned client. ___ ___ ___ _____

11. Removed and disposed of gloves and face shield. Washed hands. ___ ___ ___ _____

	S	U	NP	Comments

EVALUATION

1. Compared assessments before and after procedure.

   — — — _____

2. Observed exhaled tidal volume from mechanical ventilator.

   — — — _____

3. Auscultate for audible air leak.

   — — — _____

4. Observed for signs of excessive cuff inflation.

   — — — _____

5. Identified unexpected outcomes.

   — — — _____

RECORDING AND REPORTING

1. Recorded in nurses' notes: presence of minimal leak at end inspiration, volume of air injected into cuff, secretions obtained when suctioning, frequency of cuff care.

   — — — _____

Student _____   Date _____

Instructor _____   Date _____

PERFORMANCE CHECKLIST 15-1 CARING FOR CLIENTS WITH CHEST TUBE CONNECTED TO DISPOSABLE DRAINAGE SYSTEMS

	S	U	NP	Comments
ASSESSMENT				
1. Obtained vital signs.	___	___	___	_____
2. Observed for changes in vital signs, increased apprehension, and chest pain.	___	___	___	_____
3. Assessed client for known allergies.	___	___	___	_____
4. Reviewed client's medical record for anticoagulant therapy.	___	___	___	_____
NURSING DIAGNOSIS				
1. Developed appropriate nursing diagnoses based on assessment data.	___	___	___	_____
PLANNING				
1. Developed individualized goals for client based on nursing diagnoses. Identified expected outcomes.	___	___	___	_____
2. Determined if informed consent was obtained if required.	___	___	___	_____
3. Reviewed physician's role and responsibilities for chest tube placement.	___	___	___	_____
4. Explained procedure to client.	___	___	___	_____
5. Gathered necessary equipment and supplies.	___	___	___	_____
6. Washed hands.	___	___	___	_____
7. Prepared prescribed drainage system.	___	___	___	_____
8. Correctly taped all connections and checked systems for patency.	___	___	___	_____
9. Turned off suction source and unclamped drainage tubing before connecting client to system.	___	___	___	_____
10. Positioned client correctly.	___	___	___	_____
IMPLEMENTATION				
1. Washed hands and applied gloves.	___	___	___	_____
2. Administered parenteral medications, if ordered.	___	___	___	_____
3. Assisted physician in providing psychologic support.	___	___	___	_____
4. Showed anesthetic to physician.	___	___	___	_____
5. Held anesthetic solution bottle upside down with label facing physician.	___	___	___	_____
6. Assisted physician in connecting drainage system.	___	___	___	_____

	S	U	NP	Comments

7. Taped the tube connection between the chest and drainage tubes.

8. Assessed patency of air vents in system.

9. Coiled and secured excess tubing on mattress next to client.

10. Promoted drainage by correctly adjusting tubing to hang in a straight line from mattress to drainage chamber.

11. Recorded time that drainage began on appropriate place on system.

12. Stripped or milked chest tube if ordered or indicated.

13. Provided hemostats to remain at bedside.

14. Assisted client to comfortable position.

15. Disposed of soiled equipment and removed gloves.

16. Washed hands.

EVALUATION

1. Assessed client's physical and psychologic status.

2. Assessed client's compliance in activities of daily living related to care of the drainage system.

3. Assessed collection system for proper functioning and for type and amount of fluid drainage.

4. Assessed client's respiratory status and vital signs.

5. Identified unexpected outcomes.

RECORDING AND REPORTING

1. Recorded and reported stated allergies and anticoagulant medications client is taking.

2. Recorded baseline vital signs.

3. Recorded postoperative vital signs at appropriate time intervals.

4. Checked chest tube insertion site and dressings at appropriate time intervals.

5. Recorded chest drainage output at appropriate time intervals.

6. Documented proper functioning of system.

7. Recorded client's physical and psychologic status at appropriate time intervals.

8. Documented that client is receiving prescribed amount of suction.

9. Recorded and reported air leaks and action(s) taken.

10. Recorded client compliance to coughing, deep breathing, and activity.

11. Documented whether system was intact and time, amount, and type of drainage.

Student _____   Date _____

Instructor _____   Date _____

PERFORMANCE CHECKLIST 15-2   **REMOVING CHEST TUBES**

	S	U	NP	Comments
ASSESSMENT				
1. Identified signs that reveal lung reexpansion.	—	—	—	_____
2. Clamped chest tube 12-24 hours before removal or as ordered by physician.	—	—	—	_____
NURSING DIAGNOSIS				
1. Developed appropriate nursing diagnoses based on assessment data.	—	—	—	_____
PLANNING				
1. Developed individualized goals for client based on nursing diagnoses.	—	—	—	_____
2. Identified expected outcomes.	—	—	—	_____
3. Explained procedure to client.	—	—	—	_____
IMPLEMENTATION				
1. Administered prescribed premedication approximately 30 minutes before procedure.	—	—	—	_____
2. Assisted client to correct position.	—	—	—	_____
3. Supported client physically and emotionally while physician or APN removed dressing and clipped sutures.	—	—	—	_____
4. Remained with client while physician or APN prepared occlusive dressing.	—	—	—	_____
5. Assisted client as physician or APN asked client to take a deep breath and hold it or exhale completely and hold it.	—	—	—	_____
6. Remained with client while physician or APN pulled out chest tube.	—	—	—	_____
7. Remained with client while physician or APN applied prepared occlusive dressing.	—	—	—	_____
8. Assisted client to comfortable position.	—	—	—	_____
9. Donned gloves and removed used equipment from bedside.	—	—	—	_____
10. Removed gloves. Washed hands.	—	—	—	_____
EVALUATION				
1. Observed client for subcutaneous emphysema or respiratory distress during first few hours after removal.	—	—	—	_____

	S	U	NP	Comments

2. Assessed client's vital signs and psychologic status. ___ ___ ___ _____

3. Asked client about level of pain or comfort. ___ ___ ___ _____

4. Assessed chest dressing for drainage and patency. ___ ___ ___ _____

5. Identified unexpected outcomes. ___ ___ ___ _____

RECORDING AND REPORTING

1. Recorded removal of tube, amount of drainage, wound appearance, and client assessment. ___ ___ ___ _____

Student _____   Date _____

Instructor _____   Date _____

PERFORMANCE CHECKLIST 15-3 **POSTOPERATIVE AUTOTRANSFUSION**

	S	U	NP	Comments
ASSESSMENT				
1. Obtained vital signs.	—	—	—	_____
2. Observed for changes in vital signs, increased apprehension, and chest pain.	—	—	—	_____
3. Assessed client for known allergies.	—	—	—	_____
4. Reviewed client's medical record for anticoagulant therapy.	—	—	—	_____
NURSING DIAGNOSIS				
1. Formulated appropriate nursing diagnoses based on assessment data.	—	—	—	_____
PLANNING				
1. Developed individualized client goals based on nursing diagnoses.	—	—	—	_____
2. Identified expected outcomes.	—	—	—	_____
IMPLEMENTATION				
1. Demonstrated correct technique with system setup, including proper equipment, tight connections, maintenance of unit sterility.	—	—	—	_____
2. Performed continuous collection correctly.				
a. Pleur-Evac A-1500 bag opened properly and excessive negative pressure relieved.	—	—	—	_____
b. Demonstrated proper technique including correct clamp management for removal of initial bag and securing replacement bag.	—	—	—	_____
3. Completed reinfusion process properly.				
a. Used new microaggregate filter for each bag.	—	—	—	_____
b. Accessed bag correctly, and after priming filter, hung bag for reinfusion.	—	—	—	_____
c. Added any ordered anticoagulants.	—	—	—	_____
4. Reconnected chest drainage tube to Pleur-Evac unit properly when autotransfusion completed.	—	—	—	_____
5. Discontinued autotransfusion correctly.	—	—	—	_____
EVALUATION				
1. Monitored vital signs, hematocrit, and hemoglobin.	—	—	—	_____

	S	U	NP	Comments

2. Monitored chest drainage system and client's lung sounds.

    ___ ___ ___ _____

3. Assessed the IV infusion site for infiltration and phlebitis.

    ___ ___ ___ _____

4. Identified unexpected outcomes.

    ___ ___ ___ _____

RECORDING AND REPORTING

1. Recorded drainage, reinfusion with times, and amounts of each.

    ___ ___ ___ _____

2. Described the condition of the IV infusion site.

    ___ ___ ___ _____

3. Reported unusual findings and client's responses to nurse in charge or physician.

    ___ ___ ___ _____

Student _____   Date _____

Instructor _____   Date _____

PERFORMANCE CHECKLIST 16-1 **REMOVING A FOREIGN BODY AIRWAY OBSTRUCTION**

	S	U	NP	Comments
ASSESSMENT				
1. Identified physical signs and symptoms indicating need to perform foreign body obstruction airway maneuver (FBOAM).	___	___	___	_____
2. Identified factors influencing use of FBOAM.	___	___	___	_____
3. Identified client and family understanding of FBOAM and anticipated outcomes.	___	___	___	_____
NURSING DIAGNOSIS				
1. Developed appropriate nursing diagnoses based on assessment data.	___	___	___	_____
PLANNING				
1. Developed individualized goals for client based on nursing diagnoses.	___	___	___	_____
2. Identified expected outcomes.	___	___	___	_____
3. Explained procedure to client.	___	___	___	_____
4. Positioned client appropriately.	___	___	___	_____
5. Removed dentures or other nonpermanent dental work.	___	___	___	_____
6. Activated emergency medical services.	___	___	___	_____
IMPLEMENTATION				
1. Washed hands and applied gloves and face shield if possible.	___	___	___	_____
2. Administered finger sweep correctly.	___	___	___	_____
3. Measured pulse and respirations. If absent, began CPR.	___	___	___	_____
4. Administered appropriate maneuver to clear obstructed airway.	___	___	___	_____
a. Performed Heimlich maneuver correctly.	___	___	___	_____
b. Performed chest thrusts correctly.	___	___	___	_____
c. Performed back blows and chest thrusts for infants correctly.	___	___	___	_____
5. Repeated sequence of finger sweep and thrust maneuver as long as necessary.	___	___	___	_____
6. Removed and disposed of gloves and face shield. Washed hands.				_____

	S	U	NP	Comments

EVALUATION

1. Compared client's respiratory status before and after FBOAM.   ___ ___ ___ _____

2. If teaching caregivers, evaluated technique.   ___ ___ ___ _____

3. Identified unexpected outcomes.   ___ ___ ___ _____

RECORDING AND REPORTING

1. Recorded client assessment and maneuver performed in nurses' notes.   ___ ___ ___ _____

Student _____   Date _____

Instructor _____   Date _____

PERFORMANCE CHECKLIST 16-2   **INSERTING A NASAL AIRWAY**

	S	U	NP	Comments

ASSESSMENT

1. Identified signs and symptoms indicating need for insertion of nasal airway.

2. Determined size of nasal airway needed.

3. Assessed client's knowledge of procedure.

NURSING DIAGNOSIS

1. Developed appropriate nursing diagnoses based on assessment data.

PLANNING

1. Developed individualized goals for inserting nasal airway.

2. Identified expected outcomes.

3. Explained reasons for insertion of airway and client's participation.

4. Positioned client comfortably.

IMPLEMENTATION

1. Washed hands, applied gloves and face shield.

2. Prepared nasal airway.

3. Cleaned excess secretions from client's nares. Determined best naris for insertion.

4. Inserted nasal airway using gentle inward and downward pressure.

5. Cleaned excess lubricant from client's face and nares.

6. Secured airway, if necessary.

7. Placed client in comfortable position.

8. Removed gloves and face shield and discarded in appropriate receptacle. Washed hands.

9. Washed nasal airway at least daily with warm soapy water.

10. Assessed pressure points at end of phalange.

11. Auscultated breath sounds.

	S	U	NP	Comments

EVALUATION

1. Compared client's assessments before and after nasal airway insertion.

— — — _____

2. Observed for patency of airway.

— — — _____

3. Assessed respiratory status.

— — — _____

4. Observed nares for signs of pressure.

— — — _____

5. Identified unexpected outcomes.

— — — _____

RECORDING AND REPORTING

1. Recorded procedure and client assessment in nurses' notes.

— — — _____

Student _____ Date _____

Instructor _____ Date _____

PERFORMANCE CHECKLIST 16-3 **INSERTING AN ORAL AIRWAY**

	S	U	NP	Comments

ASSESSMENT

1. Identified signs and symptoms indicating need for insertion of oral airway.

2. Determined factors that normally influence upper airway functioning.

3. Assessed for presence of gag reflex.

4. Assessed client's knowledge of procedure.

NURSING DIAGNOSIS

1. Developed appropriate nursing diagnoses based on assessment data.

PLANNING

1. Developed individualized goals for inserting oral airway.

2. Identified unexpected outcomes.

3. Explained reasons for oral airway insertions and techniques used.

4. Positioned client correctly.

IMPLEMENTATION

1. Washed hands and applied nonsterile gloves and face shield.

2. Opened client's mouth.

3. Inserted oral airway.

4. Secured oral airway with tape if necessary.

5. Suctioned secretions, if needed.

6. Reassessed client's respiratory status.

7. Provided client hygiene after procedure.

8. Discarded tissues, washcloth, gloves, and face shield into appropriate receptacle and washed hands.

9. Administered mouth care frequently.

EVALUATION

1. Compared client's respiratory assessments before and after insertion of oral airway.

	S	U	NP	Comments
2. Assessed patency of airway.	—	—	—	_____
3. Identified unexpected outcomes.	—	—	—	_____

RECORDING AND REPORTING

1. Recorded client assessment and procedure in nurses' notes.	—	—	—	_____

Student _____   Date _____

Instructor _____   Date _____

PERFORMANCE CHECKLIST 16-4   **USING AN AMBU-BAG**

	S	U	NP	Comments

ASSESSMENT

1. Identified signs and symptoms of need for Ambu-bag manual ventilation.

2. Identified factors affecting respiratory drive.

3. Determined alert client's knowledge of procedure or caregiver's knowledge of procedure.

NURSING DIAGNOSIS

1. Developed appropriate nursing diagnoses based on assessment data.

PLANNING

1. Identified individualized goals.

2. Identified expected outcomes.

3. Explained procedure and client's participation.

4. Assisted client with positioning.

IMPLEMENTATION

1. Washed hands, applied gloves and face shield if not an emergency procedure.

2. Prepared suction apparatus if needed.

3. Provided supplemental oxygen as needed.

4. For intubated client:

   a. Removed oxygen delivery device.

   b. Instilled saline into airway appropriately.

   c. Connected Ambu-bag to artificial airway and administered 1 breath every 3-5 seconds to hyperventilate by compressing Ambu-bag with two hands.

   d. Suctioned secretions and repeated preceding steps as needed.

5. For nonintubated client:

   a. Inserted oropharyngeal airway.

   b. Placed Ambu-bag over client's mouth and nose.

   c. Hyperextended client's neck unless contraindicated.

	S	U	NP	Comments

d. Administered breaths according to CPR protocol.
     ___ ___ ___ _____

e. Suctioned client as necessary.
     ___ ___ ___ _____

6. Assessed client throughout procedure. Continued to provide supplemental ventilation and oxygen until assessment indicated no longer necessary.
     ___ ___ ___ _____

7. Repeated Steps 4-6 as needed. Replaced oxygen delivery device.
     ___ ___ ___ _____

8. Discontinued oxygen supply to bag.
     ___ ___ ___ _____

9. Repositioned client appropriately.
     ___ ___ ___ _____

10. Cleaned equipment.
     ___ ___ ___ _____

11. Removed and disposed of gloves and face shield. Washed hands.
     ___ ___ ___ _____

EVALUATION

1. Compared assessments before and after Ambu-bag use.
     ___ ___ ___ _____

2. Observed character of suctioned secretions.
     ___ ___ ___ _____

3. Provided for return demonstration if instructing caregivers.
     ___ ___ ___ _____

4. Identified unexpected outcomes.
     ___ ___ ___ _____

RECORDING AND REPORTING

1. Charted client assessment and procedure in nurses' notes.
     ___ ___ ___ _____

Student _____   Date _____

Instructor _____   Date _____

PERFORMANCE CHECKLIST 16-5 **PERFORMING CARDIOPULMONARY RESUSCITATION**

	S	U	NP	Comments

ASSESSMENT

1. Determined client's level of consciousness.   ___ ___ ___ _____

2. Determined presence of carotid pulse and respirations.   ___ ___ ___ _____

3. Activated emergency medical services.   ___ ___ ___ _____

NURSING DIAGNOSIS

1. Developed appropriate nursing diagnoses based on assessment data.   ___ ___ ___ _____

PLANNING

1. Called for assistance.   ___ ___ ___ _____

2. Developed individualized goals for client based on nursing diagnoses.   ___ ___ ___ _____

3. Identified expected outcomes.   ___ ___ ___ _____

4. Placed victim on hard surface.   ___ ___ ___ _____

5. Positioned self in correct position as one- or two-person rescuer.   ___ ___ ___ _____

IMPLEMENTATION

1. Applied gloves and face shield if available.   ___ ___ ___ _____

2. Opened airway by using head-tilt/chin-lift or jaw thrust maneuver.   ___ ___ ___ _____

3. Inserted oral airway, if available.   ___ ___ ___ _____

4. Administered artificial respiration.   ___ ___ ___ _____

5. Observed for rise and fall of chest.   ___ ___ ___ _____

6. Suctioned secretions if necessary or turned victim's head to side.   ___ ___ ___ _____

7. Correctly assessed for presence of pulse after restoring breathing.   ___ ___ ___ _____

8. Began chest compressions if pulse was absent.   ___ ___ ___ _____

9. Palpated for carotid or brachial pulse.   ___ ___ ___ _____

10. Continued CPR in absence of carotid pulse.   ___ ___ ___ _____

11. Removed and discarded gloves, face shield, and pocket mask.   ___ ___ ___ _____

	S	U	NP	Comments

EVALUATION

1. Assessed carotid pulse at 5-minute intervals.   ___ ___ ___ _____

2. Observed for spontaneous return of respirations or heart rate.   ___ ___ ___ _____

3. Documented that interruption of CPR did not exceed 5 seconds.   ___ ___ ___ _____

4. Identified unexpected outcomes.   ___ ___ ___ _____

RECORDING AND REPORTING

1. Reported location of respiratory or cardiopulmonary arrest.   ___ ___ ___ _____

2. Recorded in nurses' notes onset of arrest, assistance given, and victim's response.   ___ ___ ___ _____

Student _____   Date _____

Instructor _____   Date _____

PERFORMANCE CHECKLIST 18-1   **ADMINISTERING ORAL MEDICATIONS**

	S	U	NP	Comments
ASSESSMENT				
1. Assessed data pertinent to each medication.	—	—	—	_____
2. Assessed whether oral medications should be contraindicated for client.	—	—	—	_____
3. Assessed historical data revealing client's need for or potential response to medications.	—	—	—	_____
4. Assessed client's age.	—	—	—	_____
5. Assessed extent of client's knowledge regarding health status and medications.	—	—	—	_____
6. Asssessed client's fluid preference.	—	—	—	_____
NURSING DIAGNOSIS				
1. Developed appropriate nursing diagnoses based on assessment data.	—	—	—	_____
PLANNING				
1. Developed individualized goals for client based on nursing diagnoses.	—	—	—	_____
2. Identified expected outcomes.	—	—	—	_____
3. Checked accuracy of transcribed orders with prescriber's written order.	—	—	—	_____
4. Recopied forms that were illegible.	—	—	—	_____
IMPLEMENTATION				
Preparing Medications				
1. Washed hands.	—	—	—	_____
2. Arranged forms and supplies before preparing medications.	—	—	—	_____
3. Unlocked medicine drawer or cart.	—	—	—	_____
4. Prepared medications for one client at a time.	—	U	—	_____
5. Compared drug label with medication administration record (MAR) or form when selecting medication from supply or unit dose drawer.	—	—	—	_____
6. Calculated dosage correctly.	—	—	—	_____
7. Prepared solid tablets or capsules in medicine cup correctly.	—	—	—	_____
8. Prepared unit dose tablets or capsules correctly.	—	—	—	_____

	S	U	NP	Comments

9. Separated medications requiring preadministration assessment from other drugs.

10. Correctly prepared tablets with pill-crushing device if client had difficulty swallowing.

11. Correctly poured liquid medication without contaminating bottle caps or soiling bottle label.

12. Checked expiration date on all medications.

13. Checked narcotic record for count, if administering narcotics.

14. Compared medication and labeled container with MAR or form second time after preparing drug.

15. Compared medication and labeled container with MAR or form third time when returning stock or unused medications to shelf.

16. Arranged medications together with MAR or form on tray or cart.

17. Did not leave drugs unattended.

Administering Medications

1. Administered drugs at correct time.

2. Identified client by checking name on MAR or form with identification bracelet and asking client to state name.

3. Conducted necessary preadministration assessment.

4. Explained purpose of medications to client.

5. Assisted client to sitting or side-lying position.

6. Administered oral medications correctly depending on form.

7. Assisted client as needed with placing medication in mouth.

8. If tablet fell, discarded it and repeated procedure.

9. Remained with client and confirmed that medication had been taken.

10. Offered snack following administration for medications irritating to gastric lining.

11. Assisted client in returning to comfortable position.

12. Disposed of soiled supplies and washed hands.

13. Returned MAR or forms to medicine room.

14. Replenished supplies and cleaned work area.

Student _____   Date _____

Instructor _____   Date _____

	S	U	NP	Comments

EVALUATION

1. Evaluated client's response to medications 30 minutes after administration.

2. Determined client's or family member's level of knowledge gained about the medication.

3. Identified unexpected outcomes.

RECORDING AND REPORTING

1. Accurately recorded medications in medication record.

2. If medication was held, documented reason.

Student _____   Date _____

Instructor _____   Date _____

PERFORMANCE CHECKLIST 18-2   **ADMINISTERING MEDICATIONS BY NASOGASTRIC TUBE**

	S	U	NP	Comments
ASSESSMENT				
1. Assessed for contraindications to client receiving oral medication.	—	—	—	_____
2. Assessed client's medical history, history of allergies, medications, and diet.	—	—	—	_____
3. Reviewed assessment and laboratory data that may influence drug administration.	—	—	—	_____
4. Verified placement of nasogastric tube prior to administration of medications.	—	—	—	_____
NURSING DIAGNOSIS				
1. Developed appropriate nursing diagnoses based on assessment data.	—	—	—	_____
PLANNING				
1. Developed individualized goals for client receiving medications.	—	—	—	_____
2. Identified expected outcomes.	—	—	—	_____
3. Compared MAR or computer readout with medication label.	—	—	—	_____
4. Explained procedure to client.	—	—	—	_____
IMPLEMENTATION				
1. Washed hands.	—	—	—	_____
2. Prepared medications for administration through tube. Prepared 50-100 ml of water in graduated container.	—	—	—	_____
3. Assisted client to high Fowler's position.	—	—	—	_____
4. Applied clean gloves.	—	—	—	_____
5. Verified placement of nasogastric tube.	—	—	—	_____
6. Aspirated stomach contents, noted return, and returned aspirate to client.	—	—	—	_____
7. Prepared syringe for medication delivery.	—	—	—	_____
8. Instilled 10 ml of water and then administered medication followed by another 10 ml of water.	—	—	—	_____
9. Followed last dose of medication with 30 to 60 ml of water.	—	—	—	_____

	S	U	NP	Comments

10. Clamped off and capped end of tube. ___ ___ ___ _____

11. Removed gloves, disposed of supplies, and rinsed graduated container. Washed hands. ___ ___ ___ _____

EVALUATION

1. Returned within 30 minutes to determine client's response to medications or reinstitute continuous tube feedings. ___ ___ ___ _____

2. Identified unexpected outcomes. ___ ___ ___ _____

RECORDING AND REPORTING

1. Recorded in nurses' notes method to check tube placement, volume of aspirate, and pH of aspirate (if indicated). ___ ___ ___ _____

2. Recorded actual time of drug administration on MAR or computer printout. ___ ___ ___ _____

3. Recorded and reported if drug was withheld. ___ ___ ___ _____

Student _____   Date _____

Instructor _____   Date _____

PERFORMANCE CHECKLIST 18-3 **ADMINISTERING SKIN APPLICATIONS**

	S	U	NP	Comments
ASSESSMENT				
1. Assessed condition of client's skin.	___	___	___	_____
2. Inspected area where medication is to be applied.	___	___	___	_____
3. Assessed for presence of drug allergy.	___	___	___	_____
4. Determined amount of topical agent required and directions for use.	___	___	___	_____
5. Assessed client's knowledge regarding medication therapy.	___	___	___	_____
6. Assessed client's ability to self-administer medication.	___	___	___	_____
NURSING DIAGNOSIS				
1. Developed appropriate nursing diagnoses based on assessment data.	___	___	___	_____
PLANNING				
1. Developed individualized goals for client based on nursing diagnoses.	___	___	___	_____
2. Identified expected outcomes.	___	___	___	_____
3. Compared MAR with topical agent.	___	___	___	_____
4. Identified client correctly.	___	___	___	_____
5. Explained procedure to client.	___	___	___	_____
IMPLEMENTATION				
1. Washed hands, arranged supplies at bedside, and applied gloves.	___	___	___	_____
2. Closed door or curtain for privacy and positioned client comfortably.	___	___	___	_____
3. Washed affected area of skin before application.	___	___	___	_____
4. Allowed skin to air dry or patted lightly to dry.	___	___	___	_____
5. Applied topical agent while skin still damp if skin was dry and flaking.	___	___	___	_____
6. Removed gloves and applied new gloves.	___	___	___	_____
7. Used correct procedure when applying any of following: cream, ointment, or oil-based lotion; antianginal ointment; patch; aerosol spray; suspension-based lotion; powder.	___	___	___	_____

	S	U	NP	Comments
8. Covered skin area with dressing when ordered.	___	___	___	_____
9. Assisted client in returning to comfortable position after application.	___	___	___	_____
10. Removed gloves, properly disposed of soiled supplies, and washed hands after procedure.	___	___	___	_____

EVALUATION

1. Evaluated client's or caregiver's knowledge of prescribed medication.	___	___	___	_____
2. Had client keep a diary of dosages taken.	___	___	___	_____
3. Observed client administering medication.	___	___	___	_____
4. Evaluated condition of skin between applications.	___	___	___	_____
5. Identified unexpected outcomes.	___	___	___	_____

RECORDING AND REPORTING

1. Recorded in nurses' notes condition of skin before applying topical agent.	___	___	___	_____
2. Recorded application of topical agent.	___	___	___	_____
3. Reported any abnormalities of skin condition to nurse in charge or physician.	___	___	___	_____

Student _____ Date _____

Instructor _____ Date _____

PERFORMANCE CHECKLIST 18-4 **ADMINISTERING EYE DROPS AND OINTMENTS**

	S	U	NP	Comments

ASSESSMENT

1. Reviewed prescriber's medication order.

2. Assessed condition of eye.

3. Determined client's history of allergies.

4. Assessed client for symptoms of visual alteration.

5. Assessed client's level of consciousness.

6. Assessed client's knowledge regarding drug therapy.

7. Assessed client's ability to self-administer medication.

NURSING DIAGNOSIS

1. Developed appropriate nursing diagnoses based on assessment data.

PLANNING

1. Developed individualized goals for client based on nursing diagnoses.

2. Identified expected outcomes.

3. Compared MAR with medication label.

4. Identified client correctly.

5. Explained procedure to client.

IMPLEMENTATION

1. Washed hands, arranged supplies at bedside, and applied gloves.

2. Positioned client supine or in chair with head slightly hyperextended.

3. Washed existing crusts and drainage from eyelids before drug administration.

4. Placed cotton ball or tissue below lower lid margin.

5. Retracted lower lid downward to expose conjunctival sac.

6. Instructed client to look up.

7. Instilled eye drops correctly.

	S	U	NP	Comments
8. Instilled ointment correctly.	___	___	___	_____
9. Wiped away excess medication on eyelids.	___	___	___	_____
10. Applied eye patch when appropriate.	___	___	___	_____
11. Removed gloves, disposed of soiled supplies properly, and washed hands.	___	___	___	_____

EVALUATION

	S	U	NP	Comments
1. Evaluated client's response to medication.	___	___	___	_____
2. Evaluated effects of medication by assessing for visual changes or side effects.	___	___	___	_____
3. Determined client's level of understanding of medication.	___	___	___	_____
4. Had client demonstrate self-administration.	___	___	___	_____
5. Identified unexpected outcomes.	___	___	___	_____

RECORDING AND REPORTING

	S	U	NP	Comments
1. Recorded medication on medication record.	___	___	___	_____
2. Recorded in nurses' notes appearance of eye.	___	___	___	_____
3. Reported any undesired effects to nurse in charge or physician.	___	___	___	_____

Student _____   Date _____

Instructor _____   Date _____

PERFORMANCE CHECKLIST 18-5 **ADMINISTERING EAR DROPS**

	S	U	NP	Comments

ASSESSMENT

1. Reviewed prescriber's medication order.

2. Assessed condition of external ear.

3. Assessed client for symptoms of ear discomfort or hearing impairment.

4. Assessed client's level of cooperation.

5. Assessed client's knowledge of drug therapy.

6. Assessed client's ability to self-administer medication.

NURSING DIAGNOSIS

1. Developed appropriate diagnoses based on assessment data.

PLANNING

1. Developed individualized goals of client based on nursing diagnoses.

2. Identified expected outcomes.

3. Compared MAR with medication label.

4. Identified client correctly.

5. Explained procedure to client.

IMPLEMENTATION

1. Washed hands and arranged supplies at bedside.

2. Assisted client to side-lying position with ear to be treated facing up or to bedside chair.

3. Straightened ear canal correctly.

4. Wiped out cerumen and drainage with cotton applicator.

5. Instilled ordered number of drops.

6. With client in side-lying position applied gentle pressure to tragus.

7. Placed cotton ball in outer ear canal, as prescribed.

8. Removed cotton ball after 15 minutes, if prescribed.

	S	U	NP	Comments
9. Disposed of soiled supplies properly and washed hands.	___	___	___	_____
10. Assisted client to comfortable position.	___	___	___	_____

EVALUATION

	S	U	NP	Comments
1. Asked client whether there was discomfort during instillation.	___	___	___	_____
2. Evaluated condition of external ear between drug instillations.	___	___	___	_____
3. Evaluated client's hearing acuity.	___	___	___	_____
4. Asked client to explain technique for instilling ear drops.	___	___	___	_____
5. Had client demonstrate self-administration.	___	___	___	_____
6. Identified unexpected outcomes.	___	___	___	_____

RECORDING AND REPORTING

	S	U	NP	Comments
1. Recorded drug administration correctly on medication form.	___	___	___	_____
2. Recorded condition of ear canal in nurses' notes.	___	___	___	_____
3. Reported change in client's hearing acuity.	___	___	___	_____

Student _____   Date _____

Instructor _____   Date _____

PERFORMANCE CHECKLIST 18-6   **ADMINISTERING EAR IRRIGATIONS**

	S	U	NP	Comments

ASSESSMENT

1. Reviewed prescriber's medication order.

2. Reviewed medical record for history of ruptured tympanic membrane.

3. Inspected condition of pinna and external auditory meatus.

4. Determined if client is experiencing discomfort.

5. Assessed client's knowledge regarding medication therapy.

NURSING DIAGNOSIS

1. Developed appropriate nursing diagnoses based on assessment data.

PLANNING

1. Developed individualized goals for client based on nursing diagnoses.

2. Identified expected outcomes.

3. Instilled mineral oil into ear for 2-3 days before, if client had impacted cerumen.

4. Identified client correctly.

5. Explained procedure to client.

IMPLEMENTATION

1. Washed hands and arranged supplies at bedside.

2. Closed curtain or room door for privacy.

3. Positioned client in sitting or lying position with head turned toward affected ear.

4. Poured irrigation solution into sterile basin.

5. Gently cleaned auricle and ear canal with moistened cotton applicator.

6. Filled irrigation syringe with solution.

7. Correctly positioned ear to allow fluid to flow over length of canal.

8. Slowly instilled irrigation solution.

9. Did not occlude canal with syringe tip.

	S	U	NP	Comments
10. Dried outer ear canal with cotton ball and left cotton ball in place for 5-10 minutes.	—	—	—	_____
11. Assisted client to sitting position.	—	—	—	_____
12. Washed hands, removed gloves, and properly disposed of supplies.	—	—	—	_____

EVALUATION

	S	U	NP	Comments
1. Determined if client had discomfort during instillation.	—	—	—	_____
2. Inspected condition of meatus and canal.	—	—	—	_____
3. Assessed client's hearing acuity.	—	—	—	_____
4. Determined client's understanding of procedure and techniques for ear care.	—	—	—	_____
5. Identified unexpected outcomes.	—	—	—	_____

RECORDING AND REPORTING

	S	U	NP	Comments
1. Recorded procedure, amount of solution, time, and ear receiving irrigation in nurses' notes and/or MAR.	—	—	—	_____
2. Recorded appearance of external ear and client's hearing acuity in nurses' notes.	—	—	—	_____
3. Reported and recorded any side effects to nurse in charge or physician.	—	—	—	_____

Student _____   Date _____

Instructor _____   Date _____

PERFORMANCE CHECKLIST 18-7 **ADMINISTERING NASAL INSTILLATIONS**

	S	U	NP	Comments

ASSESSMENT

1. Reviewed prescriber's medication order.   ___ ___ ___ _____

2. Determined affected nasal sinus.   ___ ___ ___ _____

3. Assessed client's history to determine contraindication of drug.   ___ ___ ___ _____

4. Assessed condition of nares and sinuses.   ___ ___ ___ _____

5. Assessed client's knowledge regarding use of nasal instillations.   ___ ___ ___ _____

NURSING DIAGNOSIS

1. Developed appropriate nursing diagnoses based on assessment data.   ___ ___ ___ _____

PLANNING

1. Developed individualized goals for client based on nursing diagnoses.   ___ ___ ___ _____

2. Identified expected outcomes.   ___ ___ ___ _____

3. Compared MAR with medication label.   ___ ___ ___ _____

4. Identified client correctly.   ___ ___ ___ _____

5. Explained procedure to client.   ___ ___ ___ _____

IMPLEMENTATION

1. Washed hands and arranged supplies and medications at bedside.   ___ ___ ___ _____

2. Instructed client to blow nose, unless contraindicated.   ___ ___ ___ _____

3. Administered nasal drops correctly.   ___ ___ ___ _____

4. Assisted client to comfortable position after drug absorbed.   ___ ___ ___ _____

5. Disposed of soiled supplies properly and washed hands.   ___ ___ ___ _____

EVALUATION

1. Observed client for side effects of medication.   ___ ___ ___ _____

2. Evaluated client's ability to breathe through nose.   ___ ___ ___ _____

3. Inspected condition of nasal passages.   ___ ___ ___ _____

4. Asked client to review knowledge regarding use of decongestant and methods of administration.   ___ ___ ___ _____

	S	U	NP	Comments

5. Had client demonstrate self-administration.   ___ ___ ___ _____

6. Identified unexpected outcomes.   ___ ___ ___ _____

RECORDING AND REPORTING

1. Recorded medication administration correctly on medication record.   ___ ___ ___ _____

2. Recorded in nurses' notes client's response to medication.   ___ ___ ___ _____

3. Reported any unusual side effects to nurse in charge or physician.   ___ ___ ___ _____

Student _____   Date _____

Instructor _____   Date _____

PERFORMANCE CHECKLIST 18-8 **USING METERED-DOSE INHALERS**

	S	U	NP	Comments

ASSESSMENT

1. Assessed client's ability to handle inhaler.   ___ ___ ___ _____

2. Assessed client's readiness to learn.   ___ ___ ___ _____

3. Assessed client's ability to learn.   ___ ___ ___ _____

4. Assessed client's knowledge of disease and drug therapy.   ___ ___ ___ _____

5. Assessed drug schedule and number of prescribed inhalations.   ___ ___ ___ _____

6. Assessed client's technique in using inhaler (when applicable).   ___ ___ ___ _____

NURSING DIAGNOSIS

1. Developed appropriate nursing diagnoses based on assessment data.   ___ ___ ___ _____

PLANNING

1. Developed individualized learning objectives for teaching plan.   ___ ___ ___ _____

2. Identified expected outcomes.   ___ ___ ___ _____

3. Instructed client in comfortable environment.   ___ ___ ___ _____

4. Provided adequate time for teaching.   ___ ___ ___ _____

IMPLEMENTATION

1. Washed hands and arranged equipment.   ___ ___ ___ _____

2. Provided client opportunity to handle inhaler.   ___ ___ ___ _____

3. Explained metered dosage and problems of overuse, including drug side effects.   ___ ___ ___ _____

4. Explained each step in using inhaler.   ___ ___ ___ _____

5. Instructed client on proper technique for administering medication with an aero-chamber.   ___ ___ ___ _____

6. Instructed client on correct interval between inhalations.   ___ ___ ___ _____

7. Warned client against increasing frequency of inhalations.   ___ ___ ___ _____

8. Described common sensations after use of inhaler.   ___ ___ ___ _____

	S	U	NP	Comments

9. Instructed client in technique for cleansing inhaler. ___ ___ ___ _____

10. Asked if client had questions. ___ ___ ___ _____

EVALUATION

1. Had client demonstrate use of inhaler. ___ ___ ___ _____

2. Asked client to explain drug schedule. ___ ___ ___ _____

3. Asked client to explain medication side effects. ___ ___ ___ _____

4. Assessed respirations and lung sounds after medication instillation. ___ ___ ___ _____

5. Identified unexpected outcomes. ___ ___ ___ _____

RECORDING AND REPORTING

1. Recorded description of teaching session and client's response in nurses' notes. ___ ___ ___ _____

2. Recorded times used and amount (puffs). ___ ___ ___ _____

3. Reported any undesirable effects from medication. ___ ___ ___ _____

Student _____   Date _____

Instructor _____   Date _____

PERFORMANCE CHECKLIST 18-9 **ADMINISTERING VAGINAL INSTILLATIONS**

	S	U	NP	Comments

ASSESSMENT

1. Reviewed prescriber's medication order.

2. Reviewed pertinent drug information.

3. Assessed condition of external genitalia and vaginal canal.

4. Assessed client for symptoms of vaginal irritation.

5. Determined client's ability to self-administer medication.

6. Reviewed client's knowledge of drug therapy.

NURSING DIAGNOSIS

1. Developed appropriate nursing diagnoses based on assessment data.

PLANNING

1. Developed individualized goals for client based on nursing diagnoses.

2. Identified expected outcomes.

3. Compared MAR medication label.

4. Identified client correctly.

5. Explained procedure to client.

IMPLEMENTATION

1. Washed hands and arranged supplies at bedside.

2. Closed room door or curtain.

3. Assisted client to dorsal recumbent position.

4. Kept lower extremities and abdomen draped.

5. Donned disposable gloves.

6. Illuminated vaginal orifice properly.

7. Used proper procedure for inserting suppository.

8. Used proper procedure for applying cream or foam.

9. Used proper procedure for irrigation and douche.

10. Instructed client to lie flat on her back for at least 10 minutes.

	S	U	NP	Comments

11. If applicator was used, washed it with soap and water, rinsed, and stored. ___ ___ ___ _____

12. Offered client perineal pad. ___ ___ ___ _____

13. Disposed of soiled supplies and equipment. ___ ___ ___ _____

14. Removed gloves properly and discarded them. ___ ___ ___ _____

EVALUATION

1. Inspected condition of vaginal canal and external genitalia between applications. ___ ___ ___ _____

2. Evaluated client for symptoms of vaginal irritation. ___ ___ ___ _____

3. Evaluated client's understanding of medication therapy. ___ ___ ___ _____

4. Had client demonstrate self-administration. ___ ___ ___ _____

5. Identified unexpected outcomes. ___ ___ ___ _____

RECORDING AND REPORTING

1. Recorded medication correctly on medication record. ___ ___ ___ _____

2. Recorded appearance of vaginal canal and genitalia in nurses' notes, and reported any unusual findings to nurse in charge or physician. ___ ___ ___ _____

Student _____   Date _____

Instructor _____   Date _____

PERFORMANCE CHECKLIST 18-10 **ADMINISTERING RECTAL SUPPOSITORIES**

	S	U	NP	Comments

ASSESSMENT

1. Reviewed prescriber's medication order.

2. Reviewed pertinent drug information.

3. Determined whether client had history of rectal surgery or bleeding.

4. Assessed for signs and symptoms of gastrointestinal alterations.

5. Assessed client's ability to self-administer suppository.

6. Reviewed client's knowledge of drug therapy.

NURSING DIAGNOSIS

1. Developed appropriate nursing diagnoses based on assessment data.

PLANNING

1. Developed individualized goals for client based on nursing diagnoses.

2. Identified expected outcomes.

3. Compared MAR with medication label.

4. Identified client correctly.

5. Explained procedure to client.

IMPLEMENTATION

1. Washed hands and arranged supplies at bedside.

2. Closed curtain or room door for privacy.

3. Assisted client to side-lying Sims' position with upper leg flexed upward.

4. Kept client properly draped.

5. Applied disposable gloves.

6. Examined condition of anus externally and palpated rectal wall as needed; disposed of gloves properly.

7. Applied disposable gloves.

8. Removed suppository from wrapper and lubricated rounded end.

	S	U	NP	Comments

9. Instructed client to breathe slowly through mouth and relax anal sphincter.

___ ___ ___ _____

10. Retracted buttocks and inserted suppository gently through anus for proper distance.

___ ___ ___ _____

11. Cleaned excess lubricant from anal area.

___ ___ ___ _____

12. Properly disposed of gloves.

___ ___ ___ _____

13. Asked client to remain flat or on side for 5 minutes.

___ ___ ___ _____

14. Placed call light within client's reach after drug administration.

___ ___ ___ _____

15. Washed hands and disposed of supplies and equipment.

___ ___ ___ _____

EVALUATION

1. Determined whether suppository was prematurely expelled.

___ ___ ___ _____

2. Determined whether there was any discomfort during insertion.

___ ___ ___ _____

3. Evaluated effect of medication.

___ ___ ___ _____

4. Determined client's understanding of purpose of medication.

___ ___ ___ _____

5. Had client demonstrate self-administration.

___ ___ ___ _____

6. Identified unexpected outcomes.

___ ___ ___ _____

RECORDING AND REPORTING

1. Recorded medication correctly on medication record.

___ ___ ___ _____

2. Recorded and reported client's response to medication.

___ ___ ___ _____

Student _____   Date _____

Instructor _____   Date _____

PERFORMANCE CHECKLIST 19-1 **PREPARING INJECTIONS FROM AMPULES AND VIALS**

	S	U	NP	Comments
ASSESSMENT				
1. Assessed client's body build, muscle size, and weight.	__	__	__	_____
2. Considered medication and type of injection.	__	__	__	_____
PLANNING				
1. Checked MAR or computer printout.	__	__	__	_____
2. Identified expected outcomes.	__	__	__	_____
IMPLEMENTATION				
1. Washed hands.	__	__	__	_____
2. Arranged supplies at work area in medicine room.	__	__	__	_____
3. Checked medication card, form, or printout against label on ampule or vial.	__	__	__	_____
Ampule Preparation				
1. Tapped top of ampule to dislodge fluid in neck.	__	__	__	_____
2. Placed gauze pad or dry alcohol swab around ampule neck.	__	__	__	_____
3. Snapped neck of ampule away from hands.	__	__	__	_____
4. Drew up medication quickly; while holding ampule upright or upside down, inserted needle through opening in center of ampule.	__	__	__	_____
5. Aspirated medication.	__	__	__	_____
6. Kept needle tip below fluid level.	__	__	__	_____
7. Did not expel air into ampule.	__	__	__	_____
8. Expelled air from syringe correctly.	__	__	__	_____
9. Correctly expelled excess fluid within syringe into sink.	__	__	__	_____
10. Covered needle with sheath or cap after preparation and changed needle or syringe.	__	__	__	_____
11. Disposed of soiled supplies and placed ampule in special container. Cleaned work area. Washed hands.	__	__	__	_____
Vial Preparation				
1. Removed metal cap from vial to expose rubber seal.	__	__	__	_____

	S	U	NP	Comments

2. Wiped off surface of seal with alcohol swab.   ___ ___ ___ _____

3. Drew up air in syringe equivalent to volume of medication desired.   ___ ___ ___ _____

4. Inserted needle tip, bevel up, through center of rubber seal.   ___ ___ ___ _____

5. Injected air into vial while holding on to plunger.   ___ ___ ___ _____

6. With vial inverted, held vial and syringe properly.   ___ ___ ___ _____

7. Kept needle tip below fluid level.   ___ ___ ___ _____

8. Allowed air pressure to fill syringe with fluid.   ___ ___ ___ _____

9. Correctly dislodged and expelled air that accumulated in syringe barrel.   ___ ___ ___ _____

10. Removed needle from vial.   ___ ___ ___ _____

11. Correctly expelled any remaining air in syringe barrel.   ___ ___ ___ _____

12. Changed needle and cover on syringe.   ___ ___ ___ _____

13. Labeled multidose vial with date of mixing, drug concentration, and nurse's initials.   ___ ___ ___ _____

14. Disposed of soiled supplies in proper container. Cleaned work area and washed hands.   ___ ___ ___ _____

Reconstituting Medications

1. Removed cap covering vial containing powder and vial containing diluent.   ___ ___ ___ _____

2. Wiped surfaces of seals with alcohol.   ___ ___ ___ _____

3. Correctly drew up diluent into syringe.   ___ ___ ___ _____

4. Correctly injected diluent into vial with powder. Removed needle.   ___ ___ ___ _____

5. Mixed medication thoroughly.   ___ ___ ___ _____

6. Prepared to draw correct dosage of reconstituted solution into new syringe.   ___ ___ ___ _____

EVALUATION

1. Checked dosage level in syringe.   ___ ___ ___ _____

2. Identified unexpected outcomes.   ___ ___ ___ _____

Student _____   Date _____

Instructor _____   Date _____

PERFORMANCE CHECKLIST 19-2   **MIXING MEDICATIONS FROM TWO VIALS**

	S	U	NP	Comments
ASSESSMENT				
1. Assessed client's body build, muscle size, and weight.	—	—	—	_____
2. Considered medications to be mixed and type of injection.	—	—	—	_____
PLANNING				
1. Checked MAR or computer printout.	—	—	—	_____
2. Identified expected outcomes.	—	—	—	_____
IMPLEMENTATION				
1. Washed hands.	—	—	—	_____
2. Arranged supplies at work area in medicine room.	—	—	—	_____
Mixing Medications from Vials				
1. Took syringe and aspirated volume of air equal to first medication's dosage (vial A).	—	—	—	_____
2. Injected air into vial A without allowing needle to touch solution.	—	—	—	_____
3. Withdrew needle and syringe and aspirated air equal to second medication's dosage (vial B).	—	—	—	_____
4. Inserted needle into vial B, injected air, and filled syringe with proper volume of medication from vial.	—	—	—	_____
5. Withdrew needle and syringe from vial and checked dose.	—	—	—	_____
6. Determined point on scale for correct dosage of combined medications.	—	—	—	_____
7. Inserted needle into vial A and allowed solution to fill syringe to desired level.	—	—	—	_____
8. Withdrew needle and expelled excess air.	—	—	—	_____
9. Changed needle on syringe.	—	—	—	_____
10. Disposed of soiled needle and supplies in proper container.	—	—	—	_____
11. Washed hands.	—	—	—	_____
Mixing Insulin				
1. Took insulin syringe and aspirated volume of air equal to dosage to be withdrawn from modified insulin (cloudy vial).	—	—	—	_____

	S	U	NP	Comments

2. Injected air into vial of modified insulin without needle touching solution.   ___ ___ ___ _____

3. Withdrew needle and syringe from vial and aspirated air equal to dosage to be withdrawn from unmodified regular insulin (clear vial).   ___ ___ ___ _____

4. Inserted needle into vial of unmodified regular insulin (clear vial), injected air, and filled syringe with correct dosage.   ___ ___ ___ _____

5. Withdrew needle and syringe from vial and checked dose.   ___ ___ ___ _____

6. Determined point on syringe scale for correct dosage of combined medications.   ___ ___ ___ _____

7. Inserted needle into vial of modified insulin (cloudy vial), and correctly withdrew desired amount of insulin.   ___ ___ ___ _____

8. Withdrew needle and checked fluid level in syringe.   ___ ___ ___ _____

9. Disposed of soiled supplies in proper container.   ___ ___ ___ _____

10. Washed hands.   ___ ___ ___ _____

EVALUATION

1. Checked syringe scale for correct dosage of combined medications.   ___ ___ ___ _____

2. Identified unexpected outcomes.   ___ ___ ___ _____

Student _____   Date _____

Instructor _____   Date _____

PERFORMANCE CHECKLIST 19-3 **ADMINISTERING INTRADERMAL INJECTIONS**

	S	U	NP	Comments

ASSESSMENT

1. Reviewed medication order.

2. Assessed type of reaction to expect when testing skin.

3. Assessed client's history of allergies.

4. Checked date of medication expiration.

5. Assessed client's knowledge regarding procedure.

NURSING DIAGNOSIS

1. Developed appropriate nursing diagnoses based on assessment data.

PLANNING

1. Developed individualized goals for client based on nursing diagnoses.

2. Identified expected outcomes.

3. Prepared correct dosage from ampule or vial and checked dosage.

4. Correctly identified client.

5. Explained steps of procedure and expected sensations.

IMPLEMENTATION

1. Provided for client's privacy.

2. Washed hands.

3. Draped client appropriately.

4. Chose appropriate injection site and inspected skin surface for lesions or discoloration.

5. Had client flex elbow and support it on flat surface.

6. Applied disposable gloves.

7. Cleansed injection site.

8. Held swab correctly.

9. Removed needle cap correctly.

10. Held syringe comfortably with bevel of needle pointing up.

	S	U	NP	Comments

11. Stretched skin over injection site.

12. With needle at 5- to 15-degree angle, injected slowly through epidermis just below skin surface.

13. Injected medication slowly and felt normal resistance.

14. Noticed small bleb appear on skin.

15. Withdrew needle slowly with swab supporting site.

16. Did not massage site.

17. Assisted client to comfortable position.

18. Discarded uncapped needles and syringes properly.

19. Removed gloves and washed hands.

EVALUATION

1. Remained with client to observe for allergic reaction.

2. With skin pencil, drew circle around perimeter or injection site and read site within 48-72 hours of injection.

3. Encouraged client to discuss implications of skin testing.

4. Identified unexpected outcomes.

RECORDING AND REPORTING

1. Recorded test substance data correctly on medication record and nurses' notes.

2. Recorded area of injection and appearance of skin on nurses' notes.

3. Reported any undesirable effects from medication to nurse in charge or physician.

Student _____   Date _____

Instructor _____   Date _____

PERFORMANCE CHECKLIST 19-4   **ADMINISTERING SUBCUTANEOUS INJECTIONS**

	S	U	NP	Comments

ASSESSMENT

1. Reviewed medication order.

2. Gathered information pertaining to ordered drug.

3. Assessed contraindications for subcutaneous injections.

4. Assessed indications for subcutaneous injection.

5. Assessed client's medical, medication, and allergy history.

6. Considered adequacy of client's adipose tissue.

7. Assessed client's medication knowledge.

8. Observed client's behavioral reaction to receiving injection.

NURSING DIAGNOSIS

1. Developed appropriate nursing diagnoses based on assessment data.

PLANNING

1. Developed individualized goals for client based on nursing diagnoses.

2. Identified expected outcomes.

3. Checked MAR or computer printout.

4. Correctly prepared medication in syringe and checked dosage.

5. Correctly identified client receiving medication.

6. Explained procedure to client.

IMPLEMENTATION

1. Provided for client's privacy.

2. Washed hands and applied disposable gloves.

3. Kept sheet or gown draped over body parts not requiring exposure.

4. Selected appropriate injection site through inspection and palpation of tissues.

5. If daily administration required, correctly rotated injection site.

	S	U	NP	Comments

6. Accurately determined correct needle size.

7. Assisted client to comfortable position.

8. Relocated site using anatomic landmarks.

9. Cleansed site with antiseptic swab.

10. Held swab between third and fourth fingers of nondominant hand.

11. Removed needle cap correctly.

12. Held syringe comfortably in dominant hand with palm upward.

13. Injected needle quickly at correct angle.

14. Grasped lower end of syringe barrel with non-dominant hand and moved dominant hand to plunger.

15. Aspirated to check for blood return; if blood aspirated, withdrew needle; if not, injected medication slowly.

16. Withdrew needle quickly while placing swab on skin above injection site.

17. Massaged site gently, if indicated.

18. Assisted client to comfortable position.

19. Properly disposed of uncapped needle and syringe.

20. Removed gloves and washed hands.

EVALUATION

1. Evaluated for discomfort at injection site.

2. Evaluated client's response to medication.

3. Evaluated client's understanding of purpose and effects of medication.

4. Identified unexpected outcomes.

RECORDING AND REPORTING

1. Documented administration correctly on medication record.

2. Reported undesirable effects from medication to nurse in charge or physician.

3. Recorded client's response to drugs in nurses' notes when appropriate.

Student _____   Date _____

Instructor _____   Date _____

PERFORMANCE CHECKLIST 19-5 **ADMINISTERING INTRAMUSCULAR INJECTIONS**

	S	U	NP	Comments

ASSESSMENT

1. Reviewed medication order.

2. Assessed pertinent drug information.

3. Assessed contraindications for intramuscular injection.

4. Assessed client's medication, medical, and allergy history.

5. Assessed client's knowledge regarding medications.

6. Observed client's response toward receiving injection.

NURSING DIAGNOSIS

1. Developed appropriate nursing diagnoses based on assessment data.

PLANNING

1. Developed individualized goals for client based on nursing diagnoses.

2. Identified expected outcomes.

3. Prepared medication from vial or ampule and checked dosage.

4. Prepared air lock (checked agency policy).

5. Changed needle on syringe.

6. Identified client correctly.

7. Explained procedure to client.

IMPLEMENTATION

1. Provided for client's privacy.

2. Washed hands and applied gloves.

3. Exposed only injection site.

4. Assessed integrity of muscle while selecting injection site.

5. Assisted client to comfortable position according to injection site.

6. Relocated site using anatomic landmarks.

	S	U	NP	Comments

7. Cleansed injection site.

8. Held swab correctly.

9. Removed needle cap correctly.

10. Held syringe comfortably in dominant hand with palm down.

11. With nondominant hand, spread skin tightly and grasped muscle, or used Z-track method and administered injection at correct angle.

12. Released skin, and with nondominant hand, grasped lower end of syringe barrel (with Z-track method, continued to spread skin taut), then moved dominant hand to plunger.

13. Aspirated to check for blood return. If blood aspirated, withdrew needle; if not, injected medication slowly.

14. Withdrew needle quickly while placing antiseptic swab on skin above injection site (with Z-track method, kept needle inserted for 10 seconds, then withdrew and released skin).

15. Applied gentle pressure. Did not massage site.

16. Assisted client to comfortable position.

17. Discarded uncapped needle and syringe in proper receptacle.

18. Removed gloves and washed hands.

EVALUATION

1. Evaluated client for discomfort at injection site.

2. Inspected injection site.

3. Evaluated client's response to medication.

4. Evaluated client's understanding of purpose and effects of medication.

5. Identified unexpected outcomes.

RECORDING AND REPORTING

1. Documented administration correctly on medication record.

2. Reported undesirable effects from medication to nurse in charge of physician.

3. Recorded client's response to drugs in nurses' notes when appropriate.

Student _____ Date _____

Instructor _____ Date _____

PERFORMANCE CHECKLIST 19-6 **ADDING MEDICATIONS TO INTRAVENOUS FLUID CONTAINERS**

	S	U	NP	Comments

ASSESSMENT

1. Assessed order for IV solution, type of medication, and dosage.   ___ ___ ___ _____

2. Gathered information regarding drug.   ___ ___ ___ _____

3. Assessed for drug incompatibility if more than one was mixed.   ___ ___ ___ _____

4. Assessed client's fluid balance.   ___ ___ ___ _____

5. Assessed client for drug allergies.   ___ ___ ___ _____

6. Assessed condition of IV insertion site.   ___ ___ ___ _____

7. Assessed client's knowledge regarding medication.   ___ ___ ___ _____

NURSING DIAGNOSIS

1. Developed appropriate nursing diagnoses based on assessment data.   ___ ___ ___ _____

PLANNING

1. Developed individualized goals for procedure.   ___ ___ ___ _____

2. Identified expected outcomes.   ___ ___ ___ _____

3. Assembled supplies in medication room.   ___ ___ ___ _____

4. Correctly prepared medication from vial or ampule.   ___ ___ ___ _____

5. Identified client correctly.   ___ ___ ___ _____

6. Explained procedure to client.   ___ ___ ___ _____

IMPLEMENTATION

1. Washed hands.   ___ ___ ___ _____

Adding Medication to New Container

1. Located injection port on IV bag or removed cap and seal from IV bottle and located injection site.   ___ ___ ___ _____

2. Cleaned injection port or site.   ___ ___ ___ _____

3. Inserted needle of syringe through injection port or site and injected medication.   ___ ___ ___ _____

4. Withdrew syringe.   ___ ___ ___ _____

5. Mixed medications in IV solution container.   ___ ___ ___ _____

	S	U	NP	Comments

6. Labeled container correctly; applied flow strip (optional).

7. Spiked IV container and hung container correctly, regulating IV infusion at ordered rate.

Adding Medication to Existing Container

1. Prepared vented IV bottle or plastic bag by checking volume of solution, closing infusion clamps, cleaning port, inserting syringe, and injecting medication, lowering and mixing bag, and regulating infusion.

2. Completed medication label and affixed to IV container.

3. Disposed of soiled equipment properly. Did not recap needle.

4. Washed hands.

EVALUATION

1. Observed client for drug reaction.

2. Assessed client for signs and symptoms of fluid volume excess.

3. Evaluated condition of IV site and rate of infusion.

4. Assessed for signs and symptoms of IV infiltration.

5. Evaluated client's understanding of drug therapy.

6. Identified unexpected outcomes.

RECORDING AND REPORTING

1. Recorded IV solution and medication on appropriate form.

2. Reported any drug reactions to nurse in charge or physician.

Student _____   Date _____

Instructor _____   Date _____

PERFORMANCE CHECKLIST 19-7   **ADMINISTERING INTRAVENOUS MEDICATIONS BY INTERMITTENT INFUSION SETS AND MINIINFUSION PUMPS**

	S	U	NP	Comments
ASSESSMENT				
1. Checked order for IV solution, type of medication, and dosage.	___	___	___	_____
2. Collected pertinent information about drug.	___	___	___	_____
3. Assessed patency and infusion rate of main IV line.	___	___	___	_____
4. Assessed condition of IV insertion site.	___	___	___	_____
5. Assessed client's history of drug allergies.	___	___	___	_____
6. Assessed client's understanding of drug therapy.	___	___	___	_____
NURSING DIAGNOSIS				
1. Developed appropriate nursing diagnoses based on assessment data.	___	___	___	_____
PLANNING				
1. Developed individualized goals for client based on nursing diagnoses.	___	___	___	_____
2. Identified expected outcomes.	___	___	___	_____
3. Assembled supplies.	___	___	___	_____
IMPLEMENTATION				
1. Washed hands and applied gloves.	___	___	___	_____
2. Correctly identified client.	___	___	___	_____
3. Explained purpose of medication and encouraged client to report signs of discomfort at site.	___	___	___	_____
Piggyback or Tandem Infusion				
1. Connected infusion tubing to medication bag and filled tubing.	___	___	___	_____
2. Hung medication bag at proper level.	___	___	___	_____
3. Connected tubing to appropriate stopcocks or to needleless system.	___	___	___	_____
4. Cleaned injection port of main IV line with antiseptic swab.	___	___	___	_____
5. Inserted needle of secondary line into port of main line if using needles, or attached needleless device.	___	___	___	_____
6. Removed cover of stopcock and connected secondary line with main line.	___	___	___	_____
7. Regulated secondary line flow rate correctly.	___	___	___	_____

	S	U	NP	Comments

8. Checked flow regulator on primary infusion after medication infused.   ___ ___ ___ _____

9. Regulated main infusion line to desired rate, if necessary.   ___ ___ ___ _____

10. Cared for equipment properly after administration.   ___ ___ ___ _____

11. Removed gloves and washed hands.   ___ ___ ___ _____

Miniinfusor Administration

1. Connected prefilled syringe to miniinfusion tubing.   ___ ___ ___ _____

2. Filled syringe with medication, avoiding air bubbles.   ___ ___ ___ _____

3. Placed syringe into miniinfusor pump, securing syringe.   ___ ___ ___ _____

4. Correctly connected miniinfusion tubing to main IV line.   ___ ___ ___ _____

5. Hung infusion pump with syringe on IV pole and initiated infusion.   ___ ___ ___ _____

6. Assessed flow rate and patency of IV line.   ___ ___ ___ _____

7. Removed gloves and washed hands.   ___ ___ ___ _____

Volume-Control Administration Set

1. Filled Volutrol with proper volume of solution.   ___ ___ ___ _____

2. Closed clamp and assessed that clamp in air vent of Volutrol chamber was open.   ___ ___ ___ _____

3. Cleaned injection port.   ___ ___ ___ _____

4. Injected medication into Volutrol and mixed gently.   ___ ___ ___ _____

5. Regulated IV infusion.   ___ ___ ___ _____

6. Labeled Volutrol.   ___ ___ ___ _____

7. Disposed of uncapped needle and syringe in proper container.   ___ ___ ___ _____

8. Removed gloves and washed hands.   ___ ___ ___ _____

EVALUATION

1. Evaluated client's response to medication.   ___ ___ ___ _____

2. Periodically checked infusion rate and IV site.   ___ ___ ___ _____

3. Evaluated client's knowledge of purpose and side effects of medication.   ___ ___ ___ _____

4. Identified unexpected outcomes.   ___ ___ ___ _____

RECORDING AND REPORTING

1. Recorded medication data correctly on medication form.   ___ ___ ___ _____

2. Recorded diluent on I&O form.   ___ ___ ___ _____

3. Reported any adverse drug reactions to nurse in charge or physician.   ___ ___ ___ _____

Student _____   Date _____

Instructor _____   Date _____

PERFORMANCE CHECKLIST 19-8 **ADMINISTERING MEDICATIONS BY INTRAVENOUS BOLUS**

	S	U	NP	Comments
ASSESSMENT				
1. Checked order for drug, dosage, time, and route.	___	___	___	_____
2. Collected information related to drug to be given.	___	___	___	_____
3. Assessed for IV additives in existing infusion line.	___	___	___	_____
4. Assessed condition of needle insertion site.	___	___	___	_____
5. Checked client's history of allergies.	___	___	___	_____
6. Assessed client's understanding of purpose of drug therapy.	___	___	___	_____
NURSING DIAGNOSIS				
1. Developed appropriate nursing diagnoses based on assessment data.	___	___	___	_____
PLANNING				
1. Developed individualized goals for client based on nursing diagnoses.	___	___	___	_____
2. Identified expected outcomes.	___	___	___	_____
3. Assembled supplies.	___	___	___	_____
IMPLEMENTATION				
1. Washed hands and applied gloves.	___	___	___	_____
IV Push (Existing Line)				
1. Checked client's identification.	___	___	___	_____
2. Explained procedure to client and encouraged client to report any discomfort at IV site.	___	___	___	_____
3. Selected injection port of IV closest to client.	___	___	___	_____
4. Cleaned injection port with antiseptic swab.	___	___	___	_____
5. Inserted small-gauge needle of syringe correctly through port.	___	___	___	_____
6. Aspirated for blood return while occluding infusion tubing.	___	___	___	_____
7. Injected medication slowly over several minutes.	___	___	___	_____
8. Released tubing, withdrew syringe, and checked infusion rate.	___	___	___	_____

	S	U	NP	Comments

IV Push (Intravenous Lock)

1. Checked client's identification.

2. Prepared a syringe with 1 ml of normal saline.

3. Prepared syringe needed when using a heparin flush method.

4. Prepared syringe needed when using a saline flush method.

5. Correctly administered drug over several minutes after cleaning injection port, checking for blood return, flushing with saline syringe, and cleaning the port.

6. Correctly administered syringe with heparin if using heparin flush method.

7. Correctly administered syringe with saline if using saline flush method.

8. Disposed of uncapped needles and syringes in proper container.

9. Removed gloves and washed hands.

EVALUATION

1. Observed client for adverse reactions during and after administration of medication.

2. Observed IV site for swelling during injection.

3. Evaluated client's knowledge of drug's purpose and side effects.

4. Identified unexpected outcomes.

RECORDING AND REPORTING

1. Recorded drug data correctly on medication record.

2. Reported any adverse reactions to nurse in charge or physician.

Student _____ Date _____

Instructor _____ Date _____

PERFORMANCE CHECKLIST 20-1 **INITIATING INTRAVENOUS THERAPY**

	S	U	NP	Comments

ASSESSMENT
1. Identified clients whose potential for fluid and electrolyte imbalance requires IV fluid therapy, and observed for signs and symptoms indicating fluid or electrolyte imbalances. ___ ___ ___ _____

2. Reviewed client's medical record. ___ ___ ___ _____

3. Obtained information from references concerning the composition, purposes, and side effects of the IV fluids. ___ ___ ___ _____

4. Determined client's teaching needs concerning IV fluids. ___ ___ ___ _____

5. Determined any factor that increases client's risk for complications. ___ ___ ___ _____

NURSING DIAGNOSIS
1. Developed appropriate nursing diagnoses based on assessment data. ___ ___ ___ _____

PLANNING
1. Developed individualized goals for client based on nursing diagnoses. ___ ___ ___ _____

2. Identified expected outcomes. ___ ___ ___ _____

3. Prepared client and family for procedure. ___ ___ ___ _____

4. Identified accessible vein. ___ ___ ___ _____

IMPLEMENTATION
1. Washed hands. ___ ___ ___ _____

2. Organized equipment on clutter-free area. Changed client's gown to "snap" type, if available. ___ ___ ___ _____

3. Opened sterile packages aseptically. ___ ___ ___ _____

For IV Fluid Administration
1. Checked solution using "five rights" of drug administration. ___ ___ ___ _____

2. Prepared bottle or bag for entry of infusion tubing. ___ ___ ___ _____

3. Opened infusion set aseptically. ___ ___ ___ _____

4. Placed roller clamp 2-4 cm below drip chamber and moved roller clamp to "off" position. ___ ___ ___ _____

5. Correctly inserted infusion set into fluid bag. ___ ___ ___ _____

6. Correctly filled infusion tubing. ___ ___ ___ _____

For Heparin Lock
1. Used sterile technique to connect tubing and removed air form system. ___ ___ ___ _____

	S	U	NP	Comments
2. Selected appropriate IV needle or CNC.	—	—	—	_____
3. Selected distal site of vein to be used.	—	—	—	_____
4. Clipped body hair where necessary.	—	—	—	_____
5. Placed extremity in dependent position.	—	—	—	_____
6. Positioned tourniquet appropriately.	—	—	—	_____
7. Applied disposable gloves. Applied protective eyewear and mask if necessary.	—	—	—	_____
8. Placed "needle" adapter end of infusion set within reach.	—	—	—	_____
9. Selected well-dilated vein.	—	—	—	_____
10. Cleansed insertion site.	—	—	—	_____
11. Performed venipuncture correctly.	—	—	—	_____
12. Observed for blood return.	—	—	—	_____
13. Released tourniquet and connected needle to infusion set.	—	—	—	_____
14. Initiated infusion at a rate to maintain patency of IV line.	—	—	—	_____
15. Correctly secured IV catheter or needle after applying antiseptic and dressing according to policy.	—	—	—	_____
16. Adjusted correct flow rate for IV administration.	—	—	—	_____
17. Recorded date and time of IV insertion and gauge of catheter on dressing.	—	—	—	_____
18. Discarded supplies, removed gloves, and washed hands.	—	—	—	_____

EVALUATION

1. Evaluated client to determine correct infusion.	—	—	—	_____
2. Evaluated client's response to IV therapy.	—	—	—	_____
3. Identified unexpected outcomes.	—	—	—	_____
4. Assessed for signs of phlebitis.	—	—	—	_____
5. Assessed for bleeding at venipuncture site.	—	—	—	_____

RECORDING AND REPORTING

1. Recorded initiation of IV in nurses' notes and flowsheet.	—	—	—	_____
2. Recorded client's response to therapy.	—	—	—	_____
3. Reported to oncoming nursing personnel.	—	—	—	_____
4. Reported adverse reactions to physician.	—	—	—	_____

Student _____ Date _____

Instructor _____ Date _____

PERFORMANCE CHECKLIST 20-2 **INSERTING A PERIPHERALLY INSERTED CENTRAL CATHETER**

	S	U	NP	Comments
ASSESSMENT				
1. Reviewed physician's orders.	—	—	—	_____
2. Knew agency's policy regarding peripherally inserted central catheters (PICCs).	—	—	—	_____
3. Reviewed manufacturer's directions.	—	—	—	_____
4. Assessed client's understanding of and readiness for procedure.	—	—	—	_____
5. Assessed client's status and needs.	—	—	—	_____
6. Assessed for drug allergies.	—	—	—	_____
NURSING DIAGNOSIS				
1. Developed appropriate nursing diagnoses based on assessment data.	—	—	—	_____
PLANNING				
1. Developed individualized goals for client based on nursing diagnoses.	—	—	—	_____
2. Identified expected outcomes.	—	—	—	_____
3. Explained procedure to client.	—	—	—	_____
4. Verified that consent form was signed.	—	—	—	_____
5. Measured circumference of upper arm.	—	—	—	_____
IMPLEMENTATION				
1. Washed hands.	—	—	—	_____
2. Organized equipment at bedside.	—	—	—	_____
3. Instructed client to wash arms thoroughly. Assisted as necessary.	—	—	—	_____
4. Clipped hair if necessary.	—	—	—	_____
5. Identified an appropriate vein in the antecubital fossa.	—	—	—	_____
6. Positioned client correctly.	—	—	—	_____
7. Measured the distance from insertion site to proposed site for catheter tip.	—	—	—	_____
8. Put on mask, gown, and goggles.	—	—	—	_____
9. Opened sterile supplies or kit correctly.	—	—	—	_____

	S	U	NP	Comments
10. Applied sterile gloves.	___	___	___	_____
11. Prepared lidocaine (optional) and solutions for flushing.	___	___	___	_____
12. Correctly prepared insertion site.	___	___	___	_____
13. Correctly prepared catheter and tubing.	___	___	___	_____
14. Removed gloves. Reapplied tourniquet if non-sterile tourniquet used.	___	___	___	_____
15. Applied a pair of sterile gloves.	___	___	___	_____
16. Placed sterile 4×4 gauze over tourniquet or applied sterile tourniquet.	___	___	___	_____
17. Provided sterile field around venipuncture site.	___	___	___	_____
18. Administered local anesthesia if indicated. Verified placement of introducer.	___	___	___	_____
19. Ensured that vein was securely cannulated.	___	___	___	_____
20. Correctly inserted and advanced catheter through introducer needle.	___	___	___	_____
21. Released tourniquet without contaminating glove.	___	___	___	_____
22. Correctly advanced catheter the required distance.	___	___	___	_____
23. Instructed client to assume correct position.	___	___	___	_____
24. Continued to advance catheter the required distance.	___	___	___	_____
25. Correctly withdrew introducer without removing catheter.	___	___	___	_____
26. Removed needle from catheter.	___	___	___	_____
27. Removed guidewire.	___	___	___	_____
28. Verified patency of distal lumen.	___	___	___	_____
29. Attached extension tubing and cap to the lumen.	___	___	___	_____
30. Anchored hub of catheter to the skin.	___	___	___	_____
31. Placed 2×2 pads over insertion site. Covered with transparent dressing.	___	___	___	_____
32. Coiled extension tubings and secured to arm. Labeled dressing with date and time of insertion and gauge of catheter.	___	___	___	_____
33. Flushed each lumen with heparin solution.	___	___	___	_____
34. Disposed of equipment. Removed gloves and washed hands.	___	___	___	_____

Student _____   Date _____

Instructor _____   Date _____

	S	U	NP	Comments

35. Followed agency policy for x-ray examination verification of placement.

EVALUATION

1. Observed client and inquired about comfort level during insertion.

2. Inspected and palpated PICC site after insertion. Noted respiratory status.

3. Called for x-ray examination to verify placement.

4. Observed the PICC setup to determine status of system according to agency policy.

5. Observed client every hour to determine response to fluid and electrolyte therapy.

6. Weighed client daily.

7. Measured client's body temperature every 4 hours.

8. Evaluated client's knowledge of complications and maintenance of catheter.

9. Identified unexpected outcomes.

RECORDING AND REPORTING

1. Recorded PICC's gauge and length, insertion site, date and time of insertion, radiographic confirmation of location of catheter tip, presence or absence of signs and symptoms of complications.

2. Reported status of PICC, therapy being administered, and development of complications and their treatment.

Student _____   Date _____

Instructor _____   Date _____

PERFORMANCE CHECKLIST 20-3 **REGULATING INTRAVENOUS FLOW RATE**

	S	U	NP	Comments
ASSESSMENT				
1. Observed patency of the IV line and needle.	___	___	___	_____
2. Checked client's medical record for IV fluid orders.	___	___	___	_____
3. Assessed client's knowledge of how positioning affects flow rate.	___	___	___	_____
4. Verified with client how venipuncture site feels.	___	___	___	_____
NURSING DIAGNOSIS				
1. Developed appropriate nursing diagnoses based on assessment data.	___	___	___	_____
PLANNING				
1. Developed individualized goals for client based on nursing diagnoses.	___	___	___	_____
2. Identified expected outcomes.	___	___	___	_____
3. Used paper and pencil to calculate flow rate.	___	___	___	_____
4. Stated calibration in drops per milliliter of specific infusion set.	___	___	___	_____
5. Selected formula to calculate flow rate.	___	___	___	_____
IMPLEMENTATION				
1. Checked physician's orders and followed "five rights" for correct solution and additives.	___	___	___	_____
2. Calculated hourly rate in milliliters per hour (ml/hr).	___	___	___	_____
3. Placed adhesive tape on IV bottle or bag next to volume markings.	___	___	___	_____
4. Calculated drops per minute (gtt/min).	___	___	___	_____
5. Timed flow rate by watch.	___	___	___	_____
6. Followed correct procedure for using infusion controller or pump.	___	___	___	_____
7. Followed correct procedure for using volume control device.	___	___	___	_____
EVALUATION				
1. Observed client to determine effect of IV therapy.	___	___	___	_____
2. Assessed for signs of infiltration.	___	___	___	_____
3. Identified unexpected outcomes.	___	___	___	_____

	S	U	NP	Comments

RECORDING AND REPORTING

1. Recorded appropriate infusion rate.   — — — _____

2. Recorded new fluid rates in nurses' notes.   — — — _____

3. Reported appropriate information to nursing personnel.   — — — _____

Student _____   Date _____

Instructor _____   Date _____

PERFORMANCE CHECKLIST 20-4 **CHANGING INTRAVENOUS SOLUTIONS**

	S	U	NP	Comments

ASSESSMENT

1. Checked physician's orders.

2. Noted date and time when solution was last changed.

3. Determined the compatibility of all IV fluids and additives.

4. Determined client's understanding of need for continued IV therapy.

5. Determined patency of IV site.

NURSING DIAGNOSIS

1. Developed appropriate nursing diagnoses based on assessment data.

PLANNING

1. Developed individualized goals for client based on nursing diagnoses.

2. Identified expected outcomes.

3. Checked that next ordered solution was ready at least 1 hour before needed.

4. Prepared to change solution when it remained in neck of bottle or bag.

5. Explained procedure to client and family.

6. Maintained drip chamber half full.

IMPLEMENTATION

1. Washed hands.

2. Prepared solution for changing.

3. Moved roller clamp to reduce flow rate.

4. Removed old solution from IV pole.

5. Removed spike from old solution and correctly inserted spike into new solution.

6. Hung new bag or bottle of solution.

7. Checked for air in IV tubing.

8. Ensured that drip chamber contained solution.

9. Regulated flow rate to prescribed rate.

	S	U	NP	Comments

EVALUATION

1. Reassessed client to determine response to IV fluid therapy.   ___ ___ ___ _____

2. Monitored IV infusion for correct solution and additives.   ___ ___ ___ _____

3. Identified unexpected outcomes.   ___ ___ ___ _____

RECORDING AND REPORTING

1. Recorded amount and type of fluid infused and amount and type of new fluid.   ___ ___ ___ _____

Student _____   Date _____

Instructor _____   Date _____

PERFORMANCE CHECKLIST 20-5 **CHANGING INFUSION TUBING**

	S	U	NP	Comments

ASSESSMENT

1. Determined when new infusion set was warranted.

2. Observed for occlusions in IV tubing.

3. Determined client's understanding of need for continued IV infusions.

NURSING DIAGNOSIS

1. Developed appropriate nursing diagnoses based on assessment data.

PLANNING

1. Developed individualized goals for client based on nursing diagnoses.

2. Identified expected outcomes.

3. Explained procedure to client.

IMPLEMENTATION

1. Washed hands.

2. Opened new infusion set, protecting sites from contamination.

3. Applied disposable gloves.

4. Placed sterile 2 × 2 or 4 × 4 gauze on client's bed near IV puncture site.

5. Removed old dressing if required.

IV Infusion

1. Moved roller clamp to "off" position.

2. Regulated drip rate on old tubing to slow rate of infusion.

3. Compressed drip chamber and filled it while old tubing was still in place.

4. Discontinued old tubing from solution and hung drip chamber over IV pole.

5. Placed insertion spike into old IV solution opening and hung solution on IV pole.

6. Compressed and released drip chamber on new tubing.

	S	U	NP	Comments

7. Opened roller clamp, removed protective cap from needle adapter, and flushed tubing with solution.   — — — _____

8. Placed needle adapter in sterile gauze near client's IV site.   — — — _____

9. Turned roller clamp on old tubing to "off" position.   — — — _____

Heparin Lock

1. Used sterile technique to connect IV plug to tubing.   — — — _____

2. Removed air from tubing.   — — — _____

3. Removed protective cap from end and placed on sterile surface.   — — — _____

4. Stabilized hub of IV catheter or needle and gently pulled out old IV tubing; maintained stability of hub and inserted needle adapter of new tubing into hub.   — — — _____

5. Opened roller clamp on new tubing.   — — — _____

6. Regulated IV drip rate according to physician's orders and monitored hourly rate.   — — — _____

7. Applied new IV dressing if necessary.   — — — _____

8. Discarded old tubing properly.   — — — _____

9. Disposed of gloves and washed hands.   — — — _____

EVALUATION

1. Evaluated flow rate and observed connection site for leakage.   — — — _____

2. Identified unexpected outcomes.   — — — _____

RECORDING AND REPORTING

1. Recorded changing of tubing and solution on client's record.   — — — _____

2. Recorded date and time on tape below drip chamber.   — — — _____

Student _____   Date _____

Instructor _____   Date _____

PERFORMANCE CHECKLIST 20-6   **CHANGING A PERIPHERAL INTRAVENOUS DRESSING**

	S	U	NP	Comments

ASSESSMENT

1. Determined prior dressing change.

2. Observed present dressing for moisture and intactness.

3. Observed present IV system for proper functioning.

4. Inspected catheter site.

5. Monitored client's temperature.

6. Determined client's understanding of need for continued IV infusion.

NURSING DIAGNOSIS

1. Developed appropriate nursing diagnoses based on assessment data.

PLANNING

1. Developed individualized goals for client based on nursing diagnoses.

2. Identified expected outcomes.

3. Explained procedure to client.

IMPLEMENTATION

1. Washed hands and applied disposable gloves.

2. Removed old dressing.

3. Discontinued IV infusion if needed or ordered.

4. Stabilized IV catheter or needle and removed excess adhesive.

5. Cleansed venipuncture site with antiseptic solution or ointment. Allowed to dry.

6. Applied new dressing.

7. Anchored IV tube.

8. Dated new dressing.

9. Discarded equipment, removed gloves, and washed hands.

EVALUATION

1. Assessed functioning and patency of IV system.

	S	U	NP	Comments
2. Monitored client's body temperature.	—	—	—	_____
3. Identified unexpected outcomes.	—	—	—	_____

RECORDING AND REPORTING

1. Documented dressing change in nurses' notes.	—	—	—	_____
2. Notified nurse in charge of dressing change and integrity of system.	—	—	—	_____

Student _____   Date _____

Instructor _____   Date _____

PERFORMANCE CHECKLIST 20-7   **CARING FOR VASCULAR ACCESS DEVICES**

	S	U	NP	Comments
ASSESSMENT				
1. Assessed client's diagnosis, state of disease, and therapy plan by reviewing medical record.	___	___	___	_____
2. Assessed treatment schedule.	___	___	___	_____
3. Identified type of vascular access device (VAD) in place.	___	___	___	_____
4. Assessed need to use VAD for blood sampling.	___	___	___	_____
5. Assessed VAD site for skin integrity and infection.	___	___	___	_____
6. Assessed proper functioning of VAD before therapy.	___	___	___	_____
7. Assessed need for irrigation and dressing change.	___	___	___	_____
8. Assessed client's knowledge of care and maintenance of VAD.	___	___	___	_____
9. Assessed physician's order for medication, fluids, blood products, blood sampling.	___	___	___	_____
NURSING DIAGNOSIS				
1. Developed appropriate nursing diagnoses based on assessment data.	___	___	___	_____
PLANNING				
1. Developed individualized goals for client based on nursing diagnoses.	___	___	___	_____
2. Identified expected outcomes.	___	___	___	_____
3. Positioned client in supine position with head slightly elevated.	___	___	___	_____
4. Explained procedure to client.	___	___	___	_____
5. Arranged sterile equipment at bedside.	___	___	___	_____
IMPLEMENTATION				
Administration of Infusions or Sampling for Blood from Implanted Infusion Port				
1. Washed hands. Masked self and client.	___	___	___	_____
2. Prepared sterile field, opened sterile supplies.	___	___	___	_____
3. Prepared client's skin with alcohol.	___	___	___	_____
4. Prepared client's skin overlying port septum with povidone-iodine.	___	___	___	_____

	S	U	NP	Comments

5. Applied sterile gloves.

6. Assisted by another nurse, filled sterile syringe with saline solution.

7. Properly attached tubing and Huber needle and filled tubing with saline solution.

8. Applied sterile drape to port site.

9. Palpated port septum with strict aseptic technique.

10. Inserted Huber needle through skin correctly.

11. Checked for correct placement.

12. Flushed port with saline.

13. Observed for swelling.

14. Aspirated and discarded 5 ml of fluid.

15. Withdrew blood for sample, using appropriate syringe size.

16. Flushed with 2 ml heparin.

17. Refilled saline syringe and flushed port with saline.

18. Heparinized port by flushing with 5 ml heparin flush solution.

19. Secured needle with sterile gauze or transparent dressing.

20. Connected IV infusion tubing with sterile tubing.

21. Regulated IV infusion.

22. Disposed of all soiled supplies and equipment, sent specimens to laboratory, removed gloves, and washed hands.

Administration of Infusions or Sampling of Blood from Central Venous Catheter

1. Washed hands.

2. Applied gloves, gown, and goggles (per policy).

3. Cleansed injection cap or catheter hub.

4. Prepared two syringes: one with 10 ml normal saline; one with 20 ml saline.

5. Clamped catheter if removing cap.

6. With cap in place, inserted needle of syringe containing 10 ml normal saline and flushed catheter; if cap removed, connected syringe to hub, released clamp, flushed, reclamped.

Student _____   Date _____

Instructor _____   Date _____

	S	U	NP	Comments

7. Connected syringe for blood sampling, released clamp, aspirated, reclamped.

8. Attached or inserted syringe to catheter, released clamp, withdrew necessary blood for samples, reclamped.

9. Flushed with 2 ml heparin.

10. Attached or inserted syringe, filled with 20 ml normal saline, to catheter, clamped, and flushed correctly.

11. If no continuous infusion indicated, heparinized catheter.

12. Replaced new cap to end of catheter and removed clamp.

13. If IV fluids to be administered, connected IV tubing to end of catheter, maintaining aseptic technique.

14. Regulated IV infusion as ordered.

15. Taped tubing connections and pinned tubing to client's gown.

16. Correctly disposed of soiled equipment and supplies. Washed hands.

Dressing Change

1. Washed hands and applied clean gloves.

2. Masked self and client, if indicated.

3. Removed old dressing correctly.

4. Inspected placement or exit site.

5. For tunneled catheter, palpated Dacron cuff in subcutaneous tunnel.

6. Inspected catheter and hub for intactness.

7. Applied sterile gloves.

8. Cleaned placement or exit site correctly.

9. Applied povidone-iodine ointment or solution over exit site.

10. Redressed site correctly.

11. Secured tubing or needle to client's gown.

	S	U	NP	Comments

12. Labeled date, time of dressing, size of needle in place.   ___ ___ ___ _____

13. Disposed of soiled supplies, removed gloves, and washed hands.   ___ ___ ___ _____

EVALUATION

1. For continuous infusions, observed and calculated drip rate periodically.   ___ ___ ___ _____

2. Routinely assessed vital signs.   ___ ___ ___ _____

3. Observed catheter or port exit/placement site when exposed.   ___ ___ ___ _____

4. Observed catheter connection points periodically.   ___ ___ ___ _____

5. Inspected condition of catheter and tubing for malfunctioning.   ___ ___ ___ _____

6. Consulted x-ray reports for catheter placement.   ___ ___ ___ _____

7. Evaluated ability of client or family member to provide care and maintain catheter or infusion port.   ___ ___ ___ _____

8. Identified unexpected outcomes.   ___ ___ ___ _____

RECORDING AND REPORTING

1. Recorded in nurses' notes medications, blood products, and parenteral nutrition given or samples obtained.   ___ ___ ___ _____

2. Recorded condition of exit site or port implantation.   ___ ___ ___ _____

3. Recorded dressing change procedure.   ___ ___ ___ _____

4. Recorded patency of catheter, ability to draw blood, and difficulty with infusions.   ___ ___ ___ _____

5. Recorded client and family education measures.   ___ ___ ___ _____

6. Reported complications immediately to nursing or medical personnel.   ___ ___ ___ _____

Student _____ Date _____

Instructor _____ Date _____

PERFORMANCE CHECKLIST 20-8 **DISCONTINUING PERIPHERAL INTRAVENOUS ACCESS**

	S	U	NP	Comments

ASSESSMENT

1. Observed IV site for signs and symptoms of infection, infiltration, phlebitis.

2. Reviewed physician's order for discontinuation of IV.

3. Determined client's understanding of need for discontinuation of peripheral IV access.

NURSING DIAGNOSIS

1. Developed appropriate nursing diagnoses based on assessment data.

PLANNING

1. Developed individualized goals for client based on nursing diagnoses.

2. Identified expected outcomes.

3. Explained procedure to client.

IMPLEMENTATION

1. Washed hands and applied disposable gloves.

2. Turned IV tubing roller clamp to "off" position.

3. Removed IV site dressing.

4. Cleaned site with alcohol, then povidone-iodine solution.

5. Placed sterile gauze over venipuncture site and correctly removed catheter or needle. Inspected catheter for intactness.

6. Applied pressure to site for 2-3 minutes.

7. Applied folded gauze dressing with betadine ointment over site and secured with tape.

8. Discarded used supplies, removed gloves, and washed hands.

EVALUATION

1. Observed site for evidence of bleeding.

2. Observed site for redness, pain, drainage, swelling.

	S	U	NP	Comments

RECORDING AND REPORTING

1. Recorded in nurses' notes time IV discontinued and information on site assessment.

    ___ ___ ___ _____

2. Reported to nurse in charge or oncoming shift that IV was discontinued and any pertinent information related to the procedure.

    ___ ___ ___ _____

Student _____   Date _____

Instructor _____   Date _____

PERFORMANCE CHECKLIST 21-1 **INITIATING BLOOD THERAPY**

	S	U	NP	Comments
ASSESSMENT				
1. Inspected integrity and intactness of present IV line.	___	___	___	_____
2. Reviewed policy and procedure regarding administration of blood or blood products.	___	___	___	_____
3. Verified that venipuncture was performed with an 18- or 19-gauge angiocatheter.	___	___	___	_____
4. Obtained client's transfusion history.	___	___	___	_____
5. Identified indication for blood product.	___	___	___	_____
6. Reviewed baseline vital signs before initiating transfusion.	___	___	___	_____
7. Reviewed physician's order.	___	___	___	_____
NURSING DIAGNOSIS				
1. Developed appropriate nursing diagnoses based on assessment data.	___	___	___	_____
PLANNING				
1. Developed individualized goals for client based on nursing diagnoses.	___	___	___	_____
2. Identified expected outcomes.	___	___	___	_____
3. Explained procedure and its purpose to client.	___	___	___	_____
IMPLEMENTATION				
Preadministration				
1. Obtained blood from blood bank following agency protocol.	___	___	___	_____
2. Correctly verified right blood product and right client.	___	___	___	_____
3. Had client void or emptied urine collection container.	___	___	___	_____
4. Asked client to report shortness of breath, chills, headache, itching, or rash.	___	___	___	_____
5. Had client sign any necessary consent forms.	___	___	___	_____
6. Correctly recorded the verification process.	___	___	___	_____
7. Collected supplies for venipuncture, if necessary.	___	___	___	_____

	S	U	NP	Comments

Administration

1. Washed hands and applied disposable gloves.

2. Opened blood administration set.

3. Prepared Y tubing properly.

4. Initiated infusion of blood product.

5. Remained with client during first 5-15 minutes of transfusion.

6. Monitored client's vital signs appropriately.

7. Regulated infusion according to physician's orders.

8. Cleared infusion tubing with 0.9% normal saline.

9. Disposed of supplies. Removed gloves and washed hands.

EVALUATION

1. Assessed client for chills, flushing, itching, dyspnea, rash, hives, or other signs of transfusion reaction.

2. Reassessed client and assessed laboratory values to determine response to administration of blood components.

3. Monitored IV site and status of infusion.

4. Identified unexpected outcomes.

RECORDING AND REPORTING

1. Recorded type and amount of blood component administered and client's response to blood therapy on appropriate form.

2. Reported signs and symptoms of a transfusion reaction immediately.

Student _____   Date _____

Instructor _____   Date _____

PERFORMANCE CHECKLIST 21-2   **ASSISTING WITH AUTOLOGOUS BLOOD TRANSFUSION**

	S	U	NP	Comments
ASSESSMENT				
1. Determined integrity of existing IV line.	—	—	—	
2. Observed that venipuncture was performed with 18-gauge or larger angiocatheter if IV line is present.	—	—	—	
3. Obtained baseline vital signs.	—	—	—	
4. Identified factors that preclude autologous blood transfusion.	—	—	—	
NURSING DIAGNOSIS				
1. Developed appropriate nursing diagnoses based on assessment data.	—	—	—	
PLANNING				
1. Developed individualized goals for client based on nursing diagnoses.	—	—	—	
2. Identified expected outcomes.	—	—	—	
3. Explained procedure to client and family. Obtained necessary consents.	—	—	—	
IMPLEMENTATION				
1. Washed hands and put on appropriate intraoperative or postoperative attire.	—	—	—	
2. Placed collected blood into collection container or cell processing system and followed agency's or manufacturer's procedure.	—	—	—	
3. Correctly initiated blood transfusion procedure as in Skill 21-1, Implementation.	—	—	—	
EVALUATION				
1. Assessed client and laboratory values to determine response to administration of transfusion.	—	—	—	
2. Monitored IV site and infusion status when vital signs measured.	—	—	—	
3. Identified unexpected outcomes.	—	—	—	
RECORDING AND REPORTING				
1. Recorded amount of blood received by autologous blood transfusion and client's response to blood therapy.	—	—	—	

	S	U	NP	Comments
2. Reported number of units infused at change-of-shift report.	—	—	—	_____
3. Reported any deterioration in cardiac status to physician or nurse in charge.	—	—	—	_____

Student _____   Date _____

Instructor _____   Date _____

PERFORMANCE CHECKLIST 21-3 **MONITORING FOR TRANSFUSION REACTIONS**

	S	U	NP	Comments
ASSESSMENT				
1. Observed for signs of acute hemolytic reaction.	—	—	—	_____
2. Observed for signs of delayed hemolytic reaction.	—	—	—	_____
3. Observed for signs of febrile nonhemolytic reaction.	—	—	—	_____
4. Observed for signs of urticaria reaction.	—	—	—	_____
5. Observed for signs of anaphylactic reaction.	—	—	—	_____
6. Observed for signs of graft-versus-host disease.	—	—	—	_____
7. Observed for signs of circulatory overload.	—	—	—	_____
8. Observed for signs of septic shock.	—	—	—	_____
9. Observed for signs of hypothermia and cardiac dysrhythmias.	—	—	—	_____
10. Observed for signs of citrate toxicity.	—	—	—	_____
11. Observed for signs of hepatitis.	—	—	—	_____
12. Observed for signs of HIV infection.	—	—	—	_____
NURSING DIAGNOSIS				
1. Developed appropriate nursing diagnoses based on assessment data.	—	—	—	_____
PLANNING				
1. Developed individualized goals for client based on nursing diagnoses.	—	—	—	_____
2. Identified expected outcomes.	—	—	—	_____
3. Explained treatment of a reaction to client and family.	—	—	—	_____
IMPLEMENTATION				
1. Discontinued transfusion.	—	—	—	_____
2. Removed tubing with blood in it and replaced with new tubing.	—	—	—	_____
3. Maintained patent IV line, using 0.9% NaCl.	—	—	—	_____
4. Obtained two blood samples.	—	—	—	_____
5. Returned remaining blood to blood bank.	—	—	—	_____

	S	U	NP	Comments

6. Notified physician of client's transfusion reaction.

7. Monitored client's vital signs every 15 minutes.

8. Administered prescribed medications.

9. Initiated CPR if necessary.

10. Obtained first voided urine.

EVALUATION

1. Assessed client to determine improvement or changes in physiologic status.

2. Identified unexpected outcomes.

RECORDING AND REPORTING

1. Recorded in nurses' notes pertinent information regarding transfusion reaction.

2. Reported transfusion reaction immediately to nurse in charge and physician.

Student _____ Date _____

Instructor _____ Date _____

PERFORMANCE CHECKLIST 22-1 **PERFORMING NUTRITIONAL ASSESSMENT**

	S	U	NP	Comments
ASSESSMENT				
1. Determined need to perform nutritional assessment.	—	—	—	_____
2. Obtained baseline knowledge through diet history.	—	—	—	_____
3. Assessed client for usual body weight.	—	—	—	_____
4. Reviewed laboratory results.	—	—	—	_____
5. Determined medications client is taking.	—	—	—	_____
NURSING DIAGNOSIS				
1. Developed appropriate nursing diagnoses based on assessment data.	—	—	—	_____
PLANNING				
1. Identified individual goals for assessing client's nutrition.	—	—	—	_____
2. Identified expected outcomes.	—	—	—	_____
3. Prepared equipment and supplies.	—	—	—	_____
4. Explained procedure to client.	—	—	—	_____
5. Performed assessment in an environment free of distractions.	—	—	—	_____
IMPLEMENTATION				
1. Obtained complete and thorough nursing history.	—	—	—	_____
2. Initiated diet diary or 24-hour recall.	—	—	—	_____
3. Documented findings on nutritional assessment sheet.	—	—	—	_____
4. Assisted client into bed.	—	—	—	_____
5. Performed physical assessment.	—	—	—	_____
6. Assisted client to standing position.	—	—	—	_____
7. Weighed client.	—	—	—	_____
8. Obtained client's height.	—	—	—	_____
9. Calculated ideal body weight.	—	—	—	_____
10. Obtained wrist circumference.	—	—	—	_____

	S	U	NP	Comments

11. Obtained mid-upper arm circumference.

12. Obtained triceps skinfold measurements.

13. Assisted client to comfortable position.

14. Calculated mid-arm circumference.

15. Washed hands. Told client when nutritional assessment was completed.

EVALUATION

1. Reviewed history and physical examination.

2. Reviewed diet diary and 24-hour recall with client.

3. Compared client's height and weight with normal height and weight for age group.

4. Reviewed anthropometric data.

5. Compared client's laboratory data with normal values.

6. Determined client's caloric needs.

7. Determined amount of protein client requires.

8. Determined route of nutrition.

9. Chose either peripheral or central parenteral nutrition as appropriate and determined if fat was needed.

10. Identified unexpected outcomes.

RECORDING AND REPORTING

1. Documented findings and made recommendations on nutritional assessment form.

Student _____   Date _____

Instructor _____   Date _____

PERFORMANCE CHECKLIST 22-2   **ASSISTING THE ADULT CLIENT WITH ORAL NUTRITION**

	S	U	NP	Comments

ASSESSMENT

1. Assessed that GI tract is functioning and types of diet client can tolerate.

2. Assessed client's ability to swallow.

3. Assessed client's ability to feed self.

4. Assessed client's appetite, food likes, tolerance.

5. Determined food allergies before serving meal.

NURSING DIAGNOSIS

1. Developed appropriate nursing diagnoses based on assessment data.

PLANNING

1. Developed individualized goals for client based on nursing diagnoses.

2. Identified expected outcomes.

3. Prepared client's room.

4. Prepared client for meal.

IMPLEMENTATION

1. Washed hands before preparing client's tray.

2. Assessed tray for completeness and correct diet.

3. Prepared tray for client.

4. Determined how well client was eating independently.

5. Began assisting client who could not eat independently.

6. Assessed appropriate order to feed client, and cut food into bite-sized pieces.

7. Fed client.

8. Provided fluids as requested.

9. Talked with client.

10. Provided client education as appropriate.

11. Assisted client to wash hands and perform mouth care.

	S	U	NP	Comments
12. Assisted client to resting position.	___	___	___	_____
13. Returned client's tray and washed hands.	___	___	___	_____

EVALUATION

	S	U	NP	Comments
1. Observed client's ability to swallow.	___	___	___	_____
2. Assessed client's tolerance to diet.	___	___	___	_____
3. Assessed client's fluid and food intake.	___	___	___	_____
4. Weighed client daily.	___	___	___	_____
5. Assessed client's ability to assist with feeding.	___	___	___	_____
6. Identified unexpected outcomes.	___	___	___	_____

RECORDING AND REPORTING

	S	U	NP	Comments
1. Documented in client's chart: tolerance of diet, amount eaten, and intake and output.	___	___	___	_____

Student _____   Date _____

Instructor _____   Date _____

PERFORMANCE CHECKLIST 22-3   **ASPIRATION PRECAUTIONS**

	S	U	NP	Comments

ASSESSMENT

1. Performed nutritional assessment (see Skill 22-1).

2. Assessed clients who are at increased risk of aspiration for dysphagia.

3. Reported signs and symptoms of dysphagia to physician.

NURSING DIAGNOSIS

1. Developed appropriate nursing diagnoses based on assessment data.

PLANNING

1. Developed individualized goals for client based on nursing diagnoses.

2. Identified expected outcomes.

IMPLEMENTATION

1. Asked client about difficulties with swallowing or chewing various types of food.

2. Inspected mouth for pockets of food using penlight and tongue blade.

3. Positioned client upright in bed or chair.

4. Offered client thicker foods and assessed for difficulty in swallowing.

5. Proceeded to foods with thinner consistency if client tolerated thicker foods. Observed client closely for dysphagia.

6. Assisted the client to complete the meal or placed the meal in reach for self-feeding, if no signs or symptoms of dysphagia are evident.

7. Asked client to remain sitting upright for at last 30 minutes after the meal.

8. Assisted client to wash hands and perform mouth care.

9. Returned client's tray to appropriate place and washed hands.

EVALUATION

1. Assessed client's ability to ingest foods of various textures and thickness.

	S	U	NP	Comments
2. Assessed client's food and fluid intake.	——	——	——	——————————
3. Weighed client weekly.	——	——	——	——————————
4. Assessed client's oral cavity after meal to detect pockets of food.	——	——	——	——————————
5. Identified unexpected outcomes.	——	——	——	——————————

RECORDING AND REPORTING

1. Documented in client's chart: tolerance of various food textures, amount of assistance required, position during meal, absence or presence of dysphagia, and amount eaten.   —— —— —— ——————————

Student _____   Date _____

Instructor _____   Date _____

PERFORMANCE CHECKLIST 23-1 **INTUBATING THE CLIENT WITH A SMALL-BORE NASOGASTRIC OR NASOINTESTINAL FEEDING TUBE**

	S	U	NP	Comments
ASSESSMENT				
1. Assessed client's need for tube feedings.	—	—	—	_____
2. Assessed patency of nares.	—	—	—	_____
3. Assessed past medical history.	—	—	—	_____
4. Evaluated gag reflex.	—	—	—	_____
5. Assessed client's mental status.	—	—	—	_____
6. Assessed for bowel sounds.	—	—	—	_____
NURSING DIAGNOSIS				
1. Developed appropriate nursing diagnoses based on assessment data.	—	—	—	_____
PLANNING				
1. Developed individualized goals for client based on nursing diagnoses.	—	—	—	_____
2. Identified expected outcomes.	—	—	—	_____
3. Explained procedure to client.	—	—	—	_____
4. Explained to client how to communicate during procedure.	—	—	—	_____
5. Positioned client.	—	—	—	_____
6. Examined feeding tube for flaws.	—	—	—	_____
7. Determined length of tube to be inserted.	—	—	—	_____
8. Correctly prepared tube for intubation.	—	—	—	_____
9. Cut tape.	—	—	—	_____
IMPLEMENTATION				
1. Applied clean gloves.	—	—	—	_____
2. Inspected nares for irritation or obstruction.	—	—	—	_____
3. Dipped tube with surface lubricant into glass of water.	—	—	—	_____
4. Inserted tube through nostril to back of throat.	—	—	—	_____
5. Flexed client's head toward chest after tube had passed through nasopharynx.	—	—	—	_____
6. Had client swallow and advanced tube as client swallowed.	—	—	—	_____

	S	U	NP	Comments

7. Emphasized need to mouth breathe and swallow during procedure. ___ ___ ___ _____

8. Advanced tube each time client swallowed until desired length was passed. ___ ___ ___ _____

9. Did not force tube; checked for position of tube in back of throat. ___ ___ ___ _____

10. Checked placement of tube. ___ ___ ___ _____

11. Applied tincture of benzoin on tip of client's nose and tube. Allowed to dry. ___ ___ ___ _____

12. Removed gloves. Secured tube with tape. ___ ___ ___ _____

13. Positioned client on right side when possible x-ray confirmed placement. ___ ___ ___ _____

14. Obtained x-ray examination of abdomen. ___ ___ ___ _____

15. Left stylet in place until position confirmed. ___ ___ ___ _____

16. Remained with client. ___ ___ ___ _____

17. Applied gloves and administered oral hygiene. ___ ___ ___ _____

18. Removed gloves, disposed of equipment, washed hands. ___ ___ ___ _____

EVALUATION

1. Assessed client for reaction to procedure. ___ ___ ___ _____

2. Confirmed x-ray examination results. ___ ___ ___ _____

3. Identified unexpected outcomes. ___ ___ ___ _____

RECORDING AND REPORTING

1. Recorded and reported tube size/length, client's tolerance of procedure, and confirmation of placement by x-ray. ___ U NP _____

Student _____   Date _____

Instructor _____   Date _____

PERFORMANCE CHECKLIST 23-2   **VERIFYING TUBE PLACEMENT FOR A LARGE- OR SMALL-BORE FEEDING TUBE**

	S	U	NP	Comments
ASSESSMENT				
1. Identified signs and symptoms of inadvertent respiratory placement.	—	—	—	_____
2. Identified signs and symptoms that increase risk of tube dislocation.	—	—	—	_____
3. Reviewed client's record for history of prior tube placement.	—	—	—	_____
4. Observed external portion of tube for a change in length.	—	—	—	_____
NURSING DIAGNOSIS				
1. Developed appropriate nursing diagnoses based on assessment data.	—	—	—	_____
PLANNING				
1. Developed individualized goals for client based on nursing diagnoses.	—	—	—	_____
2. Identified expected outcomes.	—	—	—	_____
3. Explained procedure to client.	—	—	—	_____
IMPLEMENTATION				
1. Washed hands and applied gloves.	—	—	—	_____
2. Performed measures to verify placement of tube: injected 30 ml of air and aspirated GI contents with a syringe, measured pH of aspirated GI contents, ausculated with stethoscope over left upper quadrant of abdomen, and quickly injected 10-20 ml air via syringe into tube.	—	—	—	_____
3. Removed and disposed of gloves; washed hands.	—	—	—	_____
EVALUATION				
1. Observed client for respiratory distress.	—	—	—	_____
2. Observed flow rate of enteral formula.	—	—	—	_____
3. Identified unexpected outcomes.	—	—	—	_____
RECORDING AND REPORTING				
1. Recorded and reported information on tube, results of verification, and client's response.	—	—	—	_____

Student _____   Date _____

Instructor _____   Date _____

PERFORMANCE CHECKLIST 23-3 **ADMINISTERING ENTERAL FEEDINGS VIA NASOGASTRIC TUBE (LARGE- OR SMALL-BORE)**

	S	U	NP	Comments
ASSESSMENT				
1. Assessed client's nutritional needs.	—	—	—	_____
2. Assessed client for food allergies.	—	—	—	_____
3. Assessed client's need for enteral tube feedings.	—	—	—	_____
4. Ausculated for bowel sounds.	—	—	—	_____
5. Obtained baseline weight and laboratory values.	—	—	—	_____
6. Verified physician's order.	—	—	—	_____
NURSING DIAGNOSIS				
1. Developed appropriate nursing diagnoses based on assessment data.	—	—	—	_____
PLANNING				
1. Developed individualized goals for client based on nursing diagnoses.	—	—	—	_____
2. Identified expected outcomes.	—	—	—	_____
3. Washed hands.	—	—	—	_____
4. Prepared bag and tubing to administer formula.	—	—	—	_____
5. Explained procedure to client.	—	—	—	_____
6. Placed client in proper position.	—	—	—	_____
IMPLEMENTATION				
1. Checked placement of gastric tube.	—	—	—	_____
2. Initiated tube feeding (bolus or continuous drip method).	—	—	—	_____
3. Clamped tubing while feeding is not being administered.	—	—	—	_____
4. Administered water via tubing with or between feedings.	—	—	—	_____
5. Washed bag and tubing after feeding.	—	—	—	_____
6. Advanced tube feeding.	—	—	—	_____
EVALUATION				
1. Evaluated amount of aspirate every 4 hours.	—	—	—	_____
2. Monitored fingerstick blood glucose every 6 hours.	—	—	—	_____

	S	U	NP	Comments
3. Monitored I&O every shift.	—	—	—	_____
4. Weighed client daily.	—	—	—	_____
5. Observed laboratory values.	—	—	—	_____
6. Observed client's respiratory status.	—	—	—	_____
7. Observed client's comfort level.	—	—	—	_____
8. Identified unexpected outcomes.	—	—	—	_____

RECORDING AND REPORTING

	S	U	NP	Comments
1. Recorded amount and type of feeding.	—	—	—	_____
2. Recorded client's response to feeding, patency of tube, and any adverse effects.	—	—	—	_____
3. Reported appropriate information to oncoming nursing staff.	—	—	—	_____

Student _____   Date _____

Instructor _____   Date _____

PERFORMANCE CHECKLIST 23-4 **ADMINISTERING ENTERAL FEEDINGS VIA GASTROSTOMY TUBE**

	S	U	NP	Comments
ASSESSMENT				
1. Identified signs and symptoms of malnutrition.	___	___	___	_____
2. Assessed client for food allergies.	___	___	___	_____
3. Assessed client's need for tube feedings.	___	___	___	_____
4. Auscultated for bowel sounds.	___	___	___	_____
5. Verified physician's order.	___	___	___	_____
6. Assessed gastrostomy site.	___	___	___	_____
7. Obtained baseline weight and laboratory values.	___	___	___	_____
NURSING DIAGNOSIS				
1. Developed appropriate nursing diagnoses based on assessment data.	___	___	___	_____
PLANNING				
1. Developed individualized goals for client based on nursing diagnoses.	___	___	___	_____
2. Identified expected outcomes.	___	___	___	_____
3. Washed hands.	___	___	___	_____
4. Prepared bag and tubing to administer formula.	___	___	___	_____
5. Explained procedure to client.	___	___	___	_____
6. Placed client in correct position.	___	___	___	_____
IMPLEMENTATION				
1. Verified placement of gastric tube.	___	___	___	_____
2. Initiated feeding (bolus or continuous drip method).	___	___	___	_____
3. Clamped tubing when feeding is not being administered.	___	___	___	_____
4. Administered water via feeding tube as ordered.	___	___	___	_____
5. Rinsed bag and tubing after feeding.	___	___	___	_____
6. Advanced tube feeding.	___	___	___	_____
7. Changed gastrostomy exit site dressing as needed; inspected exit site every shift.	___	___	___	_____
8. Disposed of supplies and washed hands.	___	___	___	_____

	S	U	NP	Comments

EVALUATION

1. Evaluated client's tolerance of tube feeding.

2. Monitored fingerstick blood glucose every 6 hours.

3. Monitored I&O every shift.

4. Weighed client daily.

5. Observed laboratory values.

6. Observed stoma site.

7. Identified unexpected outcomes.

RECORDING AND REPORTING

1. Recorded amount and type of feeding.

2. Recorded client's response to feeding, patency of tube, and any adverse effects.

3. Reported appropriate information to oncoming nursing staff.

Student _____   Date _____

Instructor _____   Date _____

PERFORMANCE CHECKLIST 23-5   ADMINISTERING ENTERAL FEEDINGS VIA NASOINTESTINAL TUBE OR JEJUNOSTOMY TUBE

	S	U	NP	Comments
ASSESSMENT				
1. Identified signs and symptoms of malnutrition.	__	__	__	_____
2. Assessed client for food allergies.	__	__	__	_____
3. Assessed client's need for tube feedings.	__	__	__	_____
4. Ausculated for bowel sounds before feeding.	__	__	__	_____
5. Obtained baseline weight and laboratory values.	__	__	__	_____
6. Verified physician's orders.	__	__	__	_____
NURSING DIAGNOSIS				
1. Developed appropriate nursing diagnoses based on assessment data.	__	__	__	_____
PLANNING				
1. Developed individualized goals for client based on nursing diagnoses.	__	__	__	_____
2. Identified expected outcomes.	__	__	__	_____
3. Prepared bag and tubing to administer formula.	__	__	__	_____
4. Explained procedure to client.	__	__	__	_____
5. Placed client in proper position.	__	__	__	_____
IMPLEMENTATION				
1. Washed hands and applied clean gloves.	__	__	__	_____
2. Aspirated intestinal secretions and checked for residue. Measured pH of GI aspirate.	__	__	__	_____
3. Initiated continuous tube feeding. Flushed tube with water before and after feeding.	__	__	__	_____
4. Advanced tube feeding.	__	__	__	_____
EVALUATION				
1. Evaluated amount of aspirate every 4 hours.	__	__	__	_____
2. Monitored fingerstick glucose every 6 hours.	__	__	__	_____
3. Monitored I&O every shift.	__	__	__	_____
4. Weighed client daily.	__	__	__	_____
5. Observed laboratory values.	__	__	__	_____

	S	U	NP	Comments
6. Inspected nares for pressure.	—	—	—	_____
7. Identified unexpected outcomes.	—	—	—	_____

RECORDING AND REPORTING

1. Recorded amount and type of feeding.	—	—	—	_____
2. Recorded client's response to feeding, patency of tube, and any adverse effects.	—	—	—	_____
3. Reported appropriate information to oncoming nursing staff.	—	—	—	_____

Student _____   Date _____

Instructor _____   Date _____

PERFORMANCE CHECKLIST 24-1 **CARING FOR THE CLIENT RECEIVING CENTRAL VENOUS PLACEMENT FOR CENTRAL PARENTERAL NUTRITION**

	S	U	NP	Comments

ASSESSMENT

1. Assessed client's need for central parenteral nutrition (CPN). ___ ___ ___ _____

2. Checked physician's order for parenteral therapy. ___ ___ ___ _____

3. Assessed client's hydration status. ___ ___ ___ _____

4. Assessed client for surgical procedures or anatomical irregularities of the upper chest. ___ ___ ___ _____

NURSING DIAGNOSIS

1. Developed appropriate nursing diagnoses based on assessment data. ___ ___ ___ _____

PLANNING

1. Developed individualized goals for client based on nursing diagnoses. ___ ___ ___ _____

2. Identified expected outcomes. ___ ___ ___ _____

3. Explained procedure to client and need for CPN and follow-up care. ___ ___ ___ _____

4. Verified that consent form was signed. ___ ___ ___ _____

IMPLEMENTATION

1. Nurse and physician washed hands. ___ ___ ___ _____

2. Physician positioned client with assistance from nurse. ___ ___ ___ _____

3. Physician donned sterile attire; nurse donned cap, mask, and nonsterile gloves. ___ ___ ___ _____

4. Nurse opened central vein kit and saturated gauze. ___ ___ ___ _____

5. Physician cleansed skin with alcohol. ___ ___ ___ _____

6. Discarded gauze. ___ ___ ___ _____

7. Physician cleansed skin with povidone-iodine scrub. ___ ___ ___ _____

8. Physician wiped away excess scrub solution. ___ ___ ___ _____

9. Physician applied sterile gloves. ___ ___ ___ _____

10. Nurse opened first wrapping of central vein kit and handed to physician. ___ ___ ___ _____

	S	U	NP	Comments

11. Physician opened second wrapping and prepared sterile field. ___ ___ ___ _____

12. Physician reviewed kit and put needles on syringes. ___ ___ ___ _____

13. Nurse set up IV bag and filled tubing. ___ ___ ___ _____

14. Nurse opened sterile tubing and placed on sterile field. ___ ___ ___ _____

15. Nurse placed client in Trendelenburg position and turned client's head away from site of insertion. ___ ___ ___ _____

16. Nurse wiped off top of 1% lidocaine bottle and turned upside down. ___ ___ ___ _____

17. Physician withdrew appropriate amount of lidocaine and injected into subclavian puncture site. ___ ___ ___ _____

18. Had client perform Valsalva maneuver. ___ ___ ___ _____

19. Physician inserted subclavian IV catheter into subclavian vein. ___ ___ ___ _____

20. Nurse frequently checked client to assess tolerance to procedure. ___ ___ ___ _____

21. Nurse connected IV tubing to extension tubing and flushed with IV fluid while physician was cannulating central vein. ___ ___ ___ _____

22. Physician connected IV tubing to client's subclavian catheter after establishing rapid blood return. ___ ___ ___ _____

23. Nurse opened IV fluids wide. ___ ___ ___ _____

24. Nurse lowered IV bag below heart level. ___ ___ ___ _____

25. Nurse raised IV bag and slowed rate to 30 ml/hr until x-ray study obtained. ___ ___ ___ _____

26. Physician sutured central venous catheter in place. ___ ___ ___ _____

27. Physician removed sterile clothes and completed procedure. ___ ___ ___ _____

Applying Occlusive Dressing

1. Applied sterile gloves. ___ ___ ___ _____

2. With alcohol swab, started at catheter exit site and worked in circular motion outward approximately 2 to 3 inches (performed procedure three times). ___ ___ ___ _____

3. Repeated above steps with povidone-iodine swabs and allowed area to dry. ___ ___ ___ _____

Student _____   Date _____

Instructor _____   Date _____

	S	U	NP	Comments
4. Applied small amount of povidione-iodine ointment at catheter exit site.	___	___	___	_____
5. Applied clear, adhesive dressing over site.	___	___	___	_____
6. Assisted with x-ray examination.	___	___	___	_____
7. Connected tubing to infusion pump and set rate.	___	___	___	_____
8. Repositioned client.	___	___	___	_____
9. Disposed of supplies and washed hands.	___	___	___	_____

EVALUATION

	S	U	NP	Comments
1. Inspected site and dressing daily.	___	___	___	_____
2. Evaluated client for complications associated with parenteral nutrition.	___	___	___	_____
3. Identified unexpected outcomes.	___	___	___	_____

RECORDING AND REPORTING

	S	U	NP	Comments
1. Recorded condition of client before, during, and after the procedure.	___	___	___	_____
2. Documented presence or absence of blood return after catheter placement.	___	___	___	_____
3. Documented confirmation of central vein catheter placement.	___	___	___	_____

Student _____   Date _____

Instructor _____   Date _____

PERFORMANCE CHECKLIST 24-2 **CARING FOR THE CLIENT RECEIVING CENTRAL PARENTERAL NUTRITION (CPN)**

	S	U	NP	Comments

ASSESSMENT

1. Assessed client's nutritional status, caloric intake, laboratory values, and weight.   ___ ___ ___ _____

2. Determined if client is candidate for CPN.   ___ ___ ___ _____

3. Assessed factors influencing CPN administration.   ___ ___ ___ _____

4. Verified physician's order for CPN and flow rate.   ___ ___ ___ _____

NURSING DIAGNOSIS

1. Developed appropriate nursing diagnoses based on assessment data.   ___ ___ ___ _____

PLANNING

1. Developed individualized goals for client based on nursing diagnoses.   ___ ___ ___ _____

2. Identified expected outcomes.   ___ ___ ___ _____

3. Explained purpose of CPN.   ___ ___ ___ _____

IMPLEMENTATION

1. Washed hands and applied gloves.   ___ ___ ___ _____

2. Inspected PN solution for particulate matter or separation.   ___ ___ ___ _____

3. Placed IV tubing into intravenous infusion pump and regulated prescribed flow rate.   ___ ___ ___ _____

EVALUATION

1. Obtained daily weights.   ___ ___ ___ _____

2. Assessed for fluid retention.   ___ ___ ___ _____

3. Monitored client's glucose and laboratory parameters to determine response to CPN.   ___ ___ ___ _____

4. Inspected central venous access site.   ___ ___ ___ _____

5. Identified unexpected outcomes.   ___ ___ ___ _____

RECORDING AND REPORTING

1. Recorded condition of central venous access device, rate of infusion, I&O, vital signs, and weights.   ___ ___ ___ _____

Student _____   Date _____

Instructor _____   Date _____

PERFORMANCE CHECKLIST 24-3   CARING FOR THE CLIENT RECEIVING PERIPHERAL PARENTERAL NUTRITION WITH LIPID (FAT) EMULSION

	S	U	NP	Comments
ASSESSMENT				
1. Assessed client's needs for fat emulsion.	—	—	—	_____
2. Assessed client for essential fatty acid deficiency.	—	—	—	_____
3. Assessed appropriate IV site for fat emulsion administration.	—	—	—	_____
4. Assessed appropriate time to administer fats.	—	—	—	_____
5. Checked physician's order for volume of fat emulsion.	—	—	—	_____
NURSING DIAGNOSIS				
1. Developed appropriate nursing diagnoses based on assessment data.	—	—	—	_____
PLANNING				
1. Identified individualized goals for client based on nursing diagnoses.	—	—	—	_____
2. Identified expected outcomes.	—	—	—	_____
3. Explained why client was receiving fat emulsions.	—	—	—	_____
4. Placed client in comfortable position.	—	—	—	_____
IMPLEMENTATION				
1. Washed hands and applied gloves.	—	—	—	_____
2. Connected tubing to solution and ran fat emulsion into IV tubing.	—	—	—	_____
3. Cleaned peripheral line tubing injection port.	—	—	—	_____
4. Inserted fat emulsion infusion into injection port correctly.	—	—	—	_____
5. Set flow rate on infusion pump. Began PPN at ordered rate.	—	—	—	_____
6. Discarded supplies and washed hands.	—	—	—	_____
EVALUATION				
1. Assessed client to determine response to fat emulsion.	—	—	—	_____
2. Monitored temperature every 4 hours and regularly inspected venipuncture site.	—	—	—	_____

	S	U	NP	Comments
3. Assessed client's response to fluid volume.	—	—	—	_____
4. Identified unexpected outcomes.	—	—	—	_____

RECORDING AND REPORTING

1. Recorded I&O every shift.	—	—	—	_____
2. Recorded temperature every 4 hours.	—	—	—	_____
3. Recorded condition of IV site and status of infusion.	—	—	—	_____

Student _____   Date _____

Instructor _____   Date _____

PERFORMANCE CHECKLIST 25-1 **MEASURING AND RECORDING INTAKE AND OUTPUT**

	S	U	NP	Comments
ASSESSMENT				
1. Identified risk of insufficient fluid intake.	—	—	—	_____
2. Reviewed client's graphic chart for elevations in body temperature.	—	—	—	_____
3. Assessed for surgical wound drainage.	—	—	—	_____
4. Assessed for presence of vomiting or diarrhea.	—	—	—	_____
5. Identified presence of wound or gastric suction equipment.	—	—	—	_____
6. Assessed patency and flow rate of IV and TPN solutions.	—	—	—	_____
7. Identified conditions that could influence a client's fluid balance status.	—	—	—	_____
8. Observed for weight changes.	—	—	—	_____
9. Assessed client for signs of fluid overload or dehydration.	—	—	—	_____
10. Inspected urine color and specific gravity.	—	—	—	_____
11. Monitored hematocrit.	—	—	—	_____
12. Assess client's knowledge of purpose of procedure.	—	—	—	_____
NURSING DIAGNOSIS				
1. Developed appropriate nursing diagnoses based on assessment data.	—	—	—	_____
PLANNING				
1. Developed individualized goals for client based on nursing diagnoses.	—	—	—	_____
2. Identified expected outcomes.	—	—	—	_____
3. Selected appropriate clients whose I&O should be measured.	—	—	—	_____
4. Explained procedure.	—	—	—	_____
5. Marked containers for measuring output.	—	—	—	_____
6. Posted sign indicating I&O was instituted.	—	—	—	_____
IMPLEMENTATION				
1. Explained to client and family why I&O measurements are necessary.	—	—	—	_____

	S	U	NP	Comments

2. Provided client with copy of hospital's metric conversion chart.

3. Measured and recorded all oral and parenteral fluids and all enteral tube feedings.

4. Instructed client not to empty urinal, Foley drainage bag, bedpan, or commode.

5. Applied gloves before handling equipment or drainage.

6. Correctly measured and recorded all fluids draining from Foley catheter, nasogastric suction, wound suction at least every 8 hours.

7. Washed hands after measuring and recording output fluids.

EVALUATION

1. Reassessed client's fluid balance correctly.

2. Observed characteristics of urinary output.

3. Noted I&O balance.

4. Identified unexpected outcomes.

RECORDING AND REPORTING

1. Calculated and recorded 8-hour totals.

2. Calculated and recorded 24-hour totals.

3. Reported urine output of less than 30 ml/hr.

Student _____   Date _____

Instructor _____   Date _____

PERFORMANCE CHECKLIST 25-2   **ASSISTING A CLIENT TO USE A URINAL**

	S	U	NP	Comments

ASSESSMENT

1. Assessed client's urinary elimination patterns.

2. Assessed for incontinence.

3. Palpated client for distended bladder.

4. Assessed client's cognitive and physical status.

5. Assessed client's knowledge regarding urinal use.

NURSING DIAGNOSIS

1. Developed appropriate nursing diagnoses based on assessment data.

PLANNING

1. Developed individualized goals for client based on nursing diagnoses.

2. Identified expected outcomes.

3. Obtained appropriate assistance.

4. Explained procedure to client.

5. Set up voiding routine.

IMPLEMENTATION

1. Washed hands and applied gloves.

2. Provided privacy.

3. Assisted client into appropriate position.

4. Placed urinal properly.

5. Assessed output. Emptied, cleaned, and returned urinal.

6. Allowed client to wash hands.

7. Removed and disposed of gloves; washed hands.

EVALUATION

1. Assessed client's ability to use urinal.

2. Noted characteristics of urine.

3. Identified unexpected outcomes.

RECORDING AND REPORTING

1. Recorded client's ability to use urinal and characteristics of urinary output.

	S	U	NP	Comments
2. Recorded urinary output.	__	__	__	_____
3. Reported frequency of voiding patterns.	__	__	__	_____

Student _____   Date _____

Instructor _____   Date _____

PERFORMANCE CHECKLIST 25-3 INSERTING A STRAIGHT OR INDWELLING CATHETER

	S	U	NP	Comments

ASSESSMENT

1. Assessed client's status.   ___ ___ ___ _____

2. Reviewed client's medical record and physician's order.   ___ ___ ___ _____

3. Assessed client's knowledge of purpose for catheterization.   ___ ___ ___ _____

NURSING DIAGNOSIS

1. Developed appropriate nursing diagnoses based on assessment data.   ___ ___ ___ _____

PLANNING

1. Developed individualized goals for client based on nursing diagnoses.   ___ ___ ___ _____

2. Identified expected outcomes.   ___ ___ ___ _____

3. Explained procedure to client.   ___ ___ ___ _____

4. Obtained additional nursing personnel, if appropriate.   ___ ___ ___ _____

5. Began monitoring I&O.   ___ ___ ___ _____

IMPLEMENTATION

1. Washed hands.   ___ ___ ___ _____

2. Provided privacy.   ___ ___ ___ _____

3. Raised bed to appropriate height.   ___ ___ ___ _____

4. Positioned self correctly.   ___ ___ ___ _____

5. Raised appropriate side rail.   ___ ___ ___ _____

6. Placed pad under client.   ___ ___ ___ _____

7. Positioned client.   ___ ___ ___ _____

8. Draped client.   ___ ___ ___ _____

9. Using disposable gloves, cleansed perineal area using clean technique.   ___ ___ ___ _____

10. Prepared urinary drainage container.   ___ ___ ___ _____

11. Positioned lamp.   ___ ___ ___ _____

12. Maintained sterile asepsis while opening catheter kit.   ___ ___ ___ _____

13. Applied sterile gloves.   ___ ___ ___ _____

	S	U	NP	Comments
14. Organized supplies on sterile field.	___	___	___	_____
15. Checked integrity of inflatable balloon of indwelling catheter.	___	___	___	_____
16. Applied sterile drape over client.	___	___	___	_____
17. Placed sterile tray in easily accessible place.	___	___	___	_____
18. Applied lubricant to catheter tip.	___	___	___	_____
19. Cleansed urethral meatus correctly.	___	___	___	_____
20. Handled catheter properly.	___	___	___	_____
21. Inserted catheter correctly.	___	___	___	_____
22. Collected urine specimen if needed.	___	___	___	_____
23. Allowed bladder to empty fully.	___	___	___	_____
24. If using straight single-use catheter, withdrew it slowly and smoothly.	___	___	___	_____
25. If using indwelling catheter, inflated balloon correctly.	___	___	___	_____
26. Attached end of catheter to collecting tube.	___	___	___	_____
27. Taped catheter or applied Velcro tube holder.	___	___	___	_____
28. Maintained patent tubing.	___	___	___	_____
29. Assisted client to comfortable position. Washed and dried perineal area as needed.	___	___	___	_____
30. Removed gloves and disposed of equipment properly.	___	___	___	_____
31. Instructed client on proper positions.	___	___	___	_____
32. Cautioned client against pulling catheter.	___	___	___	_____
33. Washed hands.	___	___	___	_____

EVALUATION

1. Palpated client's bladder.	___	___	___	_____
2. Assessed client's comfort.	___	___	___	_____
3. Observed character and amount of urine.	___	___	___	_____
4. Determined that no urine was leaking from catheter or tubing.	___	___	___	_____
5. Identified unexpected outcomes.	___	___	___	_____

RECORDING AND REPORTING

| 1. Reported and recorded pertinent data: catheter description, assessment of urine, client's response to procedure. | ___ | ___ | ___ | _____ |
| 2. Initiated I&O records. | ___ | ___ | ___ | _____ |

Student _____   Date _____

Instructor _____   Date _____

PERFORMANCE CHECKLIST 25-4 **CARE OF THE INDWELLING CATHETER**

	S	U	NP	Comments
ASSESSMENT				
1. Determined how long catheter was in place.	—	—	—	_____
2. Observed for presence of discharge or encrustations.	—	—	—	_____
3. Assessed complaints of pain or discomfort.	—	—	—	_____
4. Monitored client's temperature.	—	—	—	_____
5. Determined client's fluid intake.	—	—	—	_____
6. Assessed urine color, odor, and amount.	—	—	—	_____
7. Assessed client's knowledge of procedure.	—	—	—	_____
NURSING DIAGNOSIS				
1. Developed appropriate nursing diagnoses based on assessment data.	—	—	—	_____
PLANNING				
1. Developed individualized goals for client based on nursing diagnoses.	—	—	—	_____
2. Identified expected outcomes.	—	—	—	_____
3. Explained procedure to client.	—	—	—	_____
4. Identified need for care more than every 8 hours.	—	—	—	_____
IMPLEMENTATION				
1. Washed hands.	—	—	—	_____
2. Provided privacy.	—	—	—	_____
3. Raised bed to appropriate height.	—	—	—	_____
4. Organized equipment.	—	—	—	_____
5. Positioned client correctly.	—	—	—	_____
6. Placed pad under client.	—	—	—	_____
7. Draped client.	—	—	—	_____
8. Provided perineal care (Skill 6-2).	—	—	—	_____
9. Assessed urethral meatus and surrounding tissues.	—	—	—	_____
10. Cleansed approximately 10 cm (4 in) length of catheter.	—	—	—	_____

	S	U	NP	Comments
11. Replaced adhesive tape if needed.	—	—	—	_____
12. Replaced urinary tubing and collection bag if needed.	—	—	—	_____
13. Maintained proper position of drainage tubing.	—	—	—	_____
14. Emptied collection bag as necessary.	—	—	—	_____
15. Assisted client to comfortable position.	—	—	—	_____
16. Lowered bed to lowest position.	—	—	—	_____
17. Disposed of contaminated gloves and supplies; washed hands.	—	—	—	_____

EVALUATION

	S	U	NP	Comments
1. Inspected urethra and surrounding tissue.	—	—	—	_____
2. Noted character of urine.	—	—	—	_____
3. Assessed client's temperature.	—	—	—	_____
4. Identified unexpected outcomes.	—	—	—	_____

RECORDING AND REPORTING

	S	U	NP	Comments
1. Recorded in nurses' notes when care was given and assessment of urethral meatus and urine.	—	—	—	_____
2. Reported pertinent data to appropriate health care team member(s).	—	—	—	_____

Student _____   Date _____

Instructor _____   Date _____

PERFORMANCE CHECKLIST 25-5 **OBTAINING CATHETERIZED SPECIMENS FOR RESIDUAL URINE**

	S	U	NP	Comments
ASSESSMENT				
1. Reviewed prior I&O record.	——	——	——	————————
2. Determined if client had pain or discomfort when voiding.	——	——	——	————————
3. Reviewed physician's order.	——	——	——	————————
4. Checked time of last voiding before catheterization.	——	——	——	————————
5. Assessed client's knowledge of procedure.	——	——	——	————————
NURSING DIAGNOSIS				
1. Developed appropriate nursing diagnoses based on assessment data.	——	——	——	————————
PLANNING				
1. Developed individualized goals for client based on nursing diagnoses.	——	——	——	————————
2. Identified expected outcomes.	——	——	——	————————
3. Explained procedure to client.	——	——	——	————————
IMPLEMENTATION				
1. Measured volume of urine voided.	——	——	——	————————
2. Washed hands.	——	——	——	————————
3. Catheterized client.	——	——	——	————————
4. Measured urine obtained.	——	——	——	————————
EVALUATION				
1. Compared amount of urine client voided and amount obtained on catheterization.	——	——	——	————————
2. Identified unexpected outcomes.	——	——	——	————————
RECORDING AND REPORTING				
1. Documented procedure in nurses' notes.	——	——	——	————————
2. Reported presence of unexpected outcomes.	——	——	——	————————

Student _____   Date _____

Instructor _____   Date _____

PERFORMANCE CHECKLIST 25-6   **PERFORMING CATHETER IRRIGATION**

	S	U	NP	Comments
ASSESSMENT				
1. Reviewed client's medical record.	—	—	—	
2. Assessed characteristics of urine, patency of tubing, and status of existing closed system.	—	—	—	
3. Reviewed I&O record.	—	—	—	
4. Assessed client for presence of bladder spasms and discomfort.	—	—	—	
5. Assessed client's knowledge of procedure.	—	—	—	
NURSING DIAGNOSIS				
1. Developed appropriate nursing diagnoses based on assessment data.	—	—	—	
PLANNING				
1. Developed individualized goals for client based on nursing diagnoses.	—	—	—	
2. Identified expected outcomes.	—	—	—	
3. Explained procedure to client.	—	—	—	
4. Warmed irrigant to room temperature. (Normal saline most commonly used irrigant.)	—	—	—	
IMPLEMENTATION				
1. Washed hands and applied gloves.	—	—	—	
2. Provided privacy.	—	—	—	
3. Positioned client correctly and removed tape or Velcro tube holder.	—	—	—	
4. Assessed lower abdomen for signs of bladder distention.	—	—	—	
5. Performed intermittent irrigations (closed system).	—	—	—	
6. Irrigated bladder continuously (closed system).	—	—	—	
7. Irrigated bladder (open system).	—	—	—	
8. Reanchored catheter to client.	—	—	—	
9. Assisted client to comfortable position.	—	—	—	
10. Lowered bed and side rails if appropriate.	—	—	—	
11. Disposed of contaminated supplies and gloves. Washed hands.	—	—	—	

	S	U	NP	Comments

EVALUATION

1. Accurately calculated the difference between the amount of irrigating solution instilled and the amount of drainage returned.   ___ ___ ___ _____

2. Assessed characteristics of output and urine.   ___ ___ ___ _____

3. Observed patency of catheter.   ___ ___ ___ _____

4. Identified expected outcomes.   ___ ___ ___ _____

RECORDING AND REPORTING

1. Recorded amount of solution used to irrigate and amount and consistency of drainage returned.   ___ ___ ___ _____

2. Reported occlusion, sudden bleeding, infection, or pain to physician.   ___ ___ ___ _____

Student _____   Date _____

Instructor _____   Date _____

PERFORMANCE CHECKLIST 25-7   **REMOVING A RETENTION CATHETER**

	S	U	NP	Comments

ASSESSMENT

1. Reviewed client's medical record.

2. Noted period of time catheter was in place.

3. Assessed client's knowledge of procedure.

NURSING DIAGNOSIS

1. Developed appropriate nursing diagnoses based on assessment data.

PLANNING

1. Developed individualized goals for client based on nursing diagnoses.

2. Identified expected outcomes.

3. Explained procedure to client.

4. Obtained urine hat for toilet to continue measuring I&O, if client is ambulatory.

IMPLEMENTATION

1. Washed hands and applied gloves.

2. Maintained client's privacy.

3. Raised bed and side rails to correct height.

4. Positioned client.

5. Placed waterproof pad correctly.

6. Obtained sterile urine specimen as required.

7. Removed tape or Velcro tube holder.

8. Aspirated fluid used to inflate catheter balloon.

9. Removed catheter.

10. Unhooked bag and tubing from bed.

11. Positioned client.

12. Measured contents and emptied collection bag.

13. Disposed of contaminated supplies; washed hands.

14. Repeated procedures for catheter insertion if necessary.

	S	U	NP	Comments

EVALUATION

1. Noted the time and amount of first-voided urine.   ___ ___ ___ _____

2. Noted any discomfort experienced by client.   ___ ___ ___ _____

3. Noted condition of skin.   ___ ___ ___ _____

4. Identified unexpected outcomes.   ___ ___ ___ _____

RECORDING AND REPORTING

1. Reported and recorded pertinent data to appropriate health care team member(s).   ___ ___ ___ _____

2. Recorded presence of unexpected outcomes.   ___ ___ ___ _____

3. Continued to monitor I&O as necessary.   ___ ___ ___ _____

Student _____ Date _____

Instructor _____ Date _____

PERFORMANCE CHECKLIST 25-8 **APPLYING A CONDOM CATHETER**

	S	U	NP	Comments

ASSESSMENT

1. Determined need for application of condom based on status of client.

2. Assessed client's mental status.

3. Assessed condition of penis.

4. Assessed client's knowledge of purpose of condom catheter.

NURSING DIAGNOSIS

1. Developed appropriate nursing diagnoses based on assessment data.

PLANNING

1. Developed individualized goals for client based on nursing diagnoses.

2. Identified expected outcomes.

3. Explained procedure.

4. Arranged for assistance as required.

5. Read instructions specific to condom catheter kit.

IMPLEMENTATION

1. Washed hands.

2. Provided privacy.

3. Raised bed to working height. Lowered appropriate side rail.

4. Positioned client correctly.

5. Prepared urinary drainage collection bag and tubing.

6. Put on disposable gloves and provided perineal care.

7. Clipped hair at base of penis.

8. Applied skin preparation to penis and allowed to dry.

9. Put condom on client's penis.

10. Allowed space between glans and end of condom catheter.

	S	U	NP	Comments
11. Attached Velcro or elastic to condom.	—	—	—	_____
12. Connected tubing to end of condom.	—	—	—	_____
13. Secured excess tubing.	—	—	—	_____
14. Positioned client comfortably.	—	—	—	_____
15. Raised side rail and lowered bed.	—	—	—	_____
16. Disposed of contaminated supplies and gloves. Washed hands.	—	—	—	_____

EVALUATION

	S	U	NP	Comments
1. Observed urinary drainage.	—	—	—	_____
2. Inspected penis within 30 minutes after application.	—	—	—	_____
3. Routinely assessed skin on penis and color of glans penis while condom is removed.	—	—	—	_____
4. Identified unexpected outcomes.	—	—	—	_____

RECORDING AND REPORTING

	S	U	NP	Comments
1. Recorded and reported pertinent information related to procedure.	—	—	—	_____
2. Monitored I&O as indicated.	—	—	—	_____

Student _____   Date _____

Instructor _____   Date _____

PERFORMANCE CHECKLIST 25-9   CARE OF A SUPRAPUBIC CATHETER

	S	U	NP	Comments

ASSESSMENT

1. Assessed urine in bag for amount and characteristics. — — — _____

2. Assessed dressing for drainage and intactness. — — — _____

3. Assessed catheter insertion site for signs of inflammation. Asked client if there is pain at the site. — — — _____

4. Assessed how catheter is held in place. — — — _____

5. Assessed tape site for signs of irritation. — — — _____

6. Assessed for fever. — — — _____

7. Checked for allergies. — — — _____

NURSING DIAGNOSIS

1. Developed appropriate nursing diagnoses based on assessment data. — — — _____

PLANNING

1. Developed individualized goals based on nursing diagnoses. — — — _____

2. Identified expected outcomes. — — — _____

3. Explained procedure to client. — — — _____

IMPLEMENTATION

1. Washed hands. — — — _____

2. Provided privacy. — — — _____

3. Proceeded with application of a dry sterile dressing (see Skill 38-1). — — — _____

4. Cleansed site around drain. — — — _____

5. Applied split gauze around catheter with dominant sterile gloved hand, and applied tape. — — — _____

6. Secured catheter to abdomen with tape or Velcro tube holder. — — — _____

7. Checked bag and tubing placement. — — — _____

EVALUATION

1. Asked client if there is pain or discomfort from suprapubic catheter. — — — _____

2. Observed client's urine for sediment, odor, or discoloration. — — — _____

	S	U	NP	Comments
3. Inspected dressing at least every shift.	—	—	—	_____
4. Monitored for signs of infection.	—	—	—	_____
5. Identified unexpected outcomes.	—	—	—	_____

RECORDING AND REPORTING

1. Reported and recorded dressing replacement, assessment of wound, and client's tolerance of procedure.	—	—	—	_____
2. Reported presence of unexpected outcomes.	—	—	—	_____

Student _____   Date _____

Instructor _____   Date _____

PERFORMANCE CHECKLIST 25-10 **PERITONEAL DIALYSIS AND CONTINUOUS AMBULATORY PERITONEAL DIALYSIS**

	S	U	NP	Comments
ASSESSMENT				
1. Obtained client's weight.	___	___	___	_____
2. Obtained client's vital signs.	___	___	___	_____
3. Assessed respiratory status.	___	___	___	_____
4. Measured abdominal girth.	___	___	___	_____
5. Monitored for fluid and electrolyte balance.	___	___	___	_____
6. Inspected catheter site.	___	___	___	_____
7. Measured body temperature.	___	___	___	_____
8. Reviewed agency's procedure for peritoneal dialysis (PD) or continuous ambulatory peritoneal dialysis (CAPD).	___	___	___	_____
9. Reviewed physician's orders.	___	___	___	_____
10. Obtained laboratory data as ordered.	___	___	___	_____
11. Assessed client's knowledge of procedure.	___	___	___	_____
NURSING DIAGNOSIS				
1. Developed appropriate diagnoses based on assessment data.	___	___	___	_____
PLANNING				
1. Developed individualized goals for client based on nursing diagnoses.	___	___	___	_____
2. Identified expected outcomes.	___	___	___	_____
3. Explained procedure to client.	___	___	___	_____
IMPLEMENTATION				
Initiating Manual Dialysis Exchanges				
1. Washed hands. Donned mask (nurse and client).	___	___	___	_____
2. Positioned client.	___	___	___	_____
3. Determined that all clamps on tubings were in "off" positions.	___	___	___	_____
4. Added medications as listed in physician's order.	___	___	___	_____
5. Attached two warmed dialysate bags to inflow tubing and attached to IV pole.	___	___	___	_____
6. Primed inflow tubing correctly and flushed tubing.	___	___	___	_____
7. Instilled dialysate bag #1 over prescribed time.	___	___	___	_____
8. Clamped inflow tubing for prescribed dwell time.	___	___	___	_____

	S	U	NP	Comments

9. Removed dialysate bag #1 from IV pole and placed warmed bag #3 on pole. ___ ___ ___ _____

10. Unclamped outflow tubing and allowed to drain. ___ ___ ___ _____

11. Clamped outflow tubing. ___ ___ ___ _____

12. Emptied and measured fluid in drainage bag. ___ ___ ___ _____

13. Repeated Steps 3-10 until all exchanges completed. ___ ___ ___ _____

14. Monitored client's vital signs every 15 minutes during first exchange. ___ ___ ___ _____

15. Covered catheter with sterile cap or followed guidelines specific to catheter when exchanges completed. ___ ___ ___ _____

16. Inspected catheter dressing. Reapplied transparent occlusive dressing, if indicated. ___ ___ ___ _____

17. Disposed of contaminated supplies properly and washed hands. ___ ___ ___ _____

EVALUATION

1. Obtained weight. ___ ___ ___ _____

2. Obtained dialysis fluid balance. ___ ___ ___ _____

3. Obtained vital signs, including body temperature. ___ ___ ___ _____

4. Auscultated lungs. ___ ___ ___ _____

5. Measured abdominal girth. ___ ___ ___ _____

6. Inspected catheter site. ___ ___ ___ _____

7. Inspected returned dialysate solution. ___ ___ ___ _____

8. Observed client performing CAPD. ___ ___ ___ _____

9. Assessed client's comfort level. ___ ___ ___ _____

10. Monitored lab work. ___ ___ ___ _____

11. Identified unexpected outcomes. ___ ___ ___ _____

RECORDING AND REPORTING

1. Documented client's weight, abdominal girth, dialysis fluid balance before and after PD. ___ ___ ___ _____

2. Documented client's vital signs before, during, and after dialysis. ___ ___ ___ _____

3. Documented temperature and status of catheter site. ___ ___ ___ _____

4. Recorded presence of pain or discomfort. ___ ___ ___ _____

5. Recorded color of drainage. ___ ___ ___ _____

6. Recorded condition of catheter dressing. ___ ___ ___ _____

7. Noted any unexpected outcomes and action taken by nurse and physician. ___ ___ ___ _____

Student _____ Date _____

Instructor _____ Date _____

PERFORMANCE CHECKLIST 26-1 **ASSISTING THE CLIENT TO USE A BEDPAN**

	S	U	NP	Comments
ASSESSMENT				
1. Assessed client's normal bowel elimination habits.	——	——	——	_____
2. Auscultated and palpated abdomen.	——	——	——	_____
3. Assessed client's mobility status.	——	——	——	_____
4. Determined appropriate type of bedpan to use.	——	——	——	_____
5. Assessed for rectal or abdominal pain and irritation of skin surrounding anus.	——	——	——	_____
6. Determined if stool specimen needed.	——	——	——	_____
NURSING DIAGNOSIS				
1. Developed appropriate nursing diagnoses based on assessment data.	——	——	——	_____
PLANNING				
1. Developed individualized goals for client based on nursing diagnoses.	——	——	——	_____
2. Identified expected outcomes.	——	——	——	_____
3. Explained procedure to client.	——	——	——	_____
4. If appropriate, obtained assistance from additional nursing personnel.	——	——	——	_____
IMPLEMENTATION				
1. Washed hands and applied gloves.	——	——	——	_____
2. Provided privacy.	——	——	——	_____
3. Warmed bedpan before use.	——	——	——	_____
4. Put opposite side rail up.	——	——	——	_____
5. Positioned bed at appropriate working height.	——	——	——	_____
6. Ensured that client was positioned properly.	——	——	——	_____
Mobile Client				
a. Raised client's head 60 degrees.	——	——	——	_____
b. Removed upper bed linen.	——	——	——	_____
c. Removed bedpan cover and placed bedpan in accessible location.	——	——	——	_____
d. Instructed client to flex knees and lift hips.	——	——	——	_____
e. Correctly assisted client onto bedpan.	——	——	——	_____

	S	U	NP	Comments

Immobile Client

a. Positioned bed flat or level. ___ ___ ___ _____

b. Removed upper bed linen. ___ ___ ___ _____

c. Correctly assisted client onto bedpan. ___ ___ ___ _____

d. Raised client's head 30 degrees (unless contra-indicated). ___ ___ ___ _____

7. Ensured client's comfort. ___ ___ ___ _____

8. Placed call bell and toilet tissue within client's reach. ___ ___ ___ _____

9. Ensured that bed was in lowest position with side rails up. ___ ___ ___ _____

10. Allowed client to be alone, but monitored status. ___ ___ ___ _____

11. Removed gloves and washed hands. ___ ___ ___ _____

12. Responded to client's call bell immediately. ___ ___ ___ _____

13. Positioned client's bedside chair near working side of bed for placement of bedpan. ___ ___ ___ _____

14. Collected basin of warm water. ___ ___ ___ _____

15. Removed upper linens. ___ ___ ___ _____

16. Determined if client was able to wipe perineal area. ___ ___ ___ _____

17. Removed bedpan. ___ ___ ___ _____

For Mobile Client

a. Correctly removed bedpan. ___ ___ ___ _____

b. Offered client opportunity to wash hands. ___ ___ ___ _____

For Immobile Client

a. Lowered head of bed. ___ ___ ___ _____

b. Assisted client off bedpan. ___ ___ ___ _____

c. Wiped anal area. ___ ___ ___ _____

18. Covered bedpan. ___ ___ ___ _____

19. Returned client to comfortable position. ___ ___ ___ _____

20. Positioned bed in lowest position and returned client's environment to former status. ___ ___ ___ _____

21. Wearing gloves, emptied contents of bedpan and rinsed it. Obtained stool specimen, if indicated. ___ ___ ___ _____

22. Replaced all used equipment. ___ ___ ___ _____

23. Disposed of soiled linens. ___ ___ ___ _____

24. Removed gloves and washed hands. ___ ___ ___ _____

Student _____   Date _____

Instructor _____   Date _____

	S	U	NP	Comments

EVALUATION

1. Assessed characteristics of urine and stool. ___ ___ ___ _____

2. Evaluated client's ability to use bedpan. ___ ___ ___ _____

3. Inspected condition of client's skin. ___ ___ ___ _____

4. Evaluated client's overall state of well-being. ___ ___ ___ _____

5. Identified unexpected outcomes. ___ ___ ___ _____

RECORDING AND REPORTING

1. Documented character of stool and urinary output
   if client also voids. ___ ___ ___ _____

2. Completed laboratory requisition for stool or
   urine specimen. ___ ___ ___ _____

Student _____   Date _____

Instructor _____   Date _____

PERFORMANCE CHECKLIST 26-2 **INSERTING A RECTAL TUBE**

	S	U	NP	Comments
ASSESSMENT				
1. Assessed client's status.	—	—	—	_____
2. Checked physician's order for specific instructions.	—	—	—	_____
NURSING DIAGNOSIS				
1. Developed appropriate nursing diagnoses based on assessment data.	—	—	—	_____
PLANNING				
1. Developed individualized goals for client based on nursing diagnoses.	—	—	—	_____
2. Identified expected outcomes.	—	—	—	_____
3. Explained procedure to client.	—	—	—	_____
IMPLEMENTATION				
1. Washed hands and applied gloves.	—	—	—	_____
2. Provided privacy.	—	—	—	_____
3. Raised bed to working height with opposite side rail up.	—	—	—	_____
4. Positioned client correctly.	—	—	—	_____
5. Placed waterproof pad along buttocks.	—	—	—	_____
6. Lubricated tip of rectal tube.	—	—	—	_____
7. Prepared client for insertion of tube.	—	—	—	_____
8. Inserted rectal tube slowly.	—	—	—	_____
9. Taped rectal tube to lower buttock.	—	—	—	_____
10. Left tube in place for appropriate time, lowered bed, and placed call bell within client's reach.	—	—	—	_____
11. Removed gloves and washed hands after leaving bedside.	—	—	—	_____
12. Applied gloves and removed rectal tube, cleaned client's rectal area, and assessed characteristics of drainage.	—	—	—	_____
13. Returned client to comfortable position.	—	—	—	_____
14. Disposed of used supplies.	—	—	—	_____
15. Removed gloves and washed hands.	—	—	—	_____

	S	U	NP	Comments

EVALUATION

1. Assessed client's abdomen for firmness and distention. Auscultated bowel sounds. __ __ __ _____

2. Determined client's response to procedure. __ __ __ _____

3. Identified unexpected outcomes. __ __ __ _____

RECORDING AND REPORTING

1. Documented pertinent information. __ __ __ _____

Student _____   Date _____

Instructor _____   Date _____

PERFORMANCE CHECKLIST 26-3   **REMOVING FECAL IMPACTION DIGITALLY**

	S	U	NP	Comments

ASSESSMENT

1. Assessed client's elimination status.   ___ ___ ___ _____

2. Checked client's record for physician's order.   ___ ___ ___ _____

NURSING DIAGNOSIS

1. Developed appropriate nursing diagnoses based on assessment data.   ___ ___ ___ _____

PLANNING

1. Developed individualized goals for client based on nursing diagnoses.   ___ ___ ___ _____

2. Identified expected outcomes.   ___ ___ ___ _____

3. Explained procedure to client.   ___ ___ ___ _____

IMPLEMENTATION

1. Washed hands and applied gloves.   ___ ___ ___ _____

2. Obtained assistance to position client, if needed.   ___ ___ ___ _____

3. Provided privacy.   ___ ___ ___ _____

4. Raised bed to working height with opposite rail up.   ___ ___ ___ _____

5. Draped client.   ___ ___ ___ _____

6. Placed waterproof pad under client's buttocks.   ___ ___ ___ _____

7. Placed bedpan next to client.   ___ ___ ___ _____

8. Lubricated index finger of glove.   ___ ___ ___ _____

9. Inserted index finger into rectum.   ___ ___ ___ _____

10. Gently loosened fecal mass.   ___ ___ ___ _____

11. Moved mass toward end of rectum.   ___ ___ ___ _____

12. Checked client's heart rate and looked for signs of fatigue.   ___ ___ ___ _____

13. Allowed client to rest at intervals during procedure.   ___ ___ ___ _____

14. Washed anal area after disimpaction.   ___ ___ ___ _____

15. Removed bedpan and disposed of feces. Removed and disposed of gloves.   ___ ___ ___ _____

	S	U	NP	Comments
16. Assisted client to toilet or to use a clean bedpan.	——	——	——	_____
17. Washed hands.	——	——	——	_____

EVALUATION

	S	U	NP	Comments
1. Performed rectal examination.	——	——	——	_____
2. Reassessed vital signs and compared to baseline values.	——	——	——	_____
3. Assessed bowel sounds.	——	——	——	_____
4. Assessed for soft and nontender abdomen.	——	——	——	_____
5. Identified unexpected outcomes.	——	——	——	_____

RECORDING AND REPORTING

	S	U	NP	Comments
1. Documented and reported client's tolerance, amount and consistency of stool, and any adverse effects.	——	——	——	_____

Student _____ Date _____

Instructor _____ Date _____

PERFORMANCE CHECKLIST 26-4 **ADMINISTERING AN ENEMA**

	S	U	NP	Comments
ASSESSMENT				
1. Assessed client's status.	—	—	—	_____
2. Determined client's understanding of procedure.	—	—	—	_____
3. Checked client's medical record.	—	—	—	_____
4. Reviewed physician's order.	—	—	—	_____
NURSING DIAGNOSIS				
1. Developed appropriate nursing diagnoses based on assessment data.	—	—	—	_____
PLANNING				
1. Developed individualized goals for client based on nursing diagnoses.	—	—	—	_____
2. Identified expected outcomes.	—	—	—	_____
3. Explained procedure to client.	—	—	—	_____
IMPLEMENTATION				
1. Washed hands and applied gloves.	—	—	—	_____
2. Provided privacy.	—	—	—	_____
3. Raised bed to working height with opposite side rail up.	—	—	—	_____
4. Positioned client correctly.	—	—	—	_____
5. Placed waterproof pad under hips and buttocks.	—	—	—	_____
6. Draped client.	—	—	—	_____
7. Placed bedpan within easy reach.	—	—	—	_____
8. Administered enema using prepackaged disposable container. Removed plastic cap from rectal tip and lubricated if needed, prepared client for insertion of tip, inserted tip, and squeezed out all solution.	—	—	—	_____
9. Administered enema using enema bag: prepared solution, bag, and tubing. Reclamped tubing, lubricated tip of rectal tube, prepared client for insertion of tube, and inserted tip. Held tubing until end of fluid instillation, opened regulating clamp and allowed solution to enter slowly, raised height of enema container to allow for continuous slow infusion. Lowered container if client complained of cramping, and clamped tubing after all solution was infused.	—	—	—	_____

	S	U	NP	Comments
10. Correctly removed tube.	___	___	___	_____
11. Reassured client that distention is normal and instructed client to retain fluid.	___	___	___	_____
12. Discarded enema container and tubing.	___	___	___	_____
13. Assisted client to bathroom or positioned on bedpan.	___	___	___	_____
14. Observed character of feces and solution.	___	___	___	_____
15. Assisted client to wash anal area.	___	___	___	_____
16. Removed and discarded gloves. Washed hands.	___	___	___	_____

EVALUATION

1. Inspected character of stool and fluid.	___	___	___	_____
2. Assessed condition of abdomen.	___	___	___	_____
3. Identified unexpected outcomes.	___	___	___	_____

RECORDING AND REPORTING

1. Recorded pertinent information.	___	___	___	_____
2. Reported failure of client to defecate.	___	___	___	_____

Student _____ Date _____

Instructor _____ Date _____

PERFORMANCE CHECKLIST 27-1 **POUCHING AN ENTEROSTOMY**

	S	U	NP	Comments

ASSESSMENT

1. Auscultated for bowel sounds.

2. Observed skin barrier and pouch for leakage and length of time in place.

3. Observed stoma for color and condition.

4. Observed abdominal incision for pouch placement.

5. Observed drainage from stoma; kept I&O.

6. Checked for skin irritation.

7. Avoided unnecessary changing of pouch.

8. Assessed abdomen, client's overall condition, and stoma type for best pouching system to use.

9. Assessed skin around stoma after pouch is removed.

10. Determined client's knowledge of ostomy and emotional response.

NURSING DIAGNOSIS

1. Developed appropriate nursing diagnoses based on assessment data.

PLANNING

1. Developed individualized goals for client based on nursing diagnoses.

2. Identified expected outcomes.

3. Explained steps of procedure to client.

4. Assembled equipment and provided privacy.

IMPLEMENTATION

1. Positioned client correctly.

2. Washed hands and applied gloves.

3. Placed towel or barrier under client.

4. Removed used pouch.

5. Cleansed peristomal skin, patted dry, and measured stoma.

	S	U	NP	Comments
6. Selected and prepared pouch by removing backing from barrier and adhesive.	___	___	___	_____
7. Correctly applied pouch.	___	___	___	_____
8. Applied nonallergic tape to skin barrier.	___	___	___	_____
9. Added ostomy deodorant, if desired.	___	___	___	_____
10. Secured clamp to pouch.	___	___	___	_____
11. Properly disposed of old pouch and soiled equipment.	___	___	___	_____
12. Removed gloves and washed hands.	___	___	___	_____
13. Changed pouch every 3 to 7 days unless leaking.	___	___	___	_____

EVALUATION

	S	U	NP	Comments
1. Assessed appearance of stoma, skin, and incision. Inspected pouch and skin barrier.	___	___	___	_____
2. Auscultated bowel sounds and observed character of stool.	___	___	___	_____
3. Assessed client's comfort level.	___	___	___	_____
4. Observed client's nonverbal behavior and asked if client had any questions about pouching.	___	___	___	_____
5. Identified unexpected outcomes.	___	___	___	_____

RECORDING AND REPORTING

	S	U	NP	Comments
1. Charted in nurses' notes pouching procedure and equipment used.	___	___	___	_____
2. Recorded character of effluent and appearance of stoma and skin.	___	___	___	_____
3. Reported abnormal appearance of stoma or suture line or unusual character of effluent.	___	___	___	_____
4. Reported absence of flatus for 24 to 36 hours or no stool by third day.	___	___	___	_____

Student _____   Date _____

Instructor _____   Date _____

PERFORMANCE CHECKLIST 27-2 **IRRIGATING A COLOSTOMY**

	S	U	NP	Comments

ASSESSMENT

1. Assessed frequency and character of stool, placement of stoma, and nutritional pattern.

2. Assessed time when client normally irrigates colostomy. Conferred with physician about order to irrigate new ostomy.

3. Reviewed procedural orders requiring bowel preparation.

4. Assessed client's understanding and ability to perform irrigation.

NURSING DIAGNOSIS

1. Developed appropriate nursing diagnoses based on assessment data.

PLANNING

1. Developed individualized goals for client based on nursing diagnoses.

2. Identified expected outcomes.

3. Explained procedure to client.

4. Assembled equipment and provided privacy.

IMPLEMENTATION

1. Positioned client correctly.

2. Applied gloves.

3. Filled irrigation bag with proper amount of fluid. Hung on hook at appropriate height.

4. Removed old pouch. Removed gloves and washed hands.

5. Correctly applied irrigation sleeve.

6. Applied gloves, lubricated cone tip, and held against stomal opening. Initiated flow of water.

7. Allowed water to flow in over 5-10 minutes. Clamped tubing.

8. After desired amount of water instilled, removed cone after waiting 15 seconds. Discarded gloves.

	S	U	NP	Comments

9. Allowed 15-20 minutes for initial evacuation. Applied gloves. Dried tip of sleeve and clamped bottom. Folded sleeve, discarded gloves, and allowed client to ambulate.   ___ ___ ___ _____

10. Applied gloves; unclamped sleeve, emptied contents; removed sleeve. Rinsed sleeve, hung sleeve to dry.   ___ ___ ___ _____

11. Applied new pouch or stoma covering.   ___ ___ ___ _____

12. Removed gloves and washed hands.   ___ ___ ___ _____

EVALUATION

1. Inspected volume and character of fecal material and fluid.   ___ ___ ___ _____

2. Noted client's response during irrigation.   ___ ___ ___ _____

3. Asked client to describe steps of procedure.   ___ ___ ___ _____

4. Identified unexpected outcomes.   ___ ___ ___ _____

RECORDING AND REPORTING

1. Recorded procedure, volume and type of solution administered, fluid returned, and client's tolerance in nurses' notes.   ___ ___ ___ _____

2. Recorded reapplication of pouch.   ___ ___ ___ _____

3. Reported any complications to nurse in charge or physician.   ___ ___ ___ _____

Student _____   Date _____

Instructor _____   Date _____

PERFORMANCE CHECKLIST 27-3 **POUCHING A NONCONTINENT URINARY DIVERSION**

	S	U	NP	Comments

ASSESSMENT

1. Assessed pouch and condition of skin to determine need to change pouch.

2. Observed output from stoma, stents, or catheters.

3. Assessed abdomen for best type of pouch to use.

4. Assessed bowel sounds.

5. Determined client's knowledge of ostomy, and emotional response.

NURSING DIAGNOSIS

1. Developed appropriate nursing diagnoses based on assessment data.

PLANNING

1. Developed individualized goals for client based on nursing diagnoses.

2. Identified expected outcomes.

3. Assembled equipment.

4. Closed door or curtain.

5. Explained steps of procedure to client and encouraged participation.

IMPLEMENTATION

1. Positioned client correctly.

2. Prepared pouch.

3. Washed hands and applied gloves.

4. Placed towel or barrier under client. Placed wick or gauze pad over stoma.

5. Removed old pouch.

6. Cleansed peristomal skin, patted dry.

7. Wicked stoma. Measured stoma. Applied pouch.

8. Opened drain spout and attached to urinary bag. Placed bag at foot of bed.

9. Properly disposed of used pouch and soiled equipment.

	S	U	NP	Comments
10. Removed gloves, washed hands.	——	——	——	_____
11. Changed pouch every 3 to 7 days unless leaking.	——	——	——	_____

EVALUATION

	S	U	NP	Comments
1. Noted condition of stoma, skin, and suture line. Evaluated character and volume of urine.	——	——	——	_____
2. Assessed for discomfort around stoma.	——	——	——	_____
3. Noted client's and/or significant other's willingness to view stoma and ask questions.	——	——	——	_____
4. Identified unexpected outcomes.	——	——	——	_____

RECORDING AND REPORTING

	S	U	NP	Comments
1. Recorded type of pouch, time of change, appearance of stoma and skin, and character of urine in nurses' notes.	——	——	——	_____
2. Recorded urinary output on I&O flowsheet.	——	——	——	_____
3. Noted client's or significant other's reaction to procedure in nurses' notes.	——	——	——	_____
4. Reported any abnormalities to nurse in charge or physician.	——	——	——	_____

Student _____   Date _____

Instructor _____   Date _____

PERFORMANCE CHECKLIST 27-4 CATHETERIZING A NONCONTINENT URINARY DIVERSION

	S	U	NP	Comments

ASSESSMENT

1. Determined need to obtain urine specimen.

2. Obtained physician's order.

3. Assessed client's understanding of procedure.

NURSING DIAGNOSIS

1. Developed appropriate nursing diagnoses based on assessment data.

PLANNING

1. Developed individualized goals for client based on nursing diagnoses.

2. Identified expected outcomes.

3. Assembled equipment.

4. Provided for client's privacy.

5. Explained procedure to client and timed procedure in accordance with pouch change.

IMPLEMENTATION

1. Positioned client correctly.

2. Washed hands and opened barrier. Prepared gauze wicks. Applied nonsterile gloves.

3. Removed old pouch according to Skill 27-3.

4. Removed and discarded gloves. Opened sterile catheterization set or needed equipment. Had client wick stoma while waiting, if possible.

5. Applied sterile gloves. Cleansed "face" of stoma with povidone-iodine swabs.

6. Allowed small amount of urine to flow from stoma.

7. Lubricated catheter with lubricant.

8. Placed distal end of catheter in specimen container.

9. Using dominant hand, gently inserted into stoma; instructed client to cough or turn slightly.

10. Placed specimen container below level of stoma to collect urinary drainage.

	S	U	NP	Comments
11. Withdrew catheter and placed 4 × 4 gauze pad over stoma.	—	—	—	_____
12. Secured specimen container and labeled specimen.	—	—	—	_____
13. Reapplied new pouch.	—	—	—	_____
14. Disposed of soiled pouch and equipment.	—	—	—	_____
15. Removed gloves, washed hands, and sent specimen to laboratory.	—	—	—	_____

EVALUATION

	S	U	NP	Comments
1. Compared results of culture and sensitivity with normal expected findings.	—	—	—	_____
2. Observed stoma and peristomal area for breakdown.	—	—	—	_____
3. Checked urinary pouch and skin barrier for leakage.	—	—	—	_____
4. Asked client about signs and symptoms of UTI.	—	—	—	_____
5. Identified unexpected outcomes.	—	—	—	_____

RECORDING AND REPORTING

	S	U	NP	Comments
1. Recorded specimen collection, client's tolerance of procedure, and appearance of urine, skin, and stoma.	—	—	—	_____
2. Reported results of laboratory test to nurse in charge or physician.	—	—	—	_____

Student _____ Date _____

Instructor _____ Date _____

PERFORMANCE CHECKLIST 27-5 **MAINTAINING A CONTINENT DIVERSION**

	S	U	NP	Comments

ASSESSMENT

1. Observed all tubes for intactness and patency, nature of drainage, and connection to collection system. ___ ___ ___ _____

2. Observed condition of stoma, peristomal skin, and suture lines. ___ ___ ___ _____

3. Assessed bowel and lung sounds. Assessed serum chloride and creatinine values. ___ ___ ___ _____

4. Palpated lightly around stoma, noting any signs of infection. ___ ___ ___ _____

5. Determined client's emotional response, knowledge, and understanding of urinary reservoir. Assessed client's family and other support. ___ ___ ___ _____

NURSING DIAGNOSIS

1. Formulated appropriate nursing diagnoses based on assessment data. ___ ___ ___ _____

PLANNING

1. Developed individualized goals for client based on nursing diagnoses. ___ ___ ___ _____

2. Identified expected outcomes. ___ ___ ___ _____

3. Assembled equipment. ___ ___ ___ _____

4. Provided for client's privacy. ___ ___ ___ _____

5. Explained procedure to client and encouraged participation. ___ ___ ___ _____

IMPLEMENTATION
Postoperative Care to 3 Weeks

1. Positioned client correctly. ___ ___ ___ _____

2. Washed hands and opened sterile equipment. Correctly removed lid from sterile specimen cup. Poured 20-30 ml sterile saline into cup. Opened syringe and povidone-iodine swabs. ___ ___ ___ _____

3. Applied sterile gloves and drew 20-30 ml saline into syringe. Cleansed connected point of indwelling stomal catheter and drainage tubing with swabs. ___ ___ ___ _____

4. Disconnected and irrigated stomal catheter. ___ ___ ___ _____

5. Reconnected drainage system. Recorded I&O. Changed bedside drainage bags according to policy. ___ ___ ___ _____

6. Used remaining swabs to clean "face" of stoma and to cleanse area around base of stoma. Allowed to dry and removed iodine with sterile water. ___ ___ ___ _____

	S	U	NP	Comments

7. Discarded soiled equipment; removed gloves. Labeled sterile specimen cup correctly.

Postoperative Care of 4 to 6 Weeks

1. Followed steps 1 and 2 in preceding section. (Omitted setting up sterile cup.)

2. Observed aseptic technique while unwrapping supplies.

3. Applied sterile gloves and drew 30-60 ml sterile saline into syringe. Cleansed "face" of stoma with povidone-iodine swab.

4. Lubricated catheter. Correctly inserted into stoma until urine began to drain.

5. Irrigated pouch if needed.

6. Had client cough before removing catheter.

7. Cleansed peristomal area and patted dry.

8. Covered stoma with stomal covering.

9. Discarded soiled equipment; removed gloves. Maintained sterile saline, correctly labeled.

10. Recorded urinary output and amount used for irrigation.

EVALUATION

1. Noted appearance of stoma, peristomal skin, suture lines.

2. Evaluated character and volume of urinary output.

3. Palpated for discomfort over pouch site and peristomal skin.

4. Observed client's or caregiver's willingness to participate in care.

5. Identified unexpected outcomes.

RECORDING AND REPORTING

1. Recorded time of irrigation and intubation, size of catheter used, ease of intubation, amount of N/S used, amount and character of urinary output, and client's tolerance.

2. Documented client's, family's, and significant others' responses and their level of participation in care.

3. Reported abnormalities of stoma and peristomal skin.

Student _____   Date _____

Instructor _____   Date _____

PERFORMANCE CHECKLIST 28-1 **MAINTAINING BODY ALIGNMENT**

	S	U	NP	Comments
ASSESSMENT				
1. Observed alignment of client in standing, sitting, or lying position.	—	—	—	_____
NURSING DIAGNOSIS				
1. Developed appropriate diagnoses based on assessment data.	—	—	—	_____
PLANNING				
1. Developed individualized goals for client based on nursing diagnoses.	—	—	—	_____
2. Identified expected outcomes.	—	—	—	_____
3. Instructed client or family on proper body alignment.	—	—	—	_____
IMPLEMENTATION				
1. Demonstrated to client or family correct body alignment for standing, sitting, or lying.	—	—	—	_____
2. Provided opportunity of return demonstration.	—	—	—	_____
3. Discussed with client or family hazards of prolonged immobility on body alignment and mobility.	—	—	—	_____
4. Provided client or family with community resources.	—	—	—	_____
EVALUATION				
1. Inspected skin surfaces.	—	—	—	_____
2. Had client demonstrate body alignment for standing, sitting, and lying.	—	—	—	_____
3. Asked client to describe benefits of body alignment.	—	—	—	_____
4. Identified unexpected outcomes.	—	—	—	_____
RECORDING AND REPORTING				
1. Recorded information presented to client and client's progress.	—	—	—	_____
2. Reported information taught to client at change-of-shift.	—	—	—	_____

Student _____   Date _____

Instructor _____   Date _____

PERFORMANCE CHECKLIST 28-2 **PERFORMING SAFE AND EFFICIENT LIFTING TECHNIQUES**

	S	U	NP	Comments
ASSESSMENT				
1. Assessed position of weight to be lifted.	—	—	—	_____
2. Assessed height of object to be lifted.	—	—	—	_____
3. Evaluated lifter's body position.	—	—	—	_____
4. Knew maximal weight that could be safely lifted.	—	—	—	_____
NURSING DIAGNOSIS				
1. Developed appropriate nursing diagnoses based on assessment data.	—	—	—	_____
PLANNING				
1. Developed individualized goals for client based on nursing diagnoses.	—	—	—	_____
2. Identified expected outcomes.	—	—	—	_____
3. Prepared client when lifting involved transfer.	—	—	—	_____
4. Removed excess clutter when lifting object.	—	—	—	_____
IMPLEMENTATION				
1. Lifted correctly from below center of gravity.	—	—	—	_____
2. Lifted object correctly from above center of gravity.	—	—	—	_____
EVALUATION				
1. Assessed use of safe and efficient lifting techniques.	—	—	—	_____
2. Observed environment to ensure it is free of clutter.	—	—	—	_____
3. Identified unexpected outcomes.	—	—	—	_____
RECORDING AND REPORTING				
1. Recorded type of lifting techniques taught to client or family.	—	—	—	_____
2. Reported any lifting injuries.	—	—	—	_____

Student _____   Date _____

Instructor _____   Date _____

PERFORMANCE CHECKLIST 29-1   **USING SAFE AND EFFECTIVE TRANSFER TECHNIQUES**

	S	U	NP	Comments
ASSESSMENT				
1. Correctly assessed client's physiologic capacity for transfer.	___	___	___	_____
2. Correctly assessed client for presence of weakness, dizziness, postural hypotension.	___	___	___	_____
3. Correctly assessed client's activity tolerance.	___	___	___	_____
4. Correctly assessed client's proprioceptive function.	___	___	___	_____
5. Correctly assessed client's sensory status.	___	___	___	_____
6. Assessed client for comfort.	___	___	___	_____
7. Correctly assessed client's cognitive status.	___	___	___	_____
8. Assessed client's level of motivation.	___	___	___	_____
9. Assessed previous mode of transfer, if applicable.	___	___	___	_____
10. Assessed client's risk of injury.	___	___	___	_____
NURSING DIAGNOSIS				
1. Developed appropriate nursing diagnoses based on assessment data.	___	___	___	_____
PLANNING				
1. Developed individualized goals for client based on nursing diagnoses.	___	___	___	_____
2. Identified expected outcomes.	___	___	___	_____
3. Explained procedure to client.	___	___	___	_____
IMPLEMENTATION				
1. Washed hands.	___	___	___	_____
2. Assisted client to sitting position:	___	___	___	_____
a. Placed client in supine position.	___	___	___	_____
b. Removed pillows from bed.	___	___	___	_____
c. Faced head of bed and removed pillows.	___	___	___	_____
d. Placed feet apart for broad base of support, with foot nearest bed behind other foot.	___	___	___	_____
e. Correctly placed hand under client's shoulders.	___	___	___	_____

	S	U	NP	Comments

f. Placed other hand on bed surface. ___ ___ ___ _____

g. Correctly raised client to sitting position (weight shifted to rear leg). ___ ___ ___ _____

h. Pushed against bed with hand on bed surface. ___ ___ ___ _____

3. Assisted client to a sitting position on the side of the bed: ___ ___ ___ _____

   a. Placed client in side-lying position. ___ ___ ___ _____

   b. Raised head of bed to 30 degrees. ___ ___ ___ _____

   c. Stood in correct position for transfer and turned diagonally to face client and far corner of bed. ___ ___ ___ _____

   d. Placed feet correctly. ___ ___ ___ _____

   e. Placed arm near bed under client's shoulders. ___ ___ ___ _____

   f. Placed other arm over client's thighs. ___ ___ ___ _____

   g. Moved client's lower legs and feet over side of bed and correctly pivoted leg. ___ ___ ___ _____

   h. Shifted weight to elevate client. ___ ___ ___ _____

   i. Remained in front of client until balance regained. ___ ___ ___ _____

   j. Provided physical support to weak or cognitively impaired client. ___ ___ ___ _____

4. Transferred client from bed to chair: ___ ___ ___ _____

   a. Assisted client to a sitting position on side of bed, with chair placed correctly. ___ ___ ___ _____

   b. Applied transfer belt if needed. ___ ___ ___ _____

   c. Ensured that client was wearing nonskid shoes; weight-bearing leg forward. ___ ___ ___ _____

   d. Stood with feet apart. ___ ___ ___ _____

   e. Flexed knees and hips; aligned knees with client's. ___ ___ ___ _____

   f. Correctly placed arms around client or grasped transfer belt. ___ ___ ___ _____

   g. Rocked client to standing position on count of 3. ___ ___ ___ _____

   h. Used knee to maintain stability of weak (or paralyzed) leg. ___ ___ ___ _____

   i. Pivoted on foot farther from chair. ___ ___ ___ _____

   j. Instructed client to use arm rests on chair for support. ___ ___ ___ _____

Student _____   Date _____

Instructor _____   Date _____

	S	U	NP	Comments

k. Flexed hips and knees while lowering client into chair. ___ ___ ___ _____

l. Assessed client for proper alignment in sitting position. ___ ___ ___ _____

m. Provided client with support and encouragement. ___ ___ ___ _____

5. Performed three-person carry: ___ ___ ___ _____

   a. Three nurses stood side by side, facing side of client's bed. ___ ___ ___ _____

   b. Correctly positioned at client's head, hips, thighs. ___ ___ ___ _____

   c. Used correct body mechanics for client transfer. ___ ___ ___ _____

   d. Properly positioned arms with fingers securely around client's body. ___ ___ ___ _____

   e. Client correctly log-rolled to nurses' chests. ___ ___ ___ _____

   f. Client correctly lifted with alignment maintained. ___ ___ ___ _____

   g. Nurses pivoted to stretcher in synchrony. ___ ___ ___ _____

   h. Used correct body alignment when placing client on stretcher. ___ ___ ___ _____

   i. Nurses assessed client's realignment. ___ ___ ___ _____

6. Used mechanical/hydraulic lift: ___ ___ ___ _____

   a. Moved lift to bedside. ___ ___ ___ _____

   b. Placed chair to allow adequate space to maneuver lift. ___ ___ ___ _____

   c. Raised bed to high position. ___ ___ ___ _____

   d. Kept side rail up on side opposite to nurse. ___ ___ ___ _____

   e. Rolled client away from nurse. ___ ___ ___ _____

   f. Placed hammock or a canvas strip under client to form seat. ___ ___ ___ _____

   g. Raised bed rail. ___ ___ ___ _____

   h. Went to opposite side of bed, lowered side rail. ___ ___ ___ _____

   i. Rolled client to opposite side and pulled hammock through. ___ ___ ___ _____

	S	U	NP	Comments
j. Rolled client supine onto canvas seat.	—	—	—	_____
k. Removed client's glasses, if applicable.	—	—	—	_____
l. Placed lift's horseshoe bar under bed.	—	—	—	_____
m. Lowered horizontal bar to sling level; locked valve.	—	—	—	_____
n. Attached strap hooks to holes in sling.	—	—	—	_____
o. Elevated head of bed.	—	—	—	_____
p. Folded client's arms over chest.	—	—	—	_____
q. Pumped handle until client was free of bed.	—	—	—	_____
r. Pulled lift from bed and maneuvered to chair using steering handle.	—	—	—	_____
s. Rolled base around chair.	—	—	—	_____
t. Released check valve slowly; lowered client into chair.	—	—	—	_____
u. Closed check valve.	—	—	—	_____
v. Removed straps and lift.	—	—	—	_____
w. Checked client for proper alignment.	—	—	—	_____
7. Washed hands.	—	—	—	_____

EVALUATION

	S	U	NP	Comments
1. Monitored vital signs. Asked if client felt fatigued.	—	—	—	_____
2. Observed for correct body alignment and presence of pressure points on skin.	—	—	—	_____
3. Observed client's response to transfer.	—	—	—	_____
4. Asked if client had pain during transfer.	—	—	—	_____
5. Identified unexpected outcomes.	—	—	—	_____

RECORDING AND REPORTING

	S	U	NP	Comments
1. Recorded procedure and observations.	—	—	—	_____
2. Reported any unusual occurrence to appropriate personnel.	—	—	—	_____

Student _____   Date _____

Instructor _____   Date _____

PERFORMANCE CHECKLIST 29-2 **MOVING AND POSITIONING CLIENTS IN BED**

	S	U	NP	Comments

ASSESSMENT

1. Assessed client's body alignment and comfort level.   ___ ___ ___ _____

2. Assessed for risk factors.   ___ ___ ___ _____

3. Assessed client's level of consciousness.   ___ ___ ___ _____

4. Assessed client's ability to assist with positioning.   ___ ___ ___ _____

5. Assessed for presence of tubes, incisions, and equipment.   ___ ___ ___ _____

NURSING DIAGNOSIS

1. Developed appropriate nursing diagnoses based on assessment data.   ___ ___ ___ _____

PLANNING

1. Developed individualized goals for client based on nursing diagnoses.   ___ ___ ___ _____

2. Identified expected outcomes.   ___ ___ ___ _____

3. Raised level of bed to comfortable working height.   ___ ___ ___ _____

4. Removed pillows and other objects.   ___ ___ ___ _____

5. Obtained extra assistance as needed.   ___ ___ ___ _____

6. Explained procedure to client.   ___ ___ ___ _____

IMPLEMENTATION

1. Washed hands.   ___ ___ ___ _____

2. Provided for client privacy.   ___ ___ ___ _____

3. Put bed in flat position.   ___ ___ ___ _____

4. Moved immobile client up in bed (one nurse):   ___ ___ ___ _____

   a. Placed client on back with head of bed flat; stood on one side of bed.   ___ ___ ___ _____

   b. Placed pillow at head of bed.   ___ ___ ___ _____

   c. Correctly moved client up in bed.   ___ ___ ___ _____

   d. Kept arms level with client's hips.   ___ ___ ___ _____

   e. Slid client's hip diagonally toward head of bed.   ___ ___ ___ _____

   f. Maintained proper body alignment.   ___ ___ ___ _____

	S	U	NP	Comments

g. Supported client's head on worker's arm nearest the head of bed.   ___ ___ ___ _____

h. Placed other arm under client's chest.   ___ ___ ___ _____

i. Slid client's head, shoulders, and chest toward head of bed.   ___ ___ ___ _____

j. Raised side rail next to client and repositioned self on other side of bed.   ___ ___ ___ _____

k. Repeated procedure until client reached desired height in bed.   ___ ___ ___ _____

l. Correctly centered client in middle of bed.   ___ ___ ___ _____

5. Assisted client to move up in bed (one or two nurses):   ___ ___ ___ _____

a. Placed client on back with head of bed flat.   ___ ___ ___ _____

b. Placed pillow at head of bed.   ___ ___ ___ _____

c. Faced head of bed.   ___ ___ ___ _____

d. Stood in proper position.   ___ ___ ___ _____

e. Asked client to flex knees.   ___ ___ ___ _____

f. Instructed client to flex neck.   ___ ___ ___ _____

g. Instructed client to push feet on bed surface to assist movement.   ___ ___ ___ _____

h. Maintained own body alignment.   ___ ___ ___ _____

i. Instructed client to push heels and elevate trunk.   ___ ___ ___ _____

j. Shifted weight while client elevated trunk.   ___ ___ ___ _____

6. Moved immobile client up in bed using drawsheet or pullsheet (two nurses):   ___ ___ ___ _____

a. Placed drawsheet or pullsheet under client.   ___ ___ ___ _____

b. Placed client on back with bed flat.   ___ ___ ___ _____

c. Positioned one nurse at each side of client.   ___ ___ ___ _____

d. Grasped drawsheet or pullsheet firmly near client.   ___ ___ ___ _____

e. Maintained proper body alignment while shifting weight to move client and drawsheet or pullsheet to desired position.   ___ ___ ___ _____

7. Realigned client in proper body alignment.   ___ ___ ___ _____

a. Positioned client in supported Fowler's position: ___ ___ ___ _____

Student _____ Date _____

Instructor _____ Date _____

	S	U	NP	Comments
• Elevated head of bed 45-60 degrees.	___	___	___	_____
• Rested client's head against mattress or placed small pillow underneath client's head.	___	___	___	_____
• Placed pillows appropriately to support hands and arms correctly.	___	___	___	_____
• Placed pillow at lower back.	___	___	___	_____
• Placed small pillow under thighs.	___	___	___	_____
• Placed small pillow or roll under ankles.	___	___	___	_____
• Placed footboard at bottom of client's feet.	___	___	___	_____
b. Positioned hemiplegic client in supported Fowler's position:	___	___	___	_____
• Elevated head of bed 45-60 degrees.	___	___	___	_____
• Sat client up as straight as possible.	___	___	___	_____
• Positioned client's head with chin slightly forward.	___	___	___	_____
• Supported involved arm and hand.	___	___	___	_____
• Positioned flaccid hand in normal resting position.	___	___	___	_____
• Positioned affected hand with wrist in neutral or slightly extended position.	___	___	___	_____
• Flexed knees and hips by using pillow.	___	___	___	_____
• Supported feet in dorsiflexed position.	___	___	___	_____
c. Positioned client in supine position:	___	___	___	_____
• Placed client on back with bed flat.	___	___	___	_____
• Placed small pillow or rolled towel under small of back.	___	___	___	_____
• Placed pillow under upper shoulders, neck, and head.	___	___	___	_____
• Placed trochanter rolls along hips and upper thighs.	___	___	___	_____
• Placed small pillow or roll under ankle.	___	___	___	_____
• Placed foot support to maintain feet in dorsiflexion.	___	___	___	_____
• Placed pillows under pronated forearms.	___	___	___	_____

	S	U	NP	Comments

- Placed handrolls to maintain hands in functional position.

d. Positioned hemiplegic client in supine position:

- Placed head on bed flat.

- Placed folded towel or pillow under shoulder of affected side.

- Placed affected arm properly.

- Placed affected hand properly.

- Placed folded towel under hip of involved side.

- Flexed affected knee by 30 degrees.

- Supported feet with soft pillows.

e. Positioned client in prone position:

- Placed client on abdomen with bed flat.

- Turned client's head to one side supported by a small pillow.

- Placed small pillow under client's abdomen.

- Supported arms, flexed at shoulders on pillows.

- Placed pillow under lower legs to elevate toes off bed.

f. Positioned hemiplegic client in prone position:

- Moved client toward unaffected side.

- Rolled client onto side.

- Placed pillow on client's abdomen.

- Rolled client onto abdomen.

- Turned head toward involved side.

- Positioned involved arm properly.

- Flexed knees and placed pillows correctly.

- Maintained feet at right angles.

g. Positioned client in lateral (side-lying) position:

- Lowered head of bed to comfortable level.

- Positioned client on one side of bed.

- Turned client onto one side.

Student _____ Date _____

Instructor _____ Date _____

	S	U	NP	Comments
• Placed pillow under client's head and neck.	——	——	——	_____
• Brought shoulder blade forward.	——	——	——	_____
• Positioned arms in slightly flexed position.	——	——	——	_____
• Placed pillow behind client's back.	——	——	——	_____
• Placed pillow under upper leg.	——	——	——	_____
• Placed sandbag parallel to plantar surface of foot.	——	——	——	_____
h. Positioned client in Sims' (semiprone) position:	——	——	——	_____
• Lowered head of bed completely.	——	——	——	_____
• Place client in supine position.	——	——	——	_____
• Positioned client in lateral position partially lying on abdomen.	——	——	——	_____
• Placed pillow under client's head.	——	——	——	_____
• Placed pillow under flexed upper arm to support arm level with shoulder.	——	——	——	_____
• Placed pillow under flexed upper leg to support leg level with hip.	——	——	——	_____
• Placed sandbags parallel to plantar surface of feet to maintain feet in dorsiflexion.	——	——	——	_____
8. Washed hands.	——	——	——	_____

EVALUATION

1. Observed client's body alignment and level of comfort.	——	——	——	_____
2. Measured joint ROM.	——	——	——	_____
3. Assessed for contractures or breakdown in skin integrity.	——	——	——	_____
4. Identified unexpected outcomes.	——	——	——	_____

RECORDING AND REPORTING

1. Recorded procedure in nurses' notes, including condition of skin, joint movement, client's ability to assist with repositioning.	——	——	——	_____
2. Reported observations at change of shift.	——	——	——	_____

Student _____   Date _____

Instructor _____   Date _____

PERFORMANCE CHECKLIST 30-1 **PERFORMING RANGE-OF-MOTION EXERCISES**

	S	U	NP	Comments

ASSESSMENT

1. Reviewed client's medical history and obtained physician's order if needed. ___ ___ ___ _____

2. Performed baseline assessment of joint function. ___ ___ ___ _____

3. Determined client's or caregiver's understanding of exercises. ___ ___ ___ _____

NURSING DIAGNOSIS

1. Developed appropriate nursing diagnoses based on assessment data. ___ ___ ___ _____

PLANNING

1. Developed individualized goals for performing exercises. ___ ___ ___ _____

2. Identified expected outcomes. ___ ___ ___ _____

3. Explained procedure and reason for performing ROM exercises. ___ ___ ___ _____

4. Positioned client appropriately. ___ ___ ___ _____

IMPLEMENTATION

1. Washed hands. ___ ___ ___ _____

2. Exposed only limbs to be exercised. ___ ___ ___ _____

3. Raised bed to comfortable position and stood on side of bed of joints to be exercised. ___ ___ ___ _____

4. Performed exercises slowly and gently. ___ ___ ___ _____

5. Supported joint while performing exercise. ___ ___ ___ _____

6. Performed appropriate exercises in following sequence: neck, shoulder, elbow, forearm, wrist, fingers, thumb, hip, knee, ankle, foot; discontinued exercise if client complained of discomfort, resistance was met, or muscle spasm occurred; repeated each movement 5 times. ___ ___ ___ _____

7. Repositioned client after procedure and washed hands. ___ ___ ___ _____

EVALUATION

1. Assessed client for response to exercises and degree of assistance required. ___ ___ ___ _____

2. Asked for client's subjective statements regarding the experience. ___ ___ ___ _____

	S	U	NP	Comments

3. Observed range of motion as compared to baseline. ___ ___ ___ _____

4. Asked client to independently perform exercises. ___ ___ ___ _____

5. Identified unexpected outcomes. ___ ___ ___ _____

RECORDING AND REPORTING

1. Charted in nurses' notes: joints exercised; extent to which joints could be moved; any joint abnormalities assessed; client's subjective statements regarding procedure, and nurse's objective observations of tolerance. ___ ___ ___ _____

2. Notified nurse in charge or physician if any joint abnormalities were noted. ___ ___ ___ _____

Student _____   Date _____

Instructor _____   Date _____

PERFORMANCE CHECKLIST 30-2 **PERFORMING ISOMETRIC EXERCISES**

	S	U	NP	Comments
ASSESSMENT				
1. Reviewed client's chart.	—	—	—	_____
2. Performed baseline assessment of vital signs.	—	—	—	_____
3. Assessed client's baseline muscle strength.	—	—	—	_____
4. Assessed client's or caregiver's understanding of exercises.	—	—	—	_____
NURSING DIAGNOSIS				
1. Developed appropriate nursing diagnoses based on assessment data.	—	—	—	_____
PLANNING				
1. Developed individualized goals for performing isometric exercises.	—	—	—	_____
2. Identified expected outcomes.	—	—	—	_____
3. Explained procedure and demonstrated exercises.	—	—	—	_____
4. Assisted client to comfortable position.	—	—	—	_____
IMPLEMENTATION				
1. Provided privacy.	—	—	—	_____
2. Had client perform each isometric exercise correctly.	—	—	—	_____
3. Had client perform each resistive exercise correctly.	—	—	—	_____
EVALUATION				
1. Observed client's ability to perform exercises.	—	—	—	_____
2. Determined level of energy, muscular strength, and comfort.	—	—	—	_____
3. Obtained vital signs.	—	—	—	_____
4. Identified unexpected outcomes.	—	—	—	_____
RECORDING AND REPORTING				
1. Charted in nurses' notes: type of isometric exercises used; length of time contraction held; number of repetitions for each exercise; assessment of client's muscular strength following exercises; and client's subjective statements regarding muscular strength.	—	—	—	_____
2. Reported client's tolerance of exercises to appropriate personnel.	—	—	—	_____

Student _____   Date _____

Instructor _____   Date _____

PERFORMANCE CHECKLIST 30-3 **APPLYING ELASTIC STOCKINGS**

	S	U	NP	Comments
ASSESSMENT				
1. Assessed need for application of elastic stockings.	—	—	—	_____
2. Observed for contraindications to use of elastic stockings.	—	—	—	_____
3. Obtained physician's order.	—	—	—	_____
4. Assessed client's or caregiver's understanding of applying elastic stockings.	—	—	—	_____
5. Assessed and documented condition of client's skin and circulation to the legs.	—	—	—	_____
NURSING DIAGNOSIS				
1. Developed appropriate nursing diagnoses based on assessment data.	—	—	—	_____
PLANNING				
1. Developed individualized goals for applying elastic stockings.	—	—	—	_____
2. Identified expected outcomes.	—	—	—	_____
3. Explained procedure and reasons for applying stockings.	—	—	—	_____
4. Measured stockings for proper size.	—	—	—	_____
IMPLEMENTATION				
1. Washed hands.	—	—	—	_____
2. Elevated bed to comfortable level.	—	—	—	_____
3. Positioned client in supine position.	—	—	—	_____
4. Applied talcum powder to client's legs and feet.	—	—	—	_____
5. Applied stockings correctly.	—	—	—	_____
6. Repositioned client after procedure and washed hands.	—	—	—	_____
EVALUATION				
1. Inspected stockings for fit.	—	—	—	_____
2. Observed circulatory status of lower extremities.	—	—	—	_____
3. Observed client or caregiver apply stockings.	—	—	—	_____
4. Determined client's response to procedure.	—	—	—	_____
5. Identified unexpected outcomes.	—	—	—	_____

S   U   NP   Comments

RECORDING AND REPORTING

1. Charted in nurses' progress notes: date and time of stocking application and condition of skin before application; circulatory status of lower extremities before stocking application; stocking length and size; date and time stockings removed; and condition of skin and circulatory status after removal.   ___ ___ ___   _____

2. Notified additional personnel if alteration in circulatory status of lower extremities occurred.   ___ ___ ___   _____

3. Reported signs of skin irritation to physician.   ___ ___ ___   _____

Student _____   Date _____

Instructor _____   Date _____

PERFORMANCE CHECKLIST 30-4 CHANGING CLIENT'S POSITION TO MINIMIZE OCCURRENCE OF ORTHOSTATIC HYPOTENSION

	S	U	NP	Comments
ASSESSMENT				
1. Reviewed client's chart.	—	—	—	_____
2. Obtained set of baseline vital signs.	—	—	—	_____
3. Assessed client's environment for potential safety hazards.	—	—	—	_____
NURSING DIAGNOSIS				
1. Developed appropriate nursing diagnoses based on assessment data.	—	—	—	_____
PLANNING				
1. Developed individualized goals for minimizing occurrence of orthostatic hypotension.	—	—	—	_____
2. Identified expected outcomes.	—	—	—	_____
3. Explained procedure and reasons for getting client out of bed.	—	—	—	_____
4. Assessed whether another staff member is needed with procedure.	—	—	—	_____
IMPLEMENTATION				
1. Washed hands.	—	—	—	_____
2. Placed bed in low position.	—	—	—	_____
3. Raised head of bed slowly to high Fowler's position and obtained blood pressure.	—	—	—	_____
4. Assessed client for signs of orthostatic hypotension.	—	—	—	_____
5. Assisted client to sit on side of bed and continued to assess for signs of orthostatic hypotension.	—	—	—	_____
6. Assisted client to ambulate or sit in chair.	—	—	—	_____
7. Washed hands.	—	—	—	_____
EVALUATION				
1. Assessed client for orthostatic hypotension.	—	—	—	_____
2. Rechecked client's blood pressure while sitting the first few times.	—	—	—	_____
3. Identified unexpected outcomes.	—	—	—	_____

	S	U	NP	Comments

RECORDING AND REPORTING

1. Charted in nurses' notes: supine and upright blood pressures; client's subjective statements regarding upright procedure; whether client sat in chair, length of time in chair, and how well procedure was tolerated; and whether client ambulated, distance ambulated, stability of gait, and degree of assistance needed.

2. Reported immediately if client sustained injury or was unable to tolerate procedure.

Student _____   Date _____

Instructor _____   Date _____

PERFORMANCE CHECKLIST 30-5 **ASSISTING WITH AMBULATION**

	S	U	NP	Comments
ASSESSMENT				
1. Reviewed client's chart.	___	___	___	_____
2. Assessed client's physical readiness.	___	___	___	_____
3. Assessed client's or caregiver's understanding of ambulatory technique.	___	___	___	_____
4. Determined optimal time for ambulation.	___	___	___	_____
5. Assessed degree of assistance client needed.	___	___	___	_____
NURSING DIAGNOSIS				
1. Developed appropriate nursing diagnoses based on assessment data.	___	___	___	_____
PLANNING				
1. Developed individualized goals for assisting with ambulation.	___	___	___	_____
2. Identified expected outcomes.	___	___	___	_____
3. Prepared client appropriately.	___	___	___	_____
IMPLEMENTATION				
Assisted Ambulation With One Nurse				
1. Washed hands.	___	___	___	_____
2. Applied safety belt if necessary and assisted client to standing position and observed balance.	___	___	___	_____
3. Positioned self on client's weaker side and had client take a few steps.	___	___	___	_____
4. Supported client at waist.	___	___	___	_____
5. Took a few steps forward with client and assessed for strength and balance.	___	___	___	_____
6. Allowed client to return to bed or chair if weak or dizzy.	___	___	___	_____
7. Used appropriate procedure if client began to fall.	___	___	___	_____
Assisted Ambulation With Two Nurses				
1. Followed Steps 1 and 2, Assisted Ambulation With One Nurse.	___	___	___	_____
2. Nurses stood on each side of client.	___	___	___	_____
3. Placed arms around client's waist.	___	___	___	_____

	S	U	NP	Comments

4. Stepped in unison with client.   ___ ___ ___ _____

5. Increased distance gradually.   ___ ___ ___ _____

6. Followed Steps 6 and 7, Assisted Ambulation With One Nurse.   ___ ___ ___ _____

Ambulation With Assistive Devices

1. Assisted client with crutch walking, using appropriate gait.   ___ ___ ___ _____

2. Assisted client in climbing stairs with crutches.   ___ ___ ___ _____

3. Assisted client in descending stairs with crutches.   ___ ___ ___ _____

2. Assisted client in ambulating with walker.   ___ ___ ___ _____

3. Assisted client in ambulating with cane.   ___ ___ ___ _____

EVALUATION

1. Assessed client's response to ambulation, including vital signs and energy level.   ___ ___ ___ _____

2. Assessed subjective response regarding experience.   ___ ___ ___ _____

3. Assessed gait and body alignment.   ___ ___ ___ _____

4. Observed client's ability to perform self-care activities.   ___ ___ ___ _____

5. Identified unexpected outcomes.   ___ ___ ___ _____

RECORDING AND REPORTING

1. Recorded in nurses' notes: type of gait client used; amount of assistance required; distance walked; and client's tolerance of activity.   ___ ___ ___ _____

2. Immediately reported any injury sustained during procedure, alteration in vital signs, or inability to ambulate.   ___ ___ ___ _____

Student _____   Date _____

Instructor _____   Date _____

PERFORMANCE CHECKLIST 31-1 **ASSISTING WITH CAST APPLICATION**

	S	U	NP	Comments
ASSESSMENT				
1. Assessed client's health status.	___	___	___	_____
2. Assessed client's understanding of cast application.	___	___	___	_____
3. Assessed condition of tissues to be casted.	___	___	___	_____
4. Determined client's pain status.	___	___	___	_____
5. Determined extent to which client may use casted extremity.	___	___	___	_____
NURSING DIAGNOSIS				
1. Developed appropriate nursing diagnoses based on assessment data.	___	___	___	_____
PLANNING				
1. Developed individualized goals for client based on nursing diagnoses.	___	___	___	_____
2. Identified expected outcomes.	___	___	___	_____
3. Instructed client, parent, or other assistants as needed.	___	___	___	_____
4. Administered analgesic 20-30 minutes before cast application if indicated.	___	___	___	_____
IMPLEMENTATION				
1. Washed hands and applied gloves.	___	___	___	_____
2. Positioned client appropriately.	___	___	___	_____
3. Prepared skin before casting. Explained that warmth may be felt during application.	___	___	___	_____
4. Assisted with cast application.	___	___	___	_____
5. Supplied dampened rolls of plaster or synthetic cast roll.	___	___	___	_____
6. Supplied necessary stabilizing material.	___	___	___	_____
7. Finished cast.	___	___	___	_____
8. Trimmed plaster around thumb, fingers, or toes.	___	___	___	_____
9. Facilitated drying of cast.	___	___	___	_____
10. Assisted with transfer of client, accompanied client to room, and assisted with transfer to bed if necessary.	___	___	___	_____

	S	U	NP	Comments

11. Cleaned equipment. Washed hands. ___ ___ ___ _____

12. Explained procedures of exposure for fast drying. ___ ___ ___ _____

13. Had client turn every 2 to 3 hours. ___ ___ ___ _____

14. Informed client to notify personnel of alteration in sensation or mobility. ___ ___ ___ _____

EVALUATION

1. Observed client for signs of "cast syndrome." ___ ___ ___ _____

2. Assessed neurovascular status. ___ ___ ___ _____

3. Smelled the cast edges. ___ ___ ___ _____

4. Observed client performing cast care. ___ ___ ___ _____

5. Identified unexpected outcomes. ___ ___ ___ _____

RECORDING AND REPORTING

1. Recorded application of cast and condition of skin and circulation. ___ ___ ___ _____

2. Reported abnormal or untoward progression of findings obtained from neurovascular checks. ___ ___ ___ _____

3. Reported signs of increasing anxiety, restlessness, or aerophagia to oncoming personnel. ___ ___ ___ _____

4. Recorded elevated temperature if rising. ___ ___ ___ _____

5. Recorded responses to strategies to relieve symptoms. ___ ___ ___ _____

6. Recorded all findings of neurovascular checks performed initially every 1-2 hours and gradually extended to every 3-4 hours. ___ ___ ___ _____

7. Recorded client's ability or inability to perform ADL and specific requirements for care. ___ ___ ___ _____

Student _____ Date _____

Instructor _____ Date _____

PERFORMANCE CHECKLIST 31-2 **ASSISTING WITH CAST REMOVAL**

	S	U	NP	Comments

ASSESSMENT
1. Assessed client's understanding of upcoming cast removal.
2. Assessed client's readiness for cast removal.
3. Asked client if itching or irritation under cast is felt.

NURSING DIAGNOSIS
1. Developed appropriate nursing diagnoses based on assessment data.

PLANNING
1. Developed individualized goals for client based on nursing diagnoses.
2. Identified expected outcomes.
3. Explained procedure to client and detailed physical sensations to expect.

IMPLEMENTATION
1. Applied gloves, if indicated, and assisted with cast removal.
2. Inspected underlying tissues.
3. Applied enzyme wash.
4. Cleansed tissues with water.
5. Applied lotion to skin.
6. Put joints and muscles through ROM.
7. Assisted in transfer of client for return to room or for discharge.
8. Cleaned or disposed of equipment appropriately.

EVALUATION
1. Inspected underlying skin.
2. Observed client's behavior.
3. Asked client to explain and demonstrate exercises.
4. Had client explain and perform skin care.
5. Identified unexpected outcomes.

	S	U	NP	Comments

RECORDING AND REPORTING

1. Recorded cast removal and person removing cast.   ___ ___ ___ _____

2. Recorded client's response to cast removal.   ___ ___ ___ _____

3. Recorded condition of tissue.   ___ ___ ___ _____

4. Recorded instructions given.   ___ ___ ___ _____

5. Recorded transfer of clients to room or preparations for discharge.   ___ ___ ___ _____

Student _____ Date _____

Instructor _____ Date _____

PERFORMANCE CHECKLIST 31-3 **ASSISTING WITH APPLICATION OF SKIN TRACTION**

	S	U	NP	Comments
ASSESSMENT				
1. Assessed client's health status.	___	___	___	_____
2. Assessed specific tissues to be placed in traction.	___	___	___	_____
3. Assessed client's understanding of reason for traction.	___	___	___	_____
4. Assessed client's level of pain.	___	___	___	_____
5. Assessed client's neurovascular status.	___	___	___	_____
NURSING DIAGNOSIS				
1. Developed appropriate nursing diagnoses based on assessment data.	___	___	___	_____
PLANNING				
1. Developed individualized goals for client based on nursing diagnoses.	___	___	___	_____
2. Identified expected outcomes.	___	___	___	_____
3. Explained procedure to client.	___	___	___	_____
IMPLEMENTATION				
1. Prepared client and area of body to be placed in traction.	___	___	___	_____
2. Positioned client as requested by physician.	___	___	___	_____
3. Assisted with application of specific traction equipment.	___	___	___	_____
4. Assisted with attachment of bars, ropes, and pulleys.	___	___	___	_____
5. Attached and gently lowered traction weights.	___	___	___	_____
6. Assessed client's body alignment in traction.	___	___	___	_____
7. Assessed client's initial response to traction.	___	___	___	_____
8. Elevated side rails.	___	___	___	_____
9. Assessed neurovascular status within 15 minutes after application, then every 1-2 hours for 24 hours.	___	___	___	_____
10. Returned unused materials to storage area.	___	___	___	_____
11. Washed hands.	___	___	___	_____

	S	U	NP	Comments

EVALUATION

1. Observed client's participation in self-care.

2. Observed entire traction setup.

3. Assessed condition of skin around traction.

4. Asked if client understands mobility restrictions.

5. Determined if client was having pain.

6. Conducted neurovascular checks.

7. Identified unexpected outcomes.

RECORDING AND REPORTING

1. Recorded type of traction, site, skin condition, weight applied, client's response, and other pertinent data.

2. Reported untoward findings to physician or nurse in charge.

3. Record findings of neurovascular checks.

4. Recorded traction functioning.

5. Recorded length of time client was in or out of traction.

6. Recorded client's participation in self-care.

Student _____   Date _____

Instructor _____   Date _____

PERFORMANCE CHECKLIST 31-4 ASSISTING WITH INSERTION OF PINS, WIRES, OR NAILS FOR SKELETAL TRACTION

	S	U	NP	Comments
ASSESSMENT				
1. Assessed client's health status.	—	—	—	
2. Assessed specific tissues to be placed in skeletal traction.	—	—	—	
3. Assessed client's understanding of traction.	—	—	—	
4. Assessed client's level of pain.	—	—	—	
5. Observed client's nonverbal behavior.	—	—	—	
NURSING DIAGNOSIS				
1. Developed appropriate nursing diagnoses based on assessment data.	—	—	—	
PLANNING				
1. Developed individualized goals for client based on nursing diagnoses.	—	—	—	
2. Identified expected outcomes.	—	—	—	
IMPLEMENTATION				
Traction Setup				
1. Positioned client according to physician's order.	—	—	—	
2. Assisted with skin preparation.	—	—	—	
3. Supported client's limb.	—	—	—	
4. Assisted with application of nails or pins.	—	—	—	
5. Assisted in completion of traction setup.	—	—	—	
6. Ascertained client's initial reactions or response to traction.	—	—	—	
7. Elevated side rails.	—	—	—	
8. Returned equipment and supplies.	—	—	—	
9. Washed hands.	—	—	—	
Pin Care				
1. Washed hands and applied gloves.	—	—	—	
2. Removed and discarded old dressing around pins.	—	—	—	
3. Prepared supplies and applied sterile or clean gloves (per agency policy).	—	—	—	

	S	U	NP	Comments

4. Cleaned pins correctly.

5. Removed crusts from pin site with hydrogen peroxide and saline.

6. Cleaned pin area with normal saline.

7. Applied a small amount of povidone-iodine or topical antibiotic and covered pin site with sterile gauze dressing.

8. Repeated procedure for other pin site.

9. Discarded supplies.

10. Removed and disposed of gloves. Washed hands.

EVALUATION

1. Assessed traction setup and functioning.

2. Determined client's response to traction apparatus.

3. Determined client's need for analgesics.

4. Inspected pin sites. Assessed for indications of infection.

5. Performed neurovascular checks.

6. Performed motor assessment.

7. Identified unexpected outcomes.

RECORDING AND REPORTING

1. Recorded type of traction applied, person applying traction, site, time, weights, and client's initial response.

2. Recorded client's participation in self-care.

3. Reported client's response to specific traction.

4. Reported untoward reactions or unexpected outcomes to nurse in charge or physician.

5. Recorded all findings of skin and neurovascular checks.

6. Recorded client's pain and analgesics used.

7. Documented client's ROM and ability to use trapeze.

8. Recorded indications of anxiety and client's response to interventions.

Student _____ Date _____

Instructor _____ Date _____

PERFORMANCE CHECKLIST 32-1 **PLACING A CLIENT ON A SUPPORT SURFACE MATTRESS**

	S	U	NP	Comments

ASSESSMENT

1. Determined client's risk for pressure ulcer formation using assessment tool. ___ ___ ___ _____

2. Inspected condition of client's skin. ___ ___ ___ _____

3. Assessed client's understanding of purpose of mattress. ___ ___ ___ _____

4. Assessed client's comfort level. ___ ___ ___ _____

5. Checked physician's orders. ___ ___ ___ _____

NURSING DIAGNOSIS

1. Developed appropriate nursing diagnoses based on assessment data. ___ ___ ___ _____

PLANNING

1. Developed individualized goals for client based on nursing diagnoses. ___ ___ ___ _____

2. Identified expected outcomes. ___ ___ ___ _____

3. Explained purpose and procedure to client. ___ ___ ___ _____

4. Washed hands and applied gloves (as indicated). Obtained assistance as needed. ___ ___ ___ _____

IMPLEMENTATION

1. Provided for client's privacy. ___ ___ ___ _____

2. Correctly applied support surface to bed or prepared alternate bed. ___ ___ ___ _____

Mattress Replacement

a. Applied mattress to bed frame after removing hospital mattress. ___ ___ ___ _____

b. Applied sheet over mattress. ___ ___ ___ _____

Air Mattress/Overlay

a. Applied deflated mattress over bed. ___ ___ ___ _____

b. Secured air mattress over corners of bed mattress. ___ ___ ___ _____

c. Attached connector on air mattress to inflation device and inflated mattress to proper air pressure. ___ ___ ___ _____

d. Applied sheet over air mattress. ___ ___ ___ _____

e. Checked air pump for proper cycling. ___ ___ ___ _____

	S	U	NP	Comments

Integrated Air Surface

a. Obtained and made bed.

b. Placed switch in the "Prevention" mode.

Water Mattress

a. Applied unfilled mattress flat over surface of bed mattress.

b. Secured water mattress in place.

c. Attached connector on water mattress to water source.

d. Filled mattress to recommended level.

e. Placed sheet over water mattress.

3. Positioned client comfortably and repositioned routinely.

4. Removed gloves (if worn) and washed hands.

EVALUATION

1. Inspected condition of client's skin.

2. Reassessed client's risk for pressure sore formation at routine intervals.

3. Assessed client's comfort level.

4. Evaluated inflation of mattress periodically.

5. Identified unexpected outcomes.

RECORDING AND REPORTING

1. Recorded placement of mattress and condition of client's skin in nurses' notes or skin assessment flowsheet.

2. Reported evidence of pressure sores to nurse in charge or physician.

Student _____   Date _____

Instructor _____   Date _____

PERFORMANCE CHECKLIST 32-2 **PLACING A CLIENT ON AN AIR-SUSPENSION BED**

	S	U	NP	Comments

ASSESSMENT

1. Identified clients who would benefit from air-suspension therapy.

2. Reviewed client's medical orders.

3. Assessed client for pain.

4. Assessed condition of client's skin.

5. Assessed client's level of consciousness.

6. Assessed client's and family member's understanding of purpose of bed.

7. Reviewed client's serum electrolyte levels if available.

NURSING DIAGNOSIS

1. Developed appropriate nursing diagnoses based on assessment data.

PLANNING

1. Developed individualized goals for client based on nursing diagnoses.

2. Identified expected outcomes.

3. Explained procedure and purpose of bed to client and family.

4. Washed hands, applied gloves, and prepared necessary equipment and supplies.

5. Obtained additional personnel needed to transfer client to bed.

6. Reviewed bed manufacturer's instructions.

7. Premedicated clients, as necessary, 30 minutes before transfer.

IMPLEMENTATION

1. Maintained client's privacy.

2. Explained steps of transfer.

3. Transferred client to bed using appropriate transfer techniques.

4. Turned bed on.

	S	U	NP	Comments

5. Positioned client and performed ROM exercises as appropriate.

___ ___ ___ _____

6. Set Instaflate when turning or positioning client in bed.

___ ___ ___ _____

7. In emergencies, deflated bed immediately.

___ ___ ___ _____

8. Removed gloves (if worn) and washed hands.

___ ___ ___ _____

EVALUATION

1. Inspected condition of client's skin.

___ ___ ___ _____

2. Asked client to rate sense of comfort.

___ ___ ___ _____

3. Assessed client's orientation.

___ ___ ___ _____

4. Identified unexpected outcomes.

___ ___ ___ _____

RECORDING AND REPORTING

1. Recorded transfer of client to bed, tolerance to procedure, condition of skin in nurses' notes, or skin flowsheet.

___ ___ ___ _____

2. Reported changes in condition of skin and electrolyte levels to nurse in charge or physician.

___ ___ ___ _____

3. Reported restlessness or change in orientation.

___ ___ ___ _____

Student _____   Date _____

Instructor _____   Date _____

PERFORMANCE CHECKLIST 32-3   **PLACING A CLIENT ON AN AIR-FLUIDIZED BED**

	S	U	NP	Comments

ASSESSMENT

1. Performed pressure ulcer risk assessment to identify clients who would benefit from air-fluidized therapy.

2. Reviewed client's medical orders.

3. Assessed condition of client's skin.

4. Assessed client's level of consciousness.

5. Assessed client's and family member's understanding of purpose of bed.

6. Reviewed client's serum electrolyte levels in medical record.

7. Identified clients at risk for complications of air-fluidized therapy.

NURSING DIAGNOSIS

1. Developed appropriate nursing diagnoses based on assessment data.

PLANNING

1. Developed individualized goals for client based on nursing diagnoses.

2. Identified expected outcomes.

3. Explained procedure and purpose of bed to client and family.

4. Obtained any additional personnel needed to transfer client to bed.

5. Reviewed instructions supplied by bed manufacturer.

6. Washed hands and applied gloves (as indicated).

7. Premedicated clients, as necessary, 30 minutes before transfer.

IMPLEMENTATION

1. Closed client's room door or bedside curtain.

2. Explained steps of transfer.

3. Transferred client to bed.

4. Turned fluidization cycle on and regulated temperature.

	S	U	NP	Comments

5. Positioned client and performed ROM exercises as appropriate.   ___ ___ ___ _____

6. Correctly set fluidization mode for other therapies.   ___ ___ ___ _____

7. In event of emergency, defluidized bed.   ___ ___ ___ _____

8. Removed gloves (if worn) and washed hands.   ___ ___ ___ _____

EVALUATION

1. Asked client to rate ability to sleep or rest.   ___ ___ ___ _____

2. Inspected condition of client's skin while on bed and monitored risk assessment.   ___ ___ ___ _____

3. Reviewed client's serum electrolyte levels, monitored body temperature, and noted hydration status of skin and mucous membranes.   ___ ___ ___ _____

4. Measured client's level of orientation.   ___ ___ ___ _____

5. Identified unexpected outcomes.   ___ ___ ___ _____

RECORDING AND REPORTING

1. Recorded transfer of client to bed, tolerance to procedure, and condition of skin in nurses' notes.   ___ ___ ___ _____

2. Reported changes in condition of skin and electrolyte levels to nurse in charge or physician.   ___ ___ ___ _____

3. Reported change in orientation.   ___ ___ ___ _____

Student _____ Date _____

Instructor _____ Date _____

PERFORMANCE CHECKLIST 32-4 **PLACING A CLIENT ON A BARIATRIC BED**

	S	U	NP	Comments
ASSESSMENT				
1. Identified clients who would benefit from the bariatric bed system.	—	—	—	_____
2. Assessed condition of client's skin, particularly potential pressure sites.	—	—	—	_____
3. Determined client's and family member's understanding of purpose of bed.	—	—	—	_____
4. Reviewed client's medical orders.	—	—	—	_____
NURSING DIAGNOSIS				
1. Developed appropriate nursing diagnoses based on assessment data.	—	—	—	_____
PLANNING				
1. Developed individualized goals for client based on nursing diagnoses.	—	—	—	_____
2. Identified expected outcomes.	—	—	—	_____
3. Obtained additional personnel needed to transfer client to bed.	—	—	—	_____
4. Reviewed instructions supplied by bed manufacturer.	—	—	—	_____
5. Explained procedure and purpose of bed to client and family.	—	—	—	_____
6. Premedicated client, as necessary, 30 minutes before transfer.	—	—	—	_____
IMPLEMENTATION				
1. Provided privacy.	—	—	—	_____
2. Explained steps of transfer.	—	—	—	_____
3. Washed hands and applied gloves (as indicated) before assisting client to bed using appropriate transfer techniques.	—	—	—	_____
4. Covered and positioned client, placed hand controls within reach. Attached overhead frame if needed.	—	—	—	_____
5. Removed gloves (if worn) and washed hands.	—	—	—	_____
EVALUATION				
1. Inspected condition of skin.	—	—	—	_____

	S	U	NP	Comments
2. Asked client to rate sense of comfort and safety.	___	___	___	_____
3. Evaluated client's risk for injury.	___	___	___	_____
4. Evaluated client's ability to manipulate bed.	___	___	___	_____
5. Identified unexpected outcomes.	___	___	___	_____

RECORDING AND REPORTING

	S	U	NP	Comments
1. Recorded transfer of client to bed, tolerance of procedure, and condition of skin in nurses' notes or skin assessment flowsheet.	___	___	___	_____
2. Reported changes in condition of skin to nurse in charge or physician.	___	___	___	_____

Student _____   Date _____

Instructor _____   Date _____

PERFORMANCE CHECKLIST 33-1 **HAND WASHING**

	S	U	NP	Comments

ASSESSMENT

1. Inspected surface of hands and fingers for cuts or breaks.

2. Inspected hands for heavy soiling.

3. Assessed client's risk for or extent of infection.

NURSING DIAGNOSIS

1. Developed appropriate nursing diagnoses.

PLANNING

1. Established goals for procedure.

2. Identified expected outcomes.

IMPLEMENTATION

1. Removed jewelry and pushed clothing or wrist-watch above wrist level.

2. Kept fingernails short and filed.

3. Stood at sink without touching sink with hands or uniform.

4. Regulated water flow.

5. Avoided splashing.

6. Adjusted water temperature to "warm."

7. Wet hands and lowered arms, keeping them lower than the elbows.

8. Applied antiseptic liquid soap to hands.

9. Lathered hands and applied friction to skin surfaces for 10-15 seconds on each hand; interlaced fingers and rubbed palms and back of hands in circular motion.

10. Cleaned thoroughly under fingernails.

11. Rinsed thoroughly, keeping hands below elbows.

12. Repeated Steps 10-12 but extended period of washing (optional).

13. Dried hands thoroughly, wiping from fingers up to wrists and forearms.

14. Discarded paper towel properly.

15. Turned off water at sink.

	S	U	NP	Comments
EVALUATION				
1. Inspected surface of hands.	—	—	—	_____
2. Identified unexpected outcomes.	—	—	—	_____

Student _____   Date _____

Instructor _____   Date _____

PERFORMANCE CHECKLIST 33-2 **CARING FOR CLIENTS UNDER ISOLATION PRECAUTIONS**

	S	U	NP	Comments
ASSESSMENT				
1. Reviewed precautions for client's specific isolation category.	—	—	—	_____
2. Reviewed appropriate laboratory test results.	—	—	—	_____
3. Considered types of care to be delivered to client.	—	—	—	_____
4. Assessed client's emotional status.	—	—	—	_____
5. Determined client's understanding of purpose of isolation and procedures.	—	—	—	_____
6. Determined if client allergic to latex.	—	—	—	_____
NURSING DIAGNOSIS				
1. Developed appropriate nursing diagnoses based on client's isolated status.	—	—	—	_____
PLANNING				
1. Developed individualized goals for client based on nursing diagnoses.	—	—	—	_____
2. Identified expected outcomes.	—	—	—	_____
3. Prepared equipment and supplies.	—	—	—	_____
IMPLEMENTATION				
1. Washed hands.	—	—	—	_____
2. Applied protective wear:	—	—	—	_____
a. Applied isolation gown correctly and secured ties at neck and waist.	—	—	—	_____
b. Applied disposable gloves with edges overlying gown cuffs.	—	—	—	_____
c. Applied mask or respirator securely over nose and mouth.	—	—	—	_____
d. Applied goggles if needed to fit snugly around face and eyes.	—	—	—	_____
3. Entered client's room. Arranged supplies and equipment.	—	—	—	_____
4. Explained purpose of isolation and necessary precautions to client, family, visitors.	—	—	—	_____

	S	U	NP	Comments

5. Assessed vital signs: ___ ___ ___ _____

   a. Placed clean paper towel on bedside table with additional paper towel on top. ___ ___ ___ _____

   b. Placed watch on towel for easy visibility. ___ ___ ___ _____

   c. Avoided contact of equipment with infective material while assessing vital signs. ___ ___ ___ _____

   d. Recorded vital signs on clean paper towel at bedside. ___ ___ ___ _____

   e. Returned stethoscope to clean surface, cleansed diaphragm/bell with alcohol as needed. ___ ___ ___ _____

6. Administered medications: ___ ___ ___ _____

   a. Gave oral medication in wrapper or cup. ___ ___ ___ _____

   b. Properly disposed of wrapper or cup. ___ ___ ___ _____

   c. Administered injection wearing gloves. ___ ___ ___ _____

   d. Discarded syringe and uncapped needle in proper receptacle. ___ ___ ___ _____

   e. Placed reusable syringe on clean towel for removal. ___ ___ ___ _____

7. Administered hygiene: ___ ___ ___ _____

   a. Prevented isolation gown from becoming wet. ___ ___ ___ _____

   b. Assisted client in removing gown and disposed of appropriately. ___ ___ ___ _____

   c. Removed linen from bed and disposed of appropriately. ___ ___ ___ _____

   d. Provided clean linen and towels. ___ ___ ___ _____

   e. Changed gloves if necessary. ___ ___ ___ _____

8. Collected specimens: ___ ___ ___ _____

   a. Placed specimen containers on clean paper towel in bathroom. ___ ___ ___ _____

   b. Followed procedure for specimen collection. ___ ___ ___ _____

   c. Transferred collected specimen to appropriate container without contaminating container's outer surface. Transferred specimens correctly into plastic bag held by second nurse standing outside room. ___ ___ ___ _____

   d. Checked label for accuracy. Sent specimen to laboratory. ___ ___ ___ _____

Student _____ Date _____

Instructor _____ Date _____

	S	U	NP	Comments
9. Disposed of linen and trash bags:	—	—	—	_____
a. Used appropriate bags for soiled articles.	—	—	—	_____
b. Tied bags securely.	—	—	—	_____
10. Resupplied room as needed with another care-giver handling supplies at door.	—	—	—	_____
11. Left isolation room:	—	—	—	_____
a. Removed eyewear or goggles.	—	—	—	_____
b. Untied gown at waist.	—	—	—	_____
c. Removed gloves by turning inside out, avoiding contact with contaminated surfaces. Untied and removed mask. Disposed of mask.	—	—	—	_____
d. Untied neck strings of gown. Allowed gown to fall from shoulders.	—	—	—	_____
e. Pulled gown off correctly and discarded in receptacle. Washed hands thoroughly.	—	—	—	_____
f. Picked up wristwatch and stethoscope before leaving room and noted vital signs recorded in room.	—	—	—	_____
g. Determined client's needs before leaving room.	—	—	—	_____
h. Left room and closed door.	—	—	—	_____

EVALUATION

	S	U	NP	Comments
1. While in room, determined if client has had opportunity to discuss health problems, course of treatment, and related concerns.	—	—	—	_____
2. Identified unexpected outcomes.	—	—	—	_____

RECORDING AND REPORTING

	S	U	NP	Comments
1. Documented client's response to social isolation in nurse's notes.	—	—	—	_____

Student _____   Date _____

Instructor _____   Date _____

PERFORMANCE CHECKLIST 34-1 **DONNING AND REMOVING CAP AND MASK**

	S	U	NP	Comments

ASSESSMENT

1. Determined need to apply cap or mask. ___ ___ ___ _____

2. Considered risk of transmitting infection to client. ___ ___ ___ _____

NURSING DIAGNOSIS

1. Developed appropriate nursing diagnoses based on assessment data. ___ ___ ___ _____

PLANNING

1. Developed individualized goals for client based on assessment data. ___ ___ ___ _____

2. Identified expected outcomes. ___ ___ ___ _____

3. Prepared equipment. ___ ___ ___ _____

IMPLEMENTATION
Donning Cap

1. Combed long hair back and arranged on crown of head. ___ ___ ___ _____

2. Secured hair in place. ___ ___ ___ _____

3. Applied cap over all of hair. ___ ___ ___ _____

4. Applied hood over head to cover facial hair if indicated. ___ ___ ___ _____

Donning Mask

1. Located top edge of mask. ___ ___ ___ _____

2. Held mask by top two ties with top edge of mask above nose. ___ ___ ___ _____

3. Tied top strings at top of back of head properly. ___ ___ ___ _____

4. Tied two lower strings snugly around neck with mask under chin. ___ ___ ___ _____

5. Pinched upper metal bank around bridge of nose. ___ ___ ___ _____

Disposing of Cap and Mask

1. Untied top strings of mask. ___ ___ ___ _____

2. Untied bottom strings and removed mask from face. ___ ___ ___ _____

3. Grasped outer surface of cap and lifted from hair. ___ ___ ___ _____

4. Discarded cap and mask in receptacle and washed hands. ___ ___ ___ _____

	S	U	NP	Comments

EVALUATION

1. Assessed the client for signs of infection.   ___ ___ ___ _____

2. Identified unexpected outcomes.   ___ ___ ___ _____

RECORDING AND REPORTING

1. Recorded procedure performed and client's status.   ___ ___ ___ _____

Student _____ Date _____

Instructor _____ Date _____

PERFORMANCE CHECKLIST 34-2 **PREPARING A STERILE FIELD**

	S	U	NP	Comments

ASSESSMENT

1. Verified procedure requires sterile technique.

2. Checked integrity of sterile packages.

3. Determined client's comfort and elimination needs before procedure.

4. Anticipated number and variety of supplies needed.

NURSING DIAGNOSIS

1. Developed appropriate nursing diagnoses based on assessment data.

PLANNING

1. Developed individualized goals for client based on assessment data.

2. Identified expected outcomes.

3. Prepared equipment at bedside.

4. Checked sterilization expiration dates.

5. Positioned client comfortably.

6. Explained purpose of procedure and sterile technique.

IMPLEMENTATION

1. Applied cap and mask as needed.

2. Selected clean work surface above waist level.

3. Washed hands.

Preparing Sterile Work Surface

1. Placed sterile kit or package on clean work surface above waist level.

2. Opened sterile kit, pulling paper wrapper off away from body.

3. Used opened kit or package as sterile field.

Preparing a Sterile Drape

1. Placed sterile drape pack on flat surface and opened with sterile technique.

2. Donned sterile gloves and sterile gown.

	S	U	NP	Comments

3. Using fingertips, picked up folded top edge of sterile drape. ___ ___ ___ _____

4. Lifted drape from outer cover and let it unfold without touching any object; discarded outer cover. ___ ___ ___ _____

5. With nondominant hand, grasped adjacent corner of drape; held drape straight up and away from body. ___ ___ ___ _____

6. Held the drape and positioned bottom half over work surface. ___ ___ ___ _____

7. Allowed top half of drape to be placed over work surface last. ___ ___ ___ _____

8. Gowned nurse placed top half of drape over work surface first (optional). ___ ___ ___ _____

Adding Sterile Items

1. Grasped outside wrapper of sterile package in nondominant hand and opened sterile item. ___ ___ ___ _____

2. Peeled wrapper onto the nondominant hand. ___ ___ ___ _____

3. Placed item onto sterile field without reaching over sterile field. ___ ___ ___ _____

4. Disposed of outer wrapper. ___ ___ ___ _____

Pouring Sterile Solutions

1. Verified contents and expiration date of solution. ___ ___ ___ _____

2. Removed seal and cap from bottle in an upward motion. ___ ___ ___ _____

3. Poured solution slowly, holding edge of bottle well above and away from edge and inside of sterile container. ___ ___ ___ _____

4. Discarded any remaining fluid and bottle. ___ ___ ___ _____

EVALUATION

1. Observed client for signs of local infection. ___ ___ ___ _____

2. Identified unexpected outcomes. ___ ___ ___ _____

RECORDING AND REPORTING

1. Recorded area and description of treatment site. ___ ___ ___ _____

Student _____ Date _____

Instructor _____ Date _____

PERFORMANCE CHECKLIST 34-3 **OPEN GLOVING**

	S	U	NP	Comments

ASSESSMENT

1. Considered procedure to be performed and consulted institutional policy on use of gloves. ___ ___ ___ _____

2. Considered client's risk for infection. ___ ___ ___ _____

3. Examined condition of glove package. ___ ___ ___ _____

4. Inspected condition of hands. ___ ___ ___ _____

5. Determined if client is allergic to latex. ___ ___ ___ _____

NURSING DIAGNOSIS

1. Developed appropriate nursing diagnoses based on assessment data. ___ ___ ___ _____

PLANNING

1. Developed individualized goals for client based on assessment data. ___ ___ ___ _____

2. Identified expected outcomes. ___ ___ ___ _____

3. Selected correct size and type of gloves. ___ ___ ___ _____

4. Placed glove package near work area. ___ ___ ___ _____

IMPLEMENTATION

1. Washed hands thoroughly. ___ ___ ___ _____

2. Removed outer glove wrapper. ___ ___ ___ _____

3. Opened inner package, keeping gloves on wrapper's inside surface, and laid package on surface at waist level. ___ ___ ___ _____

4. Applied powder to hands as desired. ___ ___ ___ _____

5. Identified right and left glove. ___ ___ ___ _____

6. With nondominant hand, grasped inside edge of cuff of glove for dominant hand. ___ U ___ _____

7. Carefully pulled glove over dominant hand with thumb and fingers in proper spaces. ___ ___ ___ _____

8. With gloved dominant hand, slipped fingers under cuff of second glove. ___ ___ ___ _____

9. Pulled glove over nondominant hand without contaminating gloved dominant hand. ___ ___ ___ _____

10. Interlocked fingers of gloved hands to ensure proper fit. ___ ___ ___ _____

	S	U	NP	Comments

Glove Disposal

1. Grasped outside of one cuff with other gloved hand.

2. Pulled glove off, turning it inside out. Discarded in receptacle.

3. Slid fingers of ungloved hand underneath cuff of gloved hand and pulled remaining glove off; discarded glove in receptacle.

4. Washed hands.

EVALUATION

1. Assessed client for signs of infection.

2. Identified unexpected outcomes.

RECORDING AND REPORTING

1. Recorded procedure performed and client's response and status.

Student _____   Date _____

Instructor _____   Date _____

PERFORMANCE CHECKLIST 35-1   **PREPARING THE CLIENT FOR SURGERY**

	S	U	NP	Comments

ASSESSMENT

1. Determine client's ability to answer questions.

2. Obtained nursing history.

3. Performed physical examination.

4. Identified risk factors.

5. Asked client's and family member's expectations of surgery.

6. Assessed client's preoperative orders.

NURSING DIAGNOSIS

1. Developed appropriate nursing diagnoses based on assessment data.

PLANNING

1. Developed individualized goals based on nursing diagnoses.

2. Identified expected outcomes.

3. Prepared client's chart and assembled necessary equipment.

4. Explained procedures and allowed client, family members, or significant others to ask questions.

IMPLEMENTATION

1. Oriented client to room or presurgical area.

2. Checked medical record and completed preoperative checklist.

3. Assisted with informed consent.

4. Provided preoperative teaching.

5. Instructed client on the need and rationale for NPO for 4 to 8 hours prior to surgery.

6. Provided for oral hygiene.

7. Provided privacy and instructed client to remove clothes and put on gown and cap.

8. Instructed client to remove hair appliances, jewelry, and makeup.

9. Assisted client to remove prostheses. Inventoried and stored valuables per agency policy.

	S	U	NP	Comments

10. Applied antiembolism stockings as ordered.

11. Assessed vital signs immediately before going to OR.

12. Assisted client to void prior to receiving preoperative medication.

13. Administered preoperative medications as ordered.

14. Placed client on bed rest with side rails up and call light within reach.

EVALUATION

1. Compared assessment data with client's baseline and expected normals.

2. Had client repeat preoperative instructions and demonstrate postoperative exercises.

3. Assessed client for signs and symptoms of anxiety.

4. Identified unexpected outcomes.

RECORDING AND REPORTING

1. Documented all preoperative preparations in nurses' notes and/or checklist.

2. Documented client condition on transfer to OR.

3. Reported abnormal findings, lack of signed consent form, or failure to maintain NPO status.

Student _____   Date _____

Instructor _____   Date _____

PERFORMANCE CHECKLIST 35-2   **DEMONSTRATING POSTOPERATIVE EXERCISES**

	S	U	NP	Comments

ASSESSMENT
1. Assessed client's risk for postoperative respiratory complications. —— —— —— _____

2. Assessed client's ability to cough and deep breathe. —— —— —— _____

3. Assessed client's risk for postoperative thrombus formation. —— —— —— _____

4. Assessed client's ability to move independently in bed. —— —— —— _____

5. Assessed client's willingness and ability to learn exercises. —— —— —— _____

6. Assessed family members' willingness to learn and to support client. —— —— —— _____

7. Assessed client's medical orders. —— —— —— _____

NURSING DIAGNOSIS
1. Developed appropriate nursing diagnoses based on assessment data. —— —— —— _____

PLANNING
1. Developed individualized goals for client based on nursing diagnoses. —— —— —— _____

2. Identified expected outcomes. —— —— —— _____

3. Prepared necessary equipment. —— —— —— _____

4. Provided opportunity for practice and return demonstrations. —— —— —— _____

IMPLEMENTATION
Teaching Diaphragmatic Breathing
1. Assisted client to comfortable sitting or standing position. —— —— —— _____

2. Stood or sat facing client. —— —— —— _____

3. Correctly placed hands on anterior rib cage. —— —— —— _____

4. Instructed client to take deep breaths. —— —— —— _____

5. Avoided using chest and shoulders while inhaling. —— —— —— _____

6. Held slow, deep breath for a count of 3 and exhaled. —— —— —— _____

7. Repeated breathing exercise three to five times. —— —— —— _____

8. Had client practice exercise. —— —— —— _____

Controlled Coughing
1. Explained to client importance of upright position. —— —— —— _____

2. Demonstrated two slow, deep breaths, inhaling through nose and exhaling through mouth. —— —— —— _____

	S	U	NP	Comments

3. Inhaled, held breath, and coughed.

4. Cautioned client against just clearing throat.

5. For abdominal or thoracic incision, taught client to place pillow over incisional area and hands on top of pillow.

6. Had client continue to practice coughing exercises, splinting imaginary incision.

7. Instructed client to examine characteristics of sputum.

Turning

1. Instructed client to assume supine position on right side of bed.

2. Instructed client to place left hand over incisional area to splint it.

3. Instructed client to keep left leg straight and flex right knee up and over left leg.

4. Had client grab left side rail with right hand, pull toward left, and roll onto left side.

5. Instructed client to turn every 2 hours while awake.

Leg Exercises

1. Had client assume supine position and demonstrated passive range-of-motion exercises.

2. Rotated each ankle.

3. Alternated dorsiflexion and plantar flexion of both feet.

4. Had client flex and extend knees.

5. Had client alternately raise each leg straight up from bed, keeping legs straight.

6. Had client continue to practice exercises at least every 2 hours.

EVALUATION

1. Observed client's ability to perform all four exercises independently.

2. Observed family members' ability to coach client.

3. Assessed client's chest excursion.

4. Auscultated client's lungs.

5. Assessed for Homans' sign.

6. Identified unexpected outcomes.

RECORDING AND REPORTING

1. Recorded those exercises that had been demonstrated to client and whether client could perform exercises independently.

2. Recorded physical assessment findings in nurses' notes or flowsheet.

3. Reported any problems to the next shift.

Student _____   Date _____

Instructor _____   Date _____

PERFORMANCE CHECKLIST 35-3 **PREPARING THE SURGICAL SITE**

	S	U	NP	Comments

ASSESSMENT

1. Inspected general condition of skin.

2. Assessed for allergy to iodine or shellfish.

3. Reviewed physician's order for area to be shaved.

4. Assessed for bleeding tendency.

5. Assessed client's understanding and acceptance of hair removal.

NURSING DIAGNOSIS

1. Developed appropriate nursing diagnoses based on assessment data.

PLANNING

1. Developed individual goals for client based on nursing diagnoses.

2. Identified expected outcomes.

3. Prepared needed equipment at bedside.

4. Explained procedure and rationale for shaving a larger surface area.

IMPLEMENTATION

1. Washed hands.

2. Closed room doors and bed curtains for privacy and raised bed to high position.

3. Positioned client with surgical site accessible.

4. Applied disposable gloves.

5. Depilatory hair removal:

    a. Applied depilatory cream to area.

    b. Waited required time and wiped off cream.

    c. Washed and rinsed skin.

6. Hair clipping:

    a. Lightly dried area to be clipped with towel.

    b. Held clippers in dominant hand and clipped hair in direction of growth.

    c. Rearranged drapes as necessary.

	S	U	NP	Comments

d. Lightly brushed off cut hair with towel.

e. Cleansed areas over body crevices with anti-septic solution.

7. Wet shave:

a. Placed towel or waterproof pad under area to be shaved.

b. Draped client correctly with bath blanket.

c. Adjusted lamp.

d. Lathered skin with gauze sponges dipped in antiseptic soap.

e. Correctly shaved small area at a time.

f. Rinsed razor as soap and hair accumulated on the blade; changed and discarded blades as they became dull.

g. Rearranged bath blanket as each portion of the shave was completed.

h. Used washcloth and warm water to rinse away hair and soap solution; changed water as necessary.

i. Cleansed areas over body crevices with anti-septic solution.

j. Dried body crevices.

k. Discarded waterproof towel or pad.

l. Observed skin closely for nicks or cuts.

8. Told client when procedure was completed.

9. Cleaned and disposed of equipment properly. Disposed of gloves.

10. Washed hands.

EVALUATION

1. Inspected condition of the skin.

2. Evaluated client's response to procedure.

3. Identified unexpected outcomes.

RECORDING AND REPORTING

1. Recorded procedure, area clipped or shaved, and condition of skin in nurses' notes.

2. Reported any skin alterations to physician.

Student _____   Date _____

Instructor _____   Date _____

PERFORMANCE CHECKLIST 35-4 **INSERTING AND MAINTAINING THE NASOGASTRIC TUBE**

	S	U	NP	Comments

ASSESSMENT

1. Inspected condition of client's nasal and oral cavity. ___ ___ ___ _____

2. Determined history of nasal surgery and noted if deviated nasal septum present. ___ ___ ___ _____

3. Palpated client's abdomen. ___ ___ ___ _____

4. Assessed client's level of consciousness and ability to follow instructions. ___ ___ ___ _____

NURSING DIAGNOSIS

1. Developed appropriate nursing diagnoses based on assessment data. ___ ___ ___ _____

PLANNING

1. Developed individualized goals for client based on nursing diagnoses. ___ ___ ___ _____

2. Identified expected outcomes. ___ ___ ___ _____

3. Checked medical record for surgeon's order and type of NG tube to be placed; type of suction or drainage bag. ___ ___ ___ _____

4. Prepared equipment at bedside. ___ ___ ___ _____

5. Identified client and explained procedure. ___ ___ ___ _____

IMPLEMENTATION

1. Washed hands and applied gloves. ___ ___ ___ _____

2. Positioned client in high Fowler's position with pillows behind head and shoulder. ___ ___ ___ _____

3. Provided privacy. ___ ___ ___ _____

4. Stood at correct side of bed. ___ ___ ___ _____

5. Placed bath towel over client's chest. ___ U ___ _____

6. Determined which nostril to use. ___ ___ ___ _____

7. Measured distance to insert tube using traditional or Hanson method. ___ ___ ___ _____

8. Marked length of tube to be inserted from nares to stomach. ___ ___ ___ _____

9. Prepared a piece of tape to anchor tube. ___ ___ ___ _____

S   U   NP   Comments

10. Curved tip of NG tube tightly around index finger and then released.

____ ____ ____ _____

11. Lubricated 3-4 inches of the end of tube with water-soluble lubricating jelly.

____ ____ ____ _____

12. Instructed client to extend neck and inserted tube slowly through naris with curved end pointing downward.

____ ____ ____ _____

13. Continued to pass tube along floor of nasal passage.

____ ____ ____ _____

14. If resistance met, rotated tube or withdrew tube, allowed client to rest, relubricated tube, and inserted into other naris.

____ ____ ____ _____

15. Continued tube insertion by gently rotating tube toward opposite naris; stopped tube advancement; allowed client to relax; provided tissues; explained to client that next step requires client to swallow.

____ ____ ____ _____

16. With tube above oropharynx, instructed client to flex head forward and dry swallow or suck in air through a straw; advanced the tube 1-2 inches with each swallow.

____ ____ ____ _____

17. If client began to cough, gag, or choke, stopped tube advancement; instructed client to breathe easily and take sips of water.

____ ____ ____ _____

18. If client continued to cough, pulled tube back slightly.

____ ____ ____ _____

19. If client continued to gag, checked back of pharynx.

____ ____ ____ _____

20. After client relaxed, continued to advance tube the desired distance.

____ ____ ____ _____

21. Once tube advanced, anchored tube with prepared split tape.

____ ____ ____ _____

Checking Tube Placement

1. Asked client to talk.

____ ____ ____ _____

2. Checked posterior pharynx for coiling of tube.

____ ____ ____ _____

3. Auscultated over stomach while injecting air.

____ ____ ____ _____

4. Aspirated gently back on syringe to obtain gastric contents.

____ ____ ____ _____

5. Measured pH of aspirate.

____ ____ ____ _____

6. If tube not in stomach, advanced 1-2 inches and repeated Steps 3 and 4 to check tube position.

____ ____ ____ _____

Student _____ Date _____

Instructor _____ Date _____

	S	U	NP	Comments

Anchoring Tube

1. After tube was properly inserted, either clamped end or connected to a drainage bag or suction machine.

2. Cut 4-inch piece of tape; split one end lengthwise 2 inches; placed tab of tape over bridge of nose; wrapped ½-inch strips around tube as it exited nose; avoided putting pressure on naris.

3. Fastened end of NG tube to client's gown with rubber band and safety pin; provided slack for client's movement.

4. Kept head of bed elevated 30 degrees.

5. Explained that sensation of tube should decrease.

6. Removed gloves and washed hands.

Tube Irrigation

1. Washed hands and applied gloves.

2. Checked tube placement.

3. Drew up 30 ml normal saline into Asepto or catheter-tipped syringe.

4. Clamped tube proximal to connection site for drainage or suction; disconnected tube and laid end on towel.

5. Inserted tip of syringe into end of NG tube; held syringe with tip pointed at the floor and slowly injected solution; did not force.

6. If resistance occurred, checked tube for kinks; turned client onto left side.

7. After instilling saline, aspirated with syringe to withdraw fluids; measured volume returned.

8. Reconnected NG tube to drainage or suction; if solution did not return, repeated irrigation.

9. Removed gloves and washed hands.

Discontinuation of NG Tube

1. Verified order to discontinue NG tube.

2. Washed hands and applied disposable gloves.

3. Explained procedure to client.

4. Turned off suction; disconnected NG tube from drainage bag or suction; removed tape from nose; unpinned tube from gown.

S   U   NP   Comments

5. Provided client facial tissue and placed towel across chest.

___ ___ ___ _____

6. Pulled tube out steadily and smoothly as client held breath.

___ ___ ___ _____

7. Disposed of tube and drainage unit; measured drainage.

___ ___ ___ _____

8. Cleaned nares and provided mouth care.

___ ___ ___ _____

9. Positioned client and explained fluid intake.

___ ___ ___ _____

10. Cleaned and stored equipment.

___ ___ ___ _____

11. Removed gloves and washed hands.

___ ___ ___ _____

EVALUATION

1. Observed amount and character of NG drainage.

___ ___ ___ _____

2. Palpated client's abdomen and auscultated bowel sounds.

___ ___ ___ _____

3. Inspected condition of nares and nose.

___ ___ ___ _____

4. Observed position of tubing.

___ ___ ___ _____

5. Asked if client felt pharyngeal irritation.

___ ___ ___ _____

6. Identified unexpected outcomes.

___ ___ ___ _____

RECORDING AND REPORTING

1. Recorded insertion procedure, client's tolerance, and character of drainage correctly in nurses' notes.

___ ___ ___ _____

2. Recorded tube irrigation and amount and type of aspirate correctly.

___ ___ ___ _____

3. Recorded balance of fluid instilled and aspirated on I&O sheet.

___ ___ ___ _____

4. Recorded discontinuation of tube.

___ ___ ___ _____

5. Reported absence or character of drainage and onset of abdominal distention.

___ ___ ___ _____

6. Recorded presence or absence of bowel sounds.

___ ___ ___ _____

Student _____   Date _____

Instructor _____   Date _____

PERFORMANCE CHECKLIST 35-5 **PERFORMING POSTOPERATIVE CARE OF THE SURGICAL CLIENT**

	S	U	NP	Comments
ASSESSMENT				
Immediate Recovery Period				
1. Assessed client's condition during operative procedure.	—	—	—	_____
2. Obtained report from surgeon and anesthesiologist.	—	—	—	_____
3. Considered surgery performed.	—	—	—	_____
4. Performed thorough client assessment.	—	—	—	_____
Convalescent Period				
1. Received phone report from recovery nurse.	—	—	—	_____
2. Obtained detailed report from nurse at time of client's transfer to division.	—	—	—	_____
3. Reviewed client's medical record.	—	—	—	_____
4. Reviewed surgeon's postoperative orders.	—	—	—	_____
NURSING DIAGNOSIS				
1. Developed appropriate nursing diagnoses based on assessment data.	—	—	—	_____
PLANNING				
1. Developed individualized goals for client based on nursing diagnoses.	—	—	—	_____
2. Identified expected outcomes.	—	—	—	_____
3. Prepared equipment at bedside.	—	—	—	_____
4. Explained procedures to client.	—	—	—	_____
IMPLEMENTATION				
Immediate Recovery Period				
1. Washed hands.	—	—	—	_____
2. Checked equipment setup.	—	—	—	_____
3. Immediately after client entered recovery room, attached oxygen equipment and drainage tubes and checked IV flow rates.	—	—	—	_____
4. Assessed vital signs and continued monitoring as needed.	—	—	—	_____
5. Maintained patent airway correctly.	—	—	—	_____

	S	U	NP	Comments

6. Called client by name and oriented client to surroundings. — — — _____

7. Assessed circulatory perfusion. — — — _____

8. Inspected surgical dressing and drains for bright red blood. — — — _____

9. Inspected area of surgical wound. — — — _____

10. Inspected condition of dressing. — — — _____

11. Reinforced dressing as needed. — — — _____

12. Inspected condition and contents of drainage tubes. — — — _____

13. Observed patency and intactness of urinary catheter and volume and character of urine. — — — _____

14. If NG tube was present, irrigated as needed. — — — _____

15. Monitored IV fluid infusion. — — — _____

16. Provided client mouth care. — — — _____

17. Assessed client's pain and administered analgesia as ordered. — — — _____

18. Explained to client status of recovery. — — — _____

19. Contacted physician for order to transfer client. — — — _____

Convalescent Period

1. Checked equipment setup. — — — _____

2. Transferred client to bed. — — — _____

3. Connected any existing oxygen tubing and regulated IV infusion. — — — _____

4. Assessed vital signs routinely as ordered. — — — _____

5. Maintained airway correctly. — — — _____

6. Ensured patency and intactness of all drainage tubes. — — — _____

7. Inspected condition of dressing or wound. — — — _____

8. Assessed client for bladder distention. — — — _____

9. Measured sources of fluid intake and output. — — — _____

10. Positioned client for comfort. — — — _____

11. Applied elastic stockings or pneumatic compression cuffs. — — — _____

12. Explained to client nature of observations and allowed family into room. — — — _____

Student _____   Date _____

Instructor _____   Date _____

	S	U	NP	Comments

13. Explained activities and purpose of room equipment to family.

14. Administered analgesia appropriately.

15. Provided oral hygiene.

16. Maintained support measures for functioning body systems.

17. Increased client's involvement in decision making.

18. Included family in discussion regarding discharge.

EVALUATION

1. Compared assessment findings with client's baseline and expected range.

2. Evaluated pain relief measures.

3. Monitored changes in surgical wound.

4. Monitored lung sounds.

5. Auscultated client's bowel sounds.

6. Monitored I&O.

7. Discussed client's feelings about recovery.

8. Routinely conducted needed physical assessments.

9. Identified unexpected outcomes.

RECORDING AND REPORTING

1. Recorded client's arrival at recovery room or nursing division, assessments made, nursing care initiated on nurses' notes.

2. Recorded vital signs and I&O on flowsheets.

3. Reported abnormal assessment findings and signs of complications to nurse in charge or physician.

Student _____   Date _____

Instructor _____   Date _____

PERFORMANCE CHECKLIST 36-1 **SURGICAL HAND WASHING**

	S	U	NP	Comments

ASSESSMENT

1. Checked institutional policy for length of time for hand washing.   ___ ___ ___ _____

2. Assessed condition of nails for length and presence of polish.   ___ ___ ___ _____

3. Inspected condition of hands.   ___ ___ ___ _____

NURSING DIAGNOSIS

1. Developed appropriate nursing diagnoses based on assessment data.   ___ ___ ___ _____

PLANNING

1. Developed individualized goals for client based on nursing diagnoses.   ___ ___ ___ _____

2. Identified expected outcomes.   ___ ___ ___ _____

3. Prepared needed equipment.   ___ ___ ___ _____

4. Removed all jewelry.   ___ ___ ___ _____

5. Made sure uniform was fitted or tucked at waist with sleeves above elbows.   ___ ___ ___ _____

IMPLEMENTATION

1. Applied appropriate surgical attire.   ___ ___ ___ _____

2. Wet hands and arms under lukewarm water and lathered with detergent to 2 inches above elbows.   ___ ___ ___ _____

3. Rinsed hands and arms thoroughly under running water.   ___ ___ ___ _____

4. Cleaned under surface of nails with hands under running water.   ___ ___ ___ _____

5. Wet brush and applied antimicrobial soap. Scrubbed nails of one hand with 15 strokes. Scrubbed palm, each side of thumb, posterior side of hand with 10 strokes each. Divided arm in three sections and scrubbed each 10 times. Repeated sequence for other arm.   ___ ___ ___ _____

6. Discarded brush and rinsed hands and arm thoroughly; turned off water with foot or knee pedal.   ___ ___ ___ _____

7. Used sterile towel to dry one hand thoroughly, moving from fingers to elbow.   ___ ___ ___ _____

	S	U	NP	Comments

8. Repeated drying method for other hand, using different area of towel or new sterile towel.   — — — _____

EVALUATION

1. Observed client for signs of localized wound infection.   — — — _____

2. Identified unexpected outcomes.   — — — _____

RECORDING AND REPORTING

1. Recorded area and description of surgical site postoperatively.   — — — _____

Student _____   Date _____

Instructor _____   Date _____

PERFORMANCE CHECKLIST 36-2 **DONNING A STERILE GOWN AND GLOVES (CLOSED GLOVING)**

	S	U	NP	Comments
ASSESSMENT				
1. Inspected condition of hands.	—	—	—	_____
2. Checked fingernails.	—	—	—	_____
3. Chose proper type and size of glove and gown.	—	—	—	_____
NURSING DIAGNOSIS				
1. Developed appropriate nursing diagnoses based on assessment data.	—	—	—	_____
PLANNING				
1. Developed individualized goals for client based on nursing diagnoses.	—	—	—	_____
2. Identified expected outcomes.	—	—	—	_____
3. Prepared equipment.	—	—	—	_____
IMPLEMENTATION				
Gowning				
1. Applied surgical attire before entering operating room.	—	—	—	_____
2. Performed surgical hand scrub.	—	—	—	_____
3. Asked circulating nurse to assist by opening sterile gown pack.	—	—	—	_____
4. Had circulating nurse prepare sterile glove package.	—	—	—	_____
5. Grasped gown appropriately and lifted from sterile package.	—	—	—	_____
6. Lifted gown and stepped away from table.	—	—	—	_____
7. Located neckband and grasped gown appropriately.	—	—	—	_____
8. Properly allowed gown to unfold.	—	—	—	_____
9. Inserted arms into gown and had circulating nurse bring gown over shoulders.	—	—	—	_____
10. Secured gown appropriately with assistance of circulating nurse.	—	—	—	_____
Closed Gloving				
11. Opened inner sterile glove package correctly.	—	—	—	_____

	S	U	NP	Comments

12. Picked up glove for dominant hand with non-dominant hand.

13. Placed glove on dominant palm correctly.

14. Glove cuff turned over end of dominant hand correctly.

15. Carefully extended fingers into glove.

16. Gloved nondominant hand in same manner.

17. Made sure fingers were fully extended into both gloves.

18. With wrap-around sterile gown, released fasteners on front of gown.

19. Gown flap wrapped and tied appropriately.

EVALUATION

1. Observed client for signs of localized or systemic infection.

2. Identified unexpected outcomes.

RECORDING AND REPORTING

1. Recorded area and description of surgical site postoperatively.

Student _____   Date _____

Instructor _____   Date _____

PERFORMANCE CHECKLIST 37-1 **APPLYING A DRY DRESSING**

	S	U	NP	Comments

ASSESSMENT

1. Accurately assessed size of wound.

2. Assessed location of wound.

3. Assessed client's comfort.

4. Assessed client's knowledge concerning dressing.

5. Assessed appropriateness of client and family participation.

6. Checked physician's orders.

7. Identified clients at risk for wound healing problems.

NURSING DIAGNOSIS

1. Developed appropriate nursing diagnoses based on assessment data.

PLANNING

1. Developed individualized goals for client based on nursing diagnoses.

2. Identified expected outcomes.

3. Explained procedure to client.

4. Assessed need for pain medication.

IMPLEMENTATION

1. Provided for client privacy. Washed hands. Applied gown, goggles, and mask if indicated.

2. Positioned client in comfortable manner.

3. Properly placed disposable bag. Put on clean disposable gloves.

4. Removed tape.

5. Removed dressing properly.

6. Observed drainage on dressing.

7. Properly disposed of dressing. Removed and disposed of gloves properly.

8. Opened sterile supplies properly.

9. Poured cleansing solution over gauze. Repeated procedure, if necessary.

	S	U	NP	Comments
10. Put on gloves.	—	—	—	_____
11. Inspected wound.	—	—	—	_____
12. Cleansed wound.	—	—	—	_____
13. Dried wound.	—	—	—	_____
14. Applied antiseptic ointment as ordered.	—	—	—	_____
15. Applied dressing.	—	—	—	_____
16. Secured dressing.	—	—	—	_____
17. Removed and disposed of gloves properly. Disposed of all supplies. Removed gown, mask, and goggles if worn.	—	—	—	_____
18. Positioned client comfortably.	—	—	—	_____
19. Washed hands.	—	—	—	_____

EVALUATION

1. Assessed condition of wound.	—	—	—	_____
2. Asked client if discomfort noted during procedure.	—	—	—	_____
3. Inspected condition of dressing.	—	—	—	_____
4. Asked client to describe steps and techniques of dressing change.	—	—	—	_____
5. Identified unexpected outcomes.	—	—	—	_____

RECORDING AND REPORTING

1. Reported dressing change and wound appearance appropriately.	—	—	—	_____
2. Recorded dressing change and wound appearance appropriately in nurses' notes.	—	—	—	_____
3. Recorded frequency of dressing change and supplies on care plan.	—	—	—	_____
4. Wrote date and time of dressing change on tape.	—	—	—	_____

Student _____   Date _____

Instructor _____   Date _____

PERFORMANCE CHECKLIST 37-2   **APPLYING A WET-TO-DRY DRESSING**

	S	U	NP	Comments
ASSESSMENT				
1. Assessed location and size of wound.	—	—	—	_____
2. Reviewed charts for baseline findings.	—	—	—	_____
3. Reviewed physician's orders.	—	—	—	_____
4. Assessed client's level of comfort.	—	—	—	_____
5. Assessed client's knowledge of purpose of dressing change.	—	—	—	_____
6. Assessed need for client or family member to participate in dressing wound.	—	—	—	_____
7. Identified clients at risk for wound healing.	—	—	—	_____
NURSING DIAGNOSIS				
1. Developed appropriate nursing diagnoses based on assessment data.	—	—	—	_____
PLANNING				
1. Developed individualized goals for client based on nursing diagnoses.	—	—	—	_____
2. Identified expected outcomes.	—	—	—	_____
3. Explained procedure to client.	—	—	—	_____
4. Positioned client for privacy and wound access.	—	—	—	_____
IMPLEMENTATION				
1. Provided privacy and exposed wound site.	—	—	—	_____
2. Placed disposable bag correctly.	—	—	—	_____
3. Placed disposable pad under wound site.	—	—	—	_____
4. Washed hands. Put on mask, goggles, and gown if indicated. Put on disposable gloves. Removed tape.	—	—	—	_____
5. Removed dressing.	—	—	—	_____
6. Observed drainage and condition of wound.	—	—	—	_____
7. Disposed of dressings properly.	—	—	—	_____
8. Removed and disposed of gloves.	—	—	—	_____
9. Prepared sterile dressing supplies.	—	—	—	_____
10. Poured sterile solution and added gauze.	—	—	—	_____

	S	U	NP	Comments
11. Put on sterile gloves.	___	___	___	_____
12. Inspected wound.	___	___	___	_____
13. Cleansed wound.	___	___	___	_____
14. Applied moistened gauze.	___	___	___	_____
15. Applied sterile gauze fluffs.	___	___	___	_____
16. Covered dressing with ABD pad, surgi-pad, or thick gauze.	___	___	___	_____
17. Applied tape or Montgomery ties.	___	___	___	_____
18. Removed and disposed of gloves. Removed mask, gown, and goggles.	___	___	___	_____
19. Positioned client comfortably.	___	___	___	_____
20. Washed hands.	___	___	___	_____

EVALUATION

	S	U	NP	Comments
1. Assessed client's comfort level.	___	___	___	_____
2. Observed wound for healing.	___	___	___	_____
3. Monitored status of dressing.	___	___	___	_____
4. Asked client to describe wound care method.	___	___	___	_____
5. Identified unexpected outcomes.	___	___	___	_____

RECORDING AND REPORTING

	S	U	NP	Comments
1. Reported unexpected outcomes to physician.	___	___	___	_____
2. Reported wound appearance and drainage at shift change.	___	___	___	_____
3. Recorded data on wound, drainage, and client's tolerance of procedure.	___	___	___	_____
4. Wrote date and time of dressing change on tape.	___	___	___	_____

Student _____   Date _____

Instructor _____   Date _____

PERFORMANCE CHECKLIST 37-3   **APPLYING A PRESSURE BANDAGE**

	S	U	NP	Comments

ASSESSMENT
1. Identified clients at risk for unexpected bleeding.

Phase I
1. Identified client with sudden hemorrhage and applied direct pressure.

2. Sought assistance.

Phase II
1. Rapidly observed bleeding site and size.

2. Observed objective symptoms.

NURSING DIAGNOSIS
1. Developed appropriate nursing diagnoses based on assessment data.

PLANNING
1. Developed individualized goals for client based on nursing diagnoses.

2. Identified expected outcomes.

IMPLEMENTATION
1. Washed hands and provided privacy as client's condition permitted. Applied clean gloves.

2. Pressed on site of bleeding.

3. Unwrapped roller bandage.

4. Applied bandage quickly and correctly.

5. Removed gloves and washed hands.

EVALUATION
1. Assessed client's response to treatment.

2. Identified unexpected outcomes.

RECORDING AND REPORTING
1. Immediately reported client's status to physician.

2. Recorded and implemented physician's verbal orders.

3. Made between-shift report of emergency situation.

4. Recorded findings and care administered on progress note.

Student _____   Date _____

Instructor _____   Date _____

PERFORMANCE CHECKLIST 37-4 **APPLYING A TRANSPARENT DRESSING**

	S	U	NP	Comments
ASSESSMENT				
1. Assessed size and location of wound.	—	—	—	_____
2. Reviewed physician's orders.	—	—	—	_____
3. Assessed client's level of comfort.	—	—	—	_____
4. Assessed client's knowledge level.	—	—	—	_____
5. Assessed risk for wound healing problems.	—	—	—	_____
NURSING DIAGNOSIS				
1. Developed appropriate nursing diagnoses based on assessment data.	—	—	—	_____
PLANNING				
1. Developed individualized goals for client based on nursing diagnoses.	—	—	—	_____
2. Identified expected outcomes.	—	—	—	_____
3. Explained procedure to client.	—	—	—	_____
4. Positioned client appropriately.	—	—	—	_____
IMPLEMENTATION				
1. Provided privacy and exposed wound site.	—	—	—	_____
2. Placed waterproof bag properly.	—	—	—	_____
3. Washed hands and put on disposable gloves. Put on gown, mask, and goggles.	—	—	—	_____
4. Removed old dressing.	—	—	—	_____
5. Disposed of soiled dressing properly and removed and disposed of gloves properly.	—	—	—	_____
6. Prepared sterile dressing supplies.	—	—	—	_____
7. Poured solution and soaked 4 × 4s.	—	—	—	_____
8. Put on sterile gloves (per agency policy).	—	—	—	_____
9. Cleansed wound.	—	—	—	_____
10. Dried area.	—	—	—	_____
11. Inspected wound.	—	—	—	_____
12. Applied transparent dressing.	—	—	—	_____
13. Removed and disposed of gown, mask, goggles, and gloves correctly.	—	—	—	_____

	S	U	NP	Comments
14. Positioned client comfortably.	___	___	___	_____
15. Disposed of dressing materials properly and washed hands.	___	___	___	_____

EVALUATION

1. Inspected condition of wound.	___	___	___	_____
2. Evaluated client for pain.	___	___	___	_____
3. Identified unexpected outcomes.	___	___	___	_____

RECORDING AND REPORTING

1. Recorded unexpected outcomes.	___	___	___	_____
2. Documented findings and dressing change in nurses' notes.	___	___	___	_____
3. Wrote date and time of dressing change on a sticker.	___	___	___	_____

Student _____   Date _____

Instructor _____   Date _____

PERFORMANCE CHECKLIST 37-5 **APPLYING A HYDROCOLLOID OR HYDROGEL DRESSING**

	S	U	NP	Comments

ASSESSMENT

1. Assessed location and size of wound.

2. Determined type of hydrocolloid or hydrogel dressing.

3. Reviewed orders.

4. Assessed client's comfort level.

5. Assessed client's knowledge of purpose of dressing.

6. Assessed risk for wound healing problems.

NURSING DIAGNOSIS

1. Developed appropriate nursing diagnoses based on assessment data.

PLANNING

1. Developed individualized goals for client based on nursing diagnoses.

2. Identified expected outcomes.

3. Explained procedure to client.

4. Positioned client properly.

IMPLEMENTATION

1. Maintained client's privacy.

2. Exposed wound and draped client.

3. Placed cuffed disposable waterproof bag within reach.

4. Washed hands and applied clean disposable gloves. Donned gown, mask, and goggles if indicated.

5. Removed old dressing.

6. Disposed of soiled dressing in waterproof bag. Removed disposable gloves properly.

7. Prepared sterile dressing supplies.

8. Poured saline or prescribed solution over 4 × 4s in basin.

9. Donned clean or sterile gloves.

	S	U	NP	Comments
10. Cleansed area with soaked 4 × 4s, swabbing exudate from wound.	—	—	—	_____
11. Dried area.	—	—	—	_____
12. Inspected wound.	—	—	—	_____
13. Applied hydrogel or hydrocolloid dressing according to manufacturer's directions.	—	—	—	_____
14. Removed gloves properly. Removed gown, mask, and goggles if worn.	—	—	—	_____
15. Assisted client to comfortable position.	—	—	—	_____
16. Discarded soiled dressing materials properly. Washed hands.	—	—	—	_____

EVALUATION

	S	U	NP	Comments
1. Inspected condition of wound and characteristics of wound drainage.	—	—	—	_____
2. Evaluated client's comfort level.	—	—	—	_____
3. Asked client to describe wound care.	—	—	—	_____
4. Identified unexpected outcomes.	—	—	—	_____

RECORDING AND REPORTING

	S	U	NP	Comments
1. Reported and recorded unusual observations.	—	—	—	_____
2. Recorded characteristics of wound and drainage.	—	—	—	_____
3. Wrote date, time, and initials on dressing.	—	—	—	_____

Student _____   Date _____

Instructor _____   Date _____

PERFORMANCE CHECKLIST 37-6   **APPLYING A FOAM DRESSING**

	S	U	NP	Comments

ASSESSMENT

1. Assessed location and size of wound.

2. Assessed client's level of comfort.

3. Reviewed physician's orders.

4. Assessed client's knowledge of purpose of dressing.

5. Assessed client's risk for wound healing problems.

NURSING DIAGNOSIS

1. Developed appropriate nursing diagnoses based on assessment data.

PLANNING

1. Developed individualized goals for client based on nursing diagnoses.

2. Identified expected outcomes.

3. Explained procedure to client.

4. Positioned client correctly.

IMPLEMENTATION

1. Provided privacy.

2. Exposed wound site and draped client.

3. Properly placed disposable bag.

4. Washed hands and put on clean disposable gloves. Donned gown, goggles, and mask if necessary.

5. Removed old dressing.

6. Disposed of soiled dressing. Removed and disposed of gloves properly.

7. Prepared sterile supplies.

8. Poured solution over gauze.

9. Put on gloves.

10. Cleansed area.

11. Removed excess wound moisture and dried skin around wound.

	S	U	NP	Comments
12. Inspected and measured wound.	___	___	___	_____
13. Applied foam dressing according to manufacturer's directions.	___	___	___	_____
14. Removed and disposed of gloves properly.	___	___	___	_____
15. Positioned client comfortably.	___	___	___	_____
16. Disposed of materials properly.	___	___	___	_____
17. Washed hands.	___	___	___	_____

EVALUATION

1. Inspected wound.	___	___	___	_____
2. Evaluated client's level of comfort.	___	___	___	_____
3. Asked client to describe wound care.	___	___	___	_____
4. Identified unexpected outcomes.	___	___	___	_____

RECORDING AND REPORTING

1. Reported and recorded unusual observations.	___	___	___	_____
2. Recorded characteristics of wound and drainage.	___	___	___	_____
3. Graphed wound surface area or volume of wound.	___	___	___	_____
4. Wrote time, date, and initials on new dressing or tape.	___	___	___	_____

Student _____   Date _____

Instructor _____   Date _____

PERFORMANCE CHECKLIST 37-7 **APPLYING ABSORPTION AND ALGINATE DRESSINGS**

	S	U	NP	Comments

ASSESSMENT

1. Assessed location and size of wound to be dressed. ___ ___ ___ _____

2. Reviewed physician's orders. ___ ___ ___ _____

3. Assessed client's level of comfort. ___ ___ ___ _____

4. Assessed client's knowledge of purpose of dressing. ___ ___ ___ _____

NURSING DIAGNOSIS

1. Developed appropriate nursing diagnoses based on assessment data. ___ ___ ___ _____

PLANNING

1. Developed individualized goals for client based on nursing diagnoses. ___ ___ ___ _____

2. Identified expected outcomes. ___ ___ ___ _____

3. Explained procedure to client. ___ ___ ___ _____

4. Positioned client correctly. ___ ___ ___ _____

IMPLEMENTATION

1. Provided privacy. ___ ___ ___ _____

2. Exposed wound site and draped client. ___ ___ ___ _____

3. Prepared disposable bag correctly. ___ ___ ___ _____

4. Washed hands and put on clean disposable gloves. Donned, gown, goggles, and mask if necessary. ___ ___ ___ _____

5. Removed and disposed of old dressing. Removed gloves. ___ ___ ___ _____

6. Prepared sterile dressing supplies. ___ ___ ___ _____

7. Poured solution over 4 × 4s. ___ ___ ___ _____

8. Put on sterile gloves (if required) and cleansed wound area. ___ ___ ___ _____

9. Inspected and measured wound. ___ ___ ___ _____

10. Applied absorption or alginate dressing according to manufacturer's directions. ___ ___ ___ _____

11. Removed gloves correctly and discarded. ___ ___ ___ _____

	S	U	NP	Comments
12. Assisted client to comfortable position.	___	___	___	_____
13. Discarded soiled materials correctly and washed hands.	___	___	___	_____

EVALUATION

	S	U	NP	Comments
1. Inspected conditions of wound on ongoing basis.	___	___	___	_____
2. Noted length of time before dressing needed to be changed.	___	___	___	_____
3. Identified unexpected outcomes.	___	___	___	_____

RECORDING AND REPORTING

	S	U	NP	Comments
1. Reported unusual observations immediately.	___	___	___	_____
2. Recorded wound characteristics and measurements in nurses' notes.	___	___	___	_____
3. Graphed wound surface area or volume.	___	___	___	_____
4. Wrote date, time, and initials on dressing or tape.	___	___	___	_____

Student _____   Date _____

Instructor _____   Date _____

PERFORMANCE CHECKLIST 38-1 **APPLYING AN ELASTIC BANDAGE**

	S	U	NP	Comments
ASSESSMENT				
1. Observed client's skin integrity.	—	—	—	_____
2. Observed cleanliness of dressing.	—	—	—	_____
3. Observed client's circulatory status.	—	—	—	_____
4. Reviewed client's medical record for physician's order for application of elastic bandage.	—	—	—	_____
5. Identified client's and family member's knowledge level.	—	—	—	_____
NURSING DIAGNOSIS				
1. Developed appropriate nursing diagnoses based on assessment data.	—	—	—	_____
PLANNING				
1. Developed individualized goals for client based on nursing diagnoses.	—	—	—	_____
2. Identified expected outcomes.	—	—	—	_____
3. Explained procedure to client.	—	—	—	_____
4. Taught skill to client and/or caregiver.	—	—	—	_____
IMPLEMENTATION				
1. Washed hands and applied gloves.	—	—	—	_____
2. Provided privacy.	—	—	—	_____
3. Assisted client to comfortable position.	—	—	—	_____
4. Held elastic bandage correctly.	—	—	—	_____
5. Applied bandage from distal point toward proximal boundary.	—	—	—	_____
6. Slightly stretched bandage as it was unrolled.	—	—	—	_____
7. Overlapped turns.	—	—	—	_____
8. Secured bandage.	—	—	—	_____
9. Removed gloves and washed hands.	—	—	—	_____
EVALUATION				
1. Checked circulation to the limb after application of bandage.	—	—	—	_____
2. Identified unexpected outcomes.	—	—	—	_____

	S	U	NP	Comments

RECORDING AND REPORTING

1. Correctly documented treatment and client's response. ___ ___ ___ _____

2. Reported changes in neurological or circulatory status to nurse in charge or physician. ___ ___ ___ _____

Student _____ Date _____

Instructor _____ Date _____

PERFORMANCE CHECKLIST 38-2 **APPLYING AN ABDOMINAL BINDER, T-BINDER, OR BREAST BINDER**

	S	U	NP	Comments

ASSESSMENT

1. Identified signs and symptoms of impaired respirations. ___ ___ ___ _____

2. Determined if client is allergic to tape. ___ ___ ___ _____

3. Identified level of skin integrity. ___ ___ ___ _____

4. Inspected any surgical dressing. ___ ___ ___ _____

5. Identified client's comfort level. ___ ___ ___ _____

6. Gathered necessary data regarding size of binder based on assessment. ___ ___ ___ _____

NURSING DIAGNOSIS

1. Developed appropriate nursing diagnoses based on assessment data. ___ ___ ___ _____

PLANNING

1. Developed individualized goals for client based on nursing diagnoses. ___ ___ ___ _____

2. Identified expected outcomes. ___ ___ ___ _____

3. Explained procedure to client. ___ ___ ___ _____

4. Taught skill to client and/or caregiver. ___ ___ ___ _____

IMPLEMENTATION

1. Washed hands and applied gloves. ___ ___ ___ _____

2. Provided privacy. ___ ___ ___ _____

Abdominal Binder

1. Applied abdominal binder correctly: ___ ___ ___ _____

    a. Positioned client. ___ ___ ___ _____

    b. Fanfolded binder toward midline. ___ ___ ___ _____

    c. Assisted client to correct position. ___ ___ ___ _____

    d. Placed binder ends under client. ___ ___ ___ _____

    e. Instructed client to roll over ends. ___ ___ ___ _____

    f. Smoothed ends on far side of bed. ___ ___ ___ _____

    g. Assisted client to supine position. ___ ___ ___ _____

    h. Adjusted binder. ___ ___ ___ _____

	S	U	NP	Comments

i. Closed binder correctly.   —— —— —— ——————————

j. Assessed adequacy of breathing and coughing.   —— —— —— ——————————

k. Assessed client's comfort level.   —— —— —— ——————————

l. Adjusted binder as necessary.   —— —— —— ——————————

T- or Double T-Binders

1. Applied T- or double T-binder correctly: —— —— —— ——————————

   a. Assisted client to correct position.   —— —— —— ——————————

   b. Placed horizontal band around client's waist.   —— —— —— ——————————

   c. Completed binder application correctly.   —— —— —— ——————————

   d. Assessed client's comfort level.   —— —— —— ——————————

   e. Instructed client regarding binder removal.   —— —— —— ——————————

Breast Binder

1. Applied breast binder correctly: —— —— —— ——————————

   a. Assisted client in placing arms through binder.   —— —— —— ——————————

   b. Assisted client to supine position.   —— —— —— ——————————

   c. Applied padding as necessary.   —— —— —— ——————————

   d. Secured binder with Velcro or pins.   —— —— —— ——————————

   e. Adjusted binder.   —— —— —— ——————————

   f. Instructed client in self-care.   —— —— —— ——————————

2. Removed gloves and washed hands.   —— —— —— ——————————

EVALUATION

1. Observed skin integrity.   —— —— —— ——————————

2. Noted client's comfort level.   —— —— —— ——————————

3. Assessed client's ability to cough and deep breathe.   —— —— —— ——————————

4. Identified client's need for assistance with daily activities.   —— —— —— ——————————

5. Identified unexpected outcomes.   —— —— —— ——————————

RECORDING AND REPORTING

1. Reported ineffective lung expansion immediately to physician.   —— —— —— ——————————

2. Reported skin irritation at between-shift report.   —— —— —— ——————————

3. Recorded application of binder and client assessment.   —— —— —— ——————————

Student _____   Date _____

Instructor _____   Date _____

PERFORMANCE CHECKLIST 39-1 **APPLYING A MOIST HOT COMPRESS TO AN OPEN WOUND**

	S	U	NP	Comments
ASSESSMENT				
1. Inspected and documented condition of exposed skin and wound.	—	—	—	_____
2. Assessed client's level of sensation.	—	—	—	_____
3. Checked medical record for contraindications to therapy.	—	—	—	_____
4. Checked physician's orders for compress application.	—	—	—	_____
5. Assessed client's understanding of application.	—	—	—	_____
NURSING DIAGNOSIS				
1. Developed appropriate nursing diagnoses based on assessment data.	—	—	—	_____
PLANNING				
1. Developed individualized goals for client based on nursing diagnoses.	—	—	—	_____
2. Identified expected outcomes.	—	—	—	_____
3. Prepared necessary equipment and supplies.	—	—	—	_____
4. Explained procedure and expected types of sensations to client.	—	—	—	_____
IMPLEMENTATION				
1. Provided privacy, assisted client to comfortable position, and placed waterproof pad under area to be treated.	—	—	—	_____
2. Draped client.	—	—	—	_____
3. Washed hands.	—	—	—	_____
4. Assembled equipment correctly and immersed compresses in solution.	—	—	—	_____
5. Applied disposable gloves and removed soiled dressing. Disposed of soiled gloves and dressing.	—	—	—	_____
6. Assessed condition of wound and surrounding skin.	—	—	—	_____
7. Applied sterile gloves.	—	—	—	_____
8. Removed excess moisture from compress, applied gauze lightly to wound, noted client's response, checked for redness.	—	—	—	_____

	S	U	NP	Comments

9. Packed wound snugly; covered all wound surfaces completely.

10. Covered moist compress with dry sterile dressing and bath towel.

11. Changed compress every 5 minutes or as ordered using sterile technique.

12. Optionally applied aquathermia pad over towel.

13. Asked if client felt discomfort.

14. Removed pad, towel, and compress after 30 minutes and replaced dry sterile dressing as ordered.

15. Assisted client to preferred comfortable position.

16. Disposed of soiled compress, dressings, and supplies; washed hands.

EVALUATION

1. Inspected condition of skin and wound.

2. Asked client if burning sensation was felt.

3. Had client explain and demonstrate application.

4. Identified unexpected outcomes.

RECORDING AND REPORTING

1. Recorded type, location, and duration of application.

2. Described condition of wound, skin, and client's response.

3. Described instruction given and client's ability to perform procedure.

4. Reported unusual findings to nurse in charge or physician.

Student _____   Date _____

Instructor _____   Date _____

PERFORMANCE CHECKLIST 39-2   **ASSISTING WITH WARM SOAKS AND SITZ BATHS**

	S	U	NP	Comments

ASSESSMENT

1. Assessed and documented condition of body part being immersed.

2. Assessed client's level of comfort.

3. Determined client's risk for reduced sensation.

4. Determined if client has systemic conditions contraindicating soaks or baths.

5. Assessed and documented client's blood pressure and pulse.

6. Assessed client's understanding of therapy.

7. Checked physician's order for procedure.

8. Determined client's ability to position self.

NURSING DIAGNOSIS

1. Developed appropriate nursing diagnoses based on assessment data.

PLANNING

1. Developed individualized goals for client based on nursing diagnoses.

2. Identified expected outcomes.

3. Prepared necessary equipment and supplies.

4. Explained procedure to client.

IMPLEMENTATION

1. Provided privacy and washed hands.

2. Filled basin; checked temperature of soak or bath solution.

3. Positioned client comfortably for soak.

4. Assisted while immersing client in tub or basin.

5. Covered client with bath blanket or towel.

6. Maintained constant temperature during procedure.

7. Assisted client from bath or soak and dried body part thoroughly.

	S	U	NP	Comments

8. Assisted client to chair or bed after procedure.

9. Disposed of soiled equipment and cleansed basin or tub; washed hands.

EVALUATION

1. Inspected condition of body part that was immersed.

2. Assessed client's response to therapy.

3. Assessed vital signs if client complained of dizziness or lightheadedness.

4. Asked client to demonstrate use of soak or sitz bath.

5. Identified unexpected outcomes.

RECORDING AND REPORTING

1. Recorded procedure in nurses' notes.

2. Described condition of body part immersed and client's exposure.

3. Reported client complaints and unusual observations to appropriate personnel.

4. Recorded preprocedure and postprocedure vital signs.

5. Described instruction given and client's ability to perform procedure.

Student _____   Date _____

Instructor _____   Date _____

PERFORMANCE CHECKLIST 39-3 **APPLYING AQUATHERMIA AND HEATING PADS**

	S	U	NP	Comments

ASSESSMENT

1. Assessed and documented condition of client's skin.

2. Assessed and documented level of discomfort and range of motion.

3. Assessed skin for sensitivity to temperature, touch, and pain.

4. Checked condition of electrical cords for safety hazards.

5. Reviewed physician's order for heat therapy.

6. Assessed client's knowledge of procedure.

NURSING DIAGNOSIS

1. Developed appropriate nursing diagnoses based on assessment data.

PLANNING

1. Developed individualized goals for client based on nursing diagnoses.

2. Identified expected outcomes.

3. Prepared necessary equipment and supplies.

4. Explained procedure and safety precautions to client.

IMPLEMENTATION

1. Provided privacy and washed hands.

2. Positioned client comfortably and exposed area to be treated.

3. Insulated surface of pad from client's skin with towel or pillowcase.

4. Placed pad over area to be treated; secured pad as needed.

5. Checked temperature setting of pad.

6. Monitored condition of skin and client's response every 5 minutes.

7. Removed pad after desired interval.

8. Assisted client to comfortable position; disposed of soiled linen and washed hands.

	S	U	NP	Comments

EVALUATION

1. Inspected condition of skin exposed to heat.   — — — _____

2. Determined level of client's discomfort.   — — — _____

3. Noted client's ability to move strained muscle.   — — — _____

4. Observed client apply pad.   — — — _____

5. Identified unexpected outcomes.   — — — _____

RECORDING AND REPORTING

1. Recorded procedure and client's response.   — — — _____

2. Described instruction given and client's ability to perform procedure.   — — — _____

3. Reported unusual changes in condition of skin.   — — — _____

Student _____   Date _____

Instructor _____   Date _____

PERFORMANCE CHECKLIST 39-4 **APPLYING COLD APPLICATIONS**

	S	U	NP	Comments

ASSESSMENT

1. Reviewed physician's order. — — — _____

2. Inspected and documented condition of injured or affected part. — — — _____

3. Considered time in which injury occurred. — — — _____

4. Asked client to describe pain and documented character of pain. — — — _____

5. Assessed area for sensitivity to temperature, touch, and pain. — — — _____

6. Assessed client's understanding of procedure. — — — _____

NURSING DIAGNOSIS

1. Developed appropriate nursing diagnoses based on assessment data. — — — _____

PLANNING

1. Developed individualized goals for client based on nursing diagnoses. — — — _____

2. Identified expected outcomes. — — — _____

3. Prepared necessary equipment and supplies. — — — _____

4. Explained procedure to client. — — — _____

IMPLEMENTATION

1. Provided privacy. — — — _____

2. Washed hands. — — — _____

3. Positioned client comfortably, with affected body part aligned properly and only area to be treated exposed. — — — _____

4. Placed towel or pad under area to be treated. — — — _____

5. Donned disposable gloves. — — — _____

6. Checked temperature of solution and submerged compress. Wrung out excess moisture and applied compress to affected area. — — — _____

7. Wrapped electronically controlled cooling pad around affected part, set temperature, and secured in place. — — — _____

8. Prepared ice bag or collar, wiped dry, and applied and secured over affected area. — — — _____

	S	U	NP	Comments
9. Prepared ice pack and applied over affected area.	—	—	—	_____
10. Removed and disposed of gloves.	—	—	—	_____
11. Inspected condition of skin every 5 minutes during application.	—	—	—	_____
12. Donned clean gloves, removed cooling application after 15 to 20 minutes (or as ordered), and dried area.	—	—	—	_____
13. Assisted client to comfortable position.	—	—	—	_____
14. Emptied and stored basin; disposed of used linens and gloves; washed hands.	—	—	—	_____

EVALUATION

	S	U	NP	Comments
1. Inspected condition of skin.	—	—	—	_____
2. Palpated affected area gently.	—	—	—	_____
3. Measured client's level of comfort.	—	—	—	_____
4. Asked client to demonstrate cold application and explain risks of treatment.	—	—	—	_____
5. Identified unexpected outcomes.	—	—	—	_____

RECORDING AND REPORTING

	S	U	NP	Comments
1. Recorded procedure and client's response in nurses' notes.	—	—	—	_____
2. Described instruction given and client's ability to perform procedure.	—	—	—	_____
3. Reported undesirable skin changes to nurse in charge or physician.	—	—	—	_____

Student _____   Date _____

Instructor _____   Date _____

PERFORMANCE CHECKLIST 39-5 CARING FOR CLIENTS REQUIRING HYPOTHERMIA OR HYPERTHERMIA BLANKETS

	S	U	NP	Comments

ASSESSMENT

1. Obtained vital signs, assessed neurologic and mental status and peripheral circulation.

2. Verified that less intensive measures were not effective in returning body temperature to normal.

3. Assessed client's skin on bony prominences and other susceptible areas before therapy.

4. Verified physician's orders and rechecked client's current body temperature.

NURSING DIAGNOSIS

1. Developed appropriate nursing diagnoses based on assessment data.

PLANNING

1. Developed individualized client goals based on nursing diagnoses.

2. Identified expected outcomes.

3. Explained procedure to client.

4. Prepared client for procedure.

IMPLEMENTATION

1. Washed hands and applied gloves.

2. Placed blanket on client's mattress and set on desired temperature.

3. Observed that the "cool" or "warm" light was on.

4. Verified that pad temperature limits were correctly set.

5. Placed sheet or thin blanket over the thermal blanket.

6. Lubricated rectal probe and inserted into client's rectum.

7. Placed client on blanket. Wrapped client's hands and feet in towels for hypothermia blanket.

8. Properly positioned client.

9. Double-checked fluid thermometer on blanket control panel.

S   U   NP   Comments

10. Removed gloves and washed hands.   —   —   —   _____

EVALUATION

1. Monitored client's vital signs at appropriate time intervals.

    —   —   —   _____

2. Verified accuracy of rectal probe and automatic temperature control device.

    —   —   —   _____

3. Observed the skin for injuries or changes.   —   —   —   _____

4. Determined client's level of comfort.   —   —   —   _____

5. Identified unexpected outcomes.   —   —   —   _____

RECORDING AND REPORTING

1. Recorded baseline data, when therapy was initiated, temperature control setting, and client's response to therapy.

    —   —   —   _____

2. Reported any unexpected outcomes to physician.   —   —   —   _____

Student _____ Date _____

Instructor _____ Date _____

PERFORMANCE CHECKLIST 40-1 PERFORMING WOUND IRRIGATION

	S	U	NP	Comments

ASSESSMENT

1. Reviewed client's medical record for physician's order.

2. Checked recent records of wound progress.

3. Assessed pain or comfort levels and identified symptoms of anxiety.

4. Identified history of allergies.

NURSING DIAGNOSIS

1. Developed appropriate nursing diagnoses based on assessment data.

PLANNING

1. Developed individualized goals for client based on nursing diagnoses.

2. Identified expected outcomes.

3. Explained procedure.

4. Administered premedication.

5. Positioned client.

6. Warmed irrigant.

7. Washed hands.

IMPLEMENTATION

1. Prepared refuse bag.

2. Provided privacy.

3. Applied gown and goggles if needed.

4. Put on clean gloves and removed and discarded soiled dressing. Removed and discarded gloves.

5. Prepared equipment, opened sterile supplies.

6. Put sterile gloves on.

7. Correctly irrigated wound with wide opening.

8. Correctly irrigated deep wound with small opening.

9. Correctly cleansed wound with hand-held shower.

	S	U	NP	Comments
10. Correctly cleansed wound with whirlpool.	___	___	___	_____
11. Obtained cultures.	___	___	___	_____
12. Dried wound edges with sterile gauze.	___	___	___	_____
13. Applied sterile dressing.	___	___	___	_____
14. Assisted client to comfortable position.	___	___	___	_____
15. Disposed of equipment and refuse.	___	___	___	_____
16. Removed gloves, gowns, and goggles. Washed hands.	___	___	___	_____

EVALUATION

	S	U	NP	Comments
1. Inspected dressing periodically.	___	___	___	_____
2. Assessed type of tissue in the wound bed.	___	___	___	_____
3. Evaluated skin integrity.	___	___	___	_____
4. Observed client for signs of discomfort.	___	___	___	_____
5. Observed for retained irrigant.	___	___	___	_____
6. Identified unexpected outcomes.	___	___	___	_____

RECORDING AND REPORTING

	S	U	NP	Comments
1. Reported any evidence of fresh bleeding, increase in pain, retention of irrigant, or signs of shock to physician.	___	___	___	_____
2. Reported outcomes at change of shift.	___	___	___	_____
3. Recorded wound irrigation and client's response on progress notes.	___	___	___	_____

Student _____   Date _____

Instructor _____   Date _____

PERFORMANCE CHECKLIST 40-2 **PERFORMING SUTURE AND STAPLE REMOVAL**

	S	U	NP	Comments
ASSESSMENT				
1. Identified client and reviewed physician's order.	—	—	—	_____
2. Observed healing status.	—	—	—	_____
3. Assessed client for history of allergies.	—	—	—	_____
NURSING DIAGNOSIS				
1. Developed appropriate nursing diagnoses related to suture or staple removal.	—	—	—	_____
PLANNING				
1. Developed individualized goals for client based on nursing diagnoses.	—	—	—	_____
2. Identified expected outcomes.	—	—	—	_____
3. Adjusted light on suture line.	—	—	—	_____
4. Explained procedure to client.	—	—	—	_____
5. Washed hands.	—	—	—	_____
IMPLEMENTATION				
1. Provided privacy.	—	—	—	_____
2. Positioned client.	—	—	—	_____
3. Prepared refuse bag.	—	—	—	_____
4. Prepared sterile field.	—	—	—	_____
5. Put on clean gloves, removed dressing; discarded dressing and gloves.	—	—	—	_____
6. Inspected wound.	—	—	—	_____
7. Applied sterile gloves.	—	—	—	_____
8. Cleaned sutures or staples and incision with antiseptic swabs.	—	—	—	_____
9. Removed staples:	—	—	—	_____
a. Applied staple extractor correctly.	—	—	—	_____
b. Carefully controlled staple extractor.	—	—	—	_____
c. Moved staple away from skin surface.	—	—	—	_____
d. Released handles of staple extractor, allowing staple to fall into refuse bag.	—	—	—	_____
e. Repeated Steps a-d until all staples removed.	—	—	—	_____

	S	U	NP	Comments

10. Removed intermittent sutures:

  a. Placed sterile gauze and grasped scissors and forceps correctly.

  b. Snipped sutures.

  c. Grasped knotted end with forceps and re-moved suture.

  d. Repeated Steps a-c until all sutures removed.

  e. Observed healing level.

11. Removed continuous sutures:

  a. Placed sterile gauze and grasped scissors and forceps correctly.

  b. Snipped first suture correctly.

  c. Snipped second suture on same side.

  d. Grasped knotted end and removed first line of spiral in continuous smooth action. Placed removed suture on gauze compress.

  e. Repeated Steps a-d until entire line removed.

12. Inspected incision site.

13. Cleaned suture line and applied light dressing.

14. Noted number of sutures or staples removed.

15. Routed reusable items for sterilization and washed hands.

EVALUATION

1. Assessed site of suture or staple removal.

2. Determined if client has pain along incision.

3. Identified unexpected outcomes.

RECORDING AND REPORTING

1. Notified physician immediately of abnormal findings.

2. Reported procedure at change of shift.

3. Recorded number of sutures or staples removed and wound appearance.

Student _____ Date _____

Instructor _____ Date _____

PERFORMANCE CHECKLIST 40-3   **PERFORMING DRAINAGE EVACUATION**

	S	U	NP	Comments

ASSESSMENT

1. Identified presence of closed wound drain and drainage system.

2. Identified number of wound drainage tubes.

3. Verified physician's order to determine if suction is needed.

4. Inspected system for straight tube or Y-tube arrangement.

5. Inspected system for proper functioning.

6. Secured drainage reservoirs.

7. Identified type of drainage container.

NURSING DIAGNOSIS

1. Developed appropriate nursing diagnoses based on assessment data.

PLANNING

1. Developed individualized goals for client based on nursing diagnoses.

2. Identified expected outcomes.

3. Explained procedure to client.

IMPLEMENTATION

1. Provided privacy for client.

2. Washed hands and applied gloves.

3. Placed open sterile laboratory specimen and graduate container on bed.

4. Maintained asepsis while opening and emptying evacuator; followed correct procedure for either Hemovac or Jackson-Pratt evacuator.

5. Noted characteristics of drainage.

6. Placed and secured drainage reservoirs to prevent pull on insertion sites.

7. Routed labeled specimen to laboratory.

8. Discarded soiled supplies and washed hands.

9. Changed dressing and inspected skin.

	S	U	NP	Comments

10. Discarded contaminated materials according to Centers for Disease Control (CDC) guidelines; washed hands.

— — — _____

EVALUATION

1. Evaluated presence of drainage.

— — — _____

2. Inspected wound for drainage.

— — — _____

3. Assessed client's comfort level.

— — — _____

4. Identified unexpected outcomes.

— — — _____

RECORDING AND REPORTING

1. Reported abnormal findings to physician immediately.

— — — _____

2. Reported procedure and findings at change of shift.

— — — _____

3. Recorded procedure and results in progress notes and an I&O report.

— — — _____

Student _____   Date _____

Instructor _____   Date _____

PERFORMANCE CHECKLIST 41-1   **MODIFYING SAFETY RISKS IN THE HOME ENVIRONMENT**

	S	U	NP	Comments

ASSESSMENT

1. Reviewed previous findings and/or conducted sensory and neuromuscular assessment.

2. Determined client's history of falls or other injuries in the home.

3. Reviewed risk factors for accidents in the home.

4. Conducted a complete home safety assessment.

5. Assessed the client's financial resources.

6. Assess client's and family's willingness to make changes.

NURSING DIAGNOSIS

1. Developed appropriate nursing diagnoses based on assessment data.

PLANNING

1. Developed individualized goals for client based on nursing diagnoses.

2. Identified expected outcomes.

3. Prioritized with client and family the greatest environmental risks to safety.

4. Recommended calling a reliable contractor if major home repairs are necessary.

IMPLEMENTATION

1. Took steps to reduce physical hazards that predispose to falls.

2. Made modifications to promote safe practice of activities of daily living.

3. Took steps to eliminate fire hazards.

4. Took steps to reduce chances of injury from burns.

EVALUATION

1. Had client and family member(s) identify potential safety risks.

2. Asked client to discuss plans for modifications and observed changes made on subsequent visits.

	S	U	NP	Comments

3. Asked if client experienced any injuries or falls on follow-up visit or call.

    ___   ___   ___   _____

4. Identified unexpected outcomes.

    ___   ___   ___   _____

RECORDING AND REPORTING

1. Retained copy of home safety assessment in client's home health record.

    ___   ___   ___   _____

2. Recorded any instruction given, client's response, and changes made in the home environment.

    ___   ___   ___   _____

Student _____   Date _____

Instructor _____   Date _____

PERFORMANCE CHECKLIST 41-2 **ADAPTING THE HOME SETTING FOR CLIENTS WITH COGNITIVE DEFICITS**

	S	U	NP	Comments
ASSESSMENT				
1. Conducted assessment during short session, being sensitive to client's needs or disabilities.	___	___	___	_____
2. Met with client and family in conducive environment.	___	___	___	_____
3. Asked client to describe level of health and self-care abilities.	___	___	___	_____
4. Asked how client is doing with home management.	___	___	___	_____
5. Assessed medications taken by client.	___	___	___	_____
6. Determined if client has family member or friend who assists with self-care or home management.	___	___	___	_____
7. Observed client's appearance and behavior during discussion.	___	___	___	_____
8. Observed immediate home environment.	___	___	___	_____
9. Completed a mini-mental exam if cognitive or mental status change is suspected.	___	___	___	_____
NURSING DIAGNOSIS				
1. Developed appropriate nursing diagnoses based on assessment data.	___	___	___	_____
PLANNING				
1. Developed individualized goals based on nursing diagnoses.	___	___	___	_____
2. Identified expected outcomes.	___	___	___	_____
3. Referred family to homemaker services and/or respite care if client has difficulty with self-care skills.	___	___	___	_____
4. Consulted with physician and/or occupational therapist if client has physical disability affecting fine motor skills.	___	___	___	_____
5. Considered client's level of cognitive impairment prior to implementing strategies.	___	___	___	_____
6. Determined best time of day for specific approaches.	___	___	___	_____

	S	U	NP	Comments

IMPLEMENTATION

1. Created methods to assist client to remember task performance.

2. Found ways to consolidate tasks to simple steps if client has difficulty completing tasks.

3. Assisted client and caregiver to determine a routine schedule for self-care activities and home management.

4. Instructed caregiver to focus on client's abilities rather than disabilities.

5. Had caregiver assist with setting up tasks that the client can complete.

6. Discussed options for scheduling multiple medications with client, caregiver, and physician/ primary care provider.

7. Instructed caregiver on use of simple and direct communication.

8. Kept clocks, calendars, and personal mementos situated throughout the house.

9. Had caregiver routinely orient client.

10. Encouraged regular naps or rest periods throughout the day.

11. Had caregiver encourage and support frequent visits by family and significant others.

EVALUATION

1. Asked client to review daily home management activities during follow-up visit.

2. Reviewed schedule for medication administration.

3. Asked caregiver to describe ways to increase client's success in self-care and home management activities.

4. Had caregiver show schedules of daily routines and specific approaches used.

5. Identified unexpected outcomes.

RECORDING AND REPORTING

1. Recorded assessment of client's cognitive and mental status, interventions, and client's and caregiver's responses in progress notes.

2. Reported changes in client's behavior reflecting a possible decline in cognitive or mental status to physician.

Student _____   Date _____

Instructor _____   Date _____

PERFORMANCE CHECKLIST 41-3 MEDICATION AND MEDICAL DEVICE SAFETY

	S	U	NP	Comments

ASSESSMENT

1. Assessed client's sensory, musculoskeletal, and neurological function.

2. Assessed medication regimen.

3. Asked client to identify where medications are kept in the home. Looked at each container.

4. Had client describe daily schedule for drug administration.

5. Asked client to identify where self-injection supplies are kept and disposed of, if applicable.

6. Asked client to identify where glucose monitor and supplies are stored, and where lancets are disposed of, if applicable.

7. Asked to identify where dressings are stored and disposed of, if applicable.

NURSING DIAGNOSIS

1. Developed appropriate nursing diagnoses based on assessment data.

PLANNING

1. Developed individualized goals for client based on nursing diagnoses.

2. Identified expected outcomes.

IMPLEMENTATION

1. Instructed client and caregiver on principles to ensure medications are safe to use.

2. Recommended approaches to facilitate preparation of medications.

3. Recommended approaches to ensure medications and supplies are stored properly.

4. Reviewed with client and caregiver the proper techniques for disposal of "sharps" and other medical supplies.

EVALUATION

1. Had client or caregiver describe steps to take to ensure medications are safe to use.

2. Observed client prepare and administer a medication dose.

	S	U	NP	Comments

3. Observed home setting for location of medications and supplies.

___ ___ ___ _____

4. Had client describe disposal of "sharps" and other medical supplies.

___ ___ ___ _____

5. Identified unexpected outcomes.

___ ___ ___ _____

RECORDING AND REPORTING

1. Recorded recommendations provided to client and caregiver and their responses in progress notes.

___ ___ ___ _____

Student _____   Date _____

Instructor _____   Date _____

PERFORMANCE CHECKLIST 42-1 **TEACHING CLIENTS TO MEASURE BODY TEMPERATURE, BLOOD PRESSURE, AND PULSE**

TEACHING CLIENTS TO MEASURE BODY TEMPERATURE

	S	U	NP	Comments
ASSESSMENT				
1. Assessed client's ability to hold and read thermometer.	—	—	—	_____
2. Assessed client's knowledge regarding temperature ranges, fever, and type of thermometer to use.	—	—	—	_____
3. Observed client's technique in measuring temperature if client has had prior experience.	—	—	—	_____
NURSING DIAGNOSIS				
1. Developed appropriate nursing diagnoses based on assessment data.	—	—	—	_____
PLANNING				
1. Developed individualized goals for client based on nursing diagnoses.	—	—	—	_____
2. Identified expected outcomes.	—	—	—	_____
3. Selected setting in home for client to measure temperature.	—	—	—	_____
4. Instructed client and/or caregiver on positioning technique.	—	—	—	_____
IMPLEMENTATION				
1. Demonstrated steps and stated rationale for preparation and insertion of thermometer.	—	—	—	_____
2. Assisted client in performance of each step.	—	—	—	_____
3. Discussed normal temperature ranges.	—	—	—	_____
4. Discussed factors influencing temperature.	—	—	—	_____
5. Discussed common symptoms of fever.	—	—	—	_____
6. Discussed signs and symptoms of hypothermia.	—	—	—	_____
7. Discussed importance of notifying physician concerning measures to control fever.	—	—	—	_____
8. Created written guidelines for reference.	—	—	—	_____
EVALUATION				
1. Had client measure body temperature and demonstrate ability to read thermometer without assistance.	—	—	—	_____

	S	U	NP	Comments

2. Had client discuss and identify knowledge related to temperature measurement.   — — — _____

3. Had client describe signs and symptoms of fever and hypothermia and methods for control.   — — — _____

4. Identified unexpected outcomes.   — — — _____

RECORDING AND REPORTING

1. Recorded information taught and client's response in nurses' notes.   — — — _____

2. Instructed client to maintain a written record of temperature readings.   — — — _____

TEACHING CLIENTS TO MEASURE BLOOD PRESSURE

ASSESSMENT

1. Assessed client's ability to manipulate equipment and determine reading.   — — — _____

2. Assessed client's knowledge of blood pressure ranges and symptoms and common causes of hypotension and hypertension.   — — — _____

3. Assessed client's knowledge of the significance of the BP measurement and its variations.   — — — _____

4. Asked for demonstration of technique if client has had previous experience.   — — — _____

5. Determined best site for BP measurement.   — — — _____

NURSING DIAGNOSIS

1. Developed appropriate nursing diagnoses based on assessment data.   — — — _____

PLANNING

1. Developed individualized goals for client based on nursing diagnoses.   — — — _____

2. Identified expected outcomes.   — — — _____

3. Encouraged client to perform BP measurements on a regular schedule.   — — — _____

4. Encouraged client to avoid activities that increase BP prior to measurement.   — — — _____

5. Had client perform measurement in a comfortable position and environment.   — — — _____

6. Explained procedure to client and had client rest 5 minutes before measurement.   — — — _____

7. Had client describe symptoms that would indicate a need to measure the BP.   — — — _____

IMPLEMENTATION

1. Discussed the best sites for BP measurement.   — — — _____

Student _____ Date _____
Instructor _____ Date _____

	S	U	NP	Comments

2. Demonstrated steps for skill performance. ___ ___ ___ _____

3. Described the sounds of measurement and relationship of gauge as BP reading. ___ ___ ___ _____

4. Had client manipulate all equipment. ___ ___ ___ _____

5. Had client perform the skill on nurse, family member, or caregiver. ___ ___ ___ _____

6. Had client demonstrate technique on self. ___ ___ ___ _____

7. Identified that teaching of skill may be accomplished slowly until client comfort is gained. ___ ___ ___ _____

8. Had client perform skill under observation and record reading with nurse verification. ___ ___ ___ _____

9. Used appropriate written and/or pictorial instructions. ___ ___ ___ _____

EVALUATION

1. Observed client demonstrate technique for BP measurement on at least 3 different occasions. ___ ___ ___ _____

2. Waited 1 to 2 minutes and repeated measurement if BP inaudible or difficult to obtain. ___ ___ ___ _____

3. Attempted alternative measures if BP remains inaudible or difficult to obtain. ___ ___ ___ _____

4. Identified unexpected outcomes. ___ ___ ___ _____

RECORDING AND REPORTING

1. Recorded teaching and client responses in home care record. ___ ___ ___ _____

2. Recorded BP in home care record and client's documentation system. ___ ___ ___ _____

3. Reported abnormal readings to physician. ___ ___ ___ _____

TEACHING CLIENTS TO ASSESS THEIR OWN PULSE

ASSESSMENT

1. Identified client's knowledge of purpose for assessing pulse and level of interest in performing skill. ___ ___ ___ _____

2. Assessed client's ability to feel pulsation by having client palpate own or nurse's artery. ___ ___ ___ _____

3. Asked client to demonstrate technique for assessing pulse. ___ ___ ___ _____

S   U   NP   Comments

NURSING DIAGNOSIS

1. Identified appropriate nursing diagnoses based on client's learning capabilities and needs.

PLANNING

1. Developed individualized goals for client based on nursing diagnoses.

2. Identified expected outcomes.

3. Selected setting in home for assessing pulse.

IMPLEMENTATION

1. Discussed with client best sites for assessing pulse.

2. Cautioned client against massaging neck while attempting to locate carotid pulse or attempting to locate both carotid arteries at same time (if applicable).

3. Demonstrated steps for palpating pulse.

4. Had client perform each step.

5. Discussed information relating to pulse range, purpose for monitoring pulse, and best time to monitor pulse.

6. Discussed importance of notifying physician and/or withholding medication when pulse alterations occur.

EVALUATION

1. Observed client or family member independently assess pulse.

2. Had learner take radial pulse at the same time as the nurse.

3. Had client discuss reasons for assessing pulse and normal pulse rate range.

4. Asked client to reiterate instructions on withholding medication according to pulse rate.

5. Asked client to state time of day and activity level in relation to pulse measurement and medication dosage.

6. Identified unexpected outcomes.

RECORDING AND REPORTING

1. Recorded teaching and client's response in home care record.

2. Had client maintain written record of pulse measurement and medication administration.

Student _____   Date _____

Instructor _____   Date _____

PERFORMANCE CHECKLIST 42-2   **USING HOME OXYGEN EQUIPMENT**

	S	U	NP	Comments

ASSESSMENT

1. Determined client's or family's ability to use oxygen equipment correctly in hospital and in the home.

2. Assessed the home environment for electrical power, if compressor is used.

3. Assessed client's or family's ability to observe for signs and symptoms of hypoxia.

4. Observed client's or family's use of prescribed oxygen therapy.

5. Determined approximate resource in the community for equipment and assistance.

6. Determined back-up system in the event of power failure.

NURSING DIAGNOSIS

1. Developed appropriate nursing diagnoses based on assessment data.

PLANNING

1. Developed individualized goals for client based on nursing diagnoses.

2. Identified expected outcomes.

3. Explained procedure to client and family.

IMPLEMENTATION

1. Washed hands.

2. Demonstrated steps for preparation and completion of oxygen therapy.

3. Prepared Liberator and Stroller for use.

4. Instructed client or family through each step.

5. Discussed signs and symptoms of infection, and instructed client or family when to notify physician.

6. Instructed client or family on removal of mucous plug.

7. Discussed emergency plan.

8. Washed hands.

	S	U	NP	Comments

9. Recorded teaching plan and documented client's learning.   ___ ___ ___ _____

EVALUATION

1. Evaluated client's or family's ability to use oxygen at home.   ___ ___ ___ _____

2. Identified unexpected outcomes.   ___ ___ ___ _____

RECORDING AND REPORTING

1. Recorded teaching plan in the care plan.   ___ ___ ___ _____

2. Recorded learning progress in nurses' notes.   ___ ___ ___ _____

3. Communicated learning activity with other staff.   ___ ___ ___ _____

Student _____ Date _____

Instructor _____ Date _____

PERFORMANCE CHECKLIST 42-3 **TEACHING HOME TRACHEOSTOMY CARE AND SUCTIONING**

	S	U	NP	Comments
ASSESSMENT				
1. Assessed client's ability to perform tracheostomy care and suctioning.	—	—	—	_____
2. Assessed client's or family's recognition of physical signs and symptoms indicating need to perform home tracheostomy care and suctioning.	—	—	—	_____
3. Assessed client's or family's recognition of factors that normally influence airway functioning.	—	—	—	_____
4. Assessed client's understanding of and ability to perform tracheostomy care and suctioning.	—	—	—	_____
5. Observed client or family member perform tracheostomy care and suctioning.	—	—	—	_____
NURSING DIAGNOSIS				
1. Developed appropriate nursing diagnoses based on assessment data.	—	—	—	_____
PLANNING				
1. Developed individualized goals for client based on nursing diagnoses.	—	—	—	_____
2. Identified expected outcomes.	—	—	—	_____
3. Selected setting in home for tracheostomy tube care.	—	—	—	_____
4. Demonstrated with client proper position for procedure.	—	—	—	_____
IMPLEMENTATION				
Demonstrated steps for tracheostomy tube suctioning				
1. Washed hands and applied gloves.	—	—	—	_____
2. Prepared suction equipment according to manufacturer's directions.	—	—	—	_____
3. Filled basin with ½ cup water or normal saline.	—	—	—	_____
4. Connected suction catheter to suction apparatus and ensured proper functioning.	—	—	—	_____
5. Coated distal ⅓ to ½ catheter with water-soluble lubricant.	—	—	—	_____

	S	U	NP	Comments

6. Removed oxygen or humidity source if applicable. Inserted catheter into tracheobronchial tree correctly.

     ___ ___ ___ _____

7. Applied intermittent suction correctly. Reapplied oxygen or humidity source.

     ___ ___ ___ _____

8. Rinsed secretions from catheter correctly. Repeated Steps 6-8 as needed.

     ___ ___ ___ _____

9. Suctioned nasal and oral pharynx if needed.

     ___ ___ ___ _____

10. Rinsed catheter properly.

     ___ ___ ___ _____

11. Had client take 2 to 3 deep breaths.

     ___ ___ ___ _____

12. Disconnected suction catheter, coiled and disposed of properly.

     ___ ___ ___ _____

Trachestomy Care

1. Prepared equipment and site for cleaning inner cannula.

     ___ ___ ___ _____

2. Prepared solutions of hydrogen peroxide, normal saline/water, and 4 × 4 gauze pads.

     ___ ___ ___ _____

3. Removed old tracheostomy bib or dressing and discarded.

     ___ ___ ___ _____

4. Removed and discarded gloves.

     ___ ___ ___ _____

5. Applied clean gloves.

     ___ ___ ___ _____

6. Cleansed site around stoma with presoaked 4 × 4's and damp applicators.

     ___ ___ ___ _____

7. Dried exposed outer cannula and skin.

     ___ ___ ___ _____

8. Cleaned inner cannula with nylon brush or pipe cleaners.

     ___ ___ ___ _____

9. Examined patency of cannula and repeated procedure as needed. Replaced inner cannula.

     ___ ___ ___ _____

10. Changed old tracheostomy ties.

     ___ ___ ___ _____

11. Applied fresh dressing.

     ___ ___ ___ _____

12. Cleaned and stored reusable supplies.

     ___ ___ ___ _____

13. Removed and discarded gloves.

     ___ ___ ___ _____

14. Disinfected reusable supplies at least weekly.

     ___ ___ ___ _____

15. Had client or family member perform each step with guidance from nurse.

     ___ ___ ___ _____

16. Discussed signs and symptoms of infection or inflammation and the importance of notifying physician.

     ___ ___ ___ _____

Student _____   Date _____

Instructor _____   Date _____

	S	U	NP	Comments

EVALUATION

1. Observed client demonstrate tracheostomy tube care and suctioning independently.   ___ ___ ___ _____

2. Had client state signs of stomal or respiratory infection.   ___ ___ ___ _____

3. Identified unexpected outcomes.   ___ ___ ___ _____

RECORDING AND REPORTING

1. Recorded teaching and client's response in home care record.   ___ ___ ___ _____

2. Developed a system of recording performance of care by client or family member.   ___ ___ ___ _____

Student _____   Date _____

Instructor _____   Date _____

PERFORMANCE CHECKLIST 42-4   **HELPING CLIENTS WITH SELF-MEDICATION**

	S	U	NP	Comments
ASSESSMENT				
1. Assessed client's knowledge of drug therapy and drug interactions.	___	___	___	_____
2. Assessed family member's knowledge of client's drug therapy.	___	___	___	_____
3. Assessed client's sensory function.	___	___	___	_____
4. Assessed client's mobility limitations.	___	___	___	_____
5. Assessed client's reading ability.	___	___	___	_____
6. Assessed client's readiness to learn.	___	___	___	_____
7. Assessed client's beliefs regarding drug therapy.	___	___	___	_____
8. Checked type and number of drugs prescribed.	___	___	___	_____
9. Assessed client's resources for obtaining medications.	___	___	___	_____
NURSING DIAGNOSIS				
1. Developed appropriate nursing diagnoses based on assessment data.	___	___	___	_____
PLANNING				
1. Developed individualized goals for client based on nursing diagnoses.	___	___	___	_____
2. Identified expected outcomes.	___	___	___	_____
3. Prepared environment for teaching session.	___	___	___	_____
4. Provided useful teaching materials that complemented client's learning capacity.	___	___	___	_____
5. Had client wear glasses or hearing aid during teaching session, if appropriate.	___	___	___	_____
6. Consulted with physician about medications prescribed.	___	___	___	_____
7. Included family in teaching program.	___	___	___	_____
IMPLEMENTATION				
1. Presented information in clear, concise manner.	___	___	___	_____
2. Offered frequent opportunities for client to ask questions.	___	___	___	_____
3. Presented content pertaining to drug information, drug safety, and illness prevention.	___	___	___	_____

	S	U	NP	Comments

4. Taught sessions that were short and frequent.

5. Provided special learning aids for dosage schedule routine.

6. Assisted client in practicing preparation of medications.

7. Arranged with pharmacy to have large-print labels for medication bottles.

8. Arranged for pharmacy to deliver prescriptions (as needed) and provide containers client can open independently.

EVALUATION

1. Had client or family member independently prepare dosages for all medications.

2. Had client or family member explain content presented in teaching session.

3. Identified client's problem-solving initiatives.

4. Offered additional opportunity for client to ask questions.

5. Identified unexpected outcomes.

RECORDING AND REPORTING

1. Documented instruction in nurses' notes.

2. Developed a system of recording medication administration.

Student _____   Date _____

Instructor _____   Date _____

PERFORMANCE CHECKLIST 42-5   **ENTERAL NUTRITION IN THE HOME**

	S	U	NP	Comments
ASSESSMENT				
1. Assessed client's health status for stability.	___	___	___	_____
2. Assessed client or caregiver's abilities and resources.	___	___	___	_____
3. Assessed environmental conditions in the client's home.	___	___	___	_____
4. Assessed client or caregiver's understanding of the purpose of enteral nutrition.	___	___	___	_____
5. Assessed client or caregiver's understanding of storage, management, and acquisition of supplies.	___	___	___	_____
6. Assessed client or caregiver's ability to administer feedings.	___	___	___	_____
7. Assessed client or caregiver's understanding of measures needed to prevent complications.	___	___	___	_____
8. Assessed client or caregiver's understanding of tube occlusion and handling of formulas.	___	___	___	_____
9. Assessed client or caregiver's understanding of the management of complications.	___	___	___	_____
NURSING DIAGNOSIS				
1. Developed appropriate nursing diagnoses based on assessment data.	___	___	___	_____
PLANNING				
1. Developed individualized goals based on nursing diagnoses.	___	___	___	_____
2. Identified expected outcomes.	___	___	___	_____
IMPLEMENTATION				
1. Washed hands.	___	___	___	_____
2. Discussed client or caregiver's understanding of enteral feeding and nutritional health.	___	___	___	_____
3. Demonstrated identification of placement of nasal tubes.	___	___	___	_____
4. Observed client or caregiver demonstrate determination of tube placement.	___	___	___	_____
5. Observed client or caregiver aspirating gastric contents.	___	___	___	_____

	S	U	NP	Comments
6. Observed client or caregiver prepare and administer feeding and clean and store supplies.	—	—	—	_____
7. Observed client or caregiver administering medication and flushing tube.	—	—	—	_____
8. Discussed and observed use of infusion pump, if indicated.	—	—	—	_____
9. Discussed measures to stabilize the feeding tube and protect skin integrity.	—	—	—	_____
10. Discussed measures to prevent tube occlusion and aspiration.	—	—	—	_____
11. Discussed whom to contact for equipment, supplies, or in case of equipment failure.	—	—	—	_____
12. Discussed emergency plan in the event of aspiration.	—	—	—	_____
13. Discussed whom to contact and when for signs of diarrhea, constipation, or weight loss.	—	—	—	_____
14. Washed hands.	—	—	—	_____

EVALUATION

	S	U	NP	Comments
1. Asked client to state purpose of home enteral nutrition therapy.	—	—	—	_____
2. Observed client or caregiver performing technique.	—	—	—	_____
3. Asked client or caregiver to state measures to prevent complications.	—	—	—	_____
4. Asked client about community contacts for supplies, equipment, and emergency care.	—	—	—	_____
5. Identified unexpected outcomes.	—	—	—	_____

RECORDING AND REPORTING

	S	U	NP	Comments
1. Documented teaching and client's response in home care record.	—	—	—	_____
2. Documented specifics of enteral feeding plan.	—	—	—	_____
3. Reviewed home documentation by client or caregiver on enteral feeding and client status.	—	—	—	_____

Student _____   Date _____

Instructor _____   Date _____

PERFORMANCE CHECKLIST 43-1   COLLECTING A MIDSTREAM (CLEAN-VOIDED) URINE SPECIMEN

	S	U	NP	Comments

ASSESSMENT

1. Assessed client's ability to use toilet facilities independently.   ___ ___ ___ _____

2. Referred to medical record for history of urinary infection.   ___ ___ ___ _____

3. Assessed client's risk for urinary tract infection.   ___ ___ ___ _____

4. Assessed signs and symptoms of urinary tract infection.   ___ ___ ___ _____

5. Assessed client's level of understanding of test.   ___ ___ ___ _____

6. Referred to agency policy for specimen collection procedure.   ___ ___ ___ _____

NURSING DIAGNOSIS

1. Developed appropriate nursing diagnoses based on assessment data.   ___ ___ ___ _____

PLANNING

1. Developed individualized goals for client based on nursing diagnoses.   ___ ___ ___ _____

2. Identified expected outcomes.   ___ ___ ___ _____

3. Offered client fluids before specimen collection.   ___ ___ ___ _____

4. Explained procedure to client.   ___ ___ ___ _____

5. Used visual aids to explain procedure to client.   ___ ___ ___ _____

IMPLEMENTATION

1. Washed hands.   ___ ___ ___ _____

2. Provided client privacy.   ___ ___ ___ _____

3. Assisted client as needed with perineal care.   ___ ___ ___ _____

4. Assisted bedridden client onto bedpan.   ___ ___ ___ _____

5. Opened sterile collection kit correctly.   ___ ___ ___ _____

6. Applied sterile gloves.   ___ ___ ___ _____

7. Prepared sterile collection kit with specimen container.   ___ ___ ___ _____

8. Opened specimen container correctly.   ___ ___ ___ _____

9. Assisted or allowed client to cleanse perineum.   ___ ___ ___ _____

	S	U	NP	Comments

10. Removed specimen container before flow of urine stopped.

11. Secured specimen container top tightly.

12. Cleaned urine from outer surface of specimen container.

13. Disposed of soiled supplies, removed and discarded gloves. Washed hands.

14. Labeled specimen and attached laboratory requisition.

15. Sent specimen to laboratory within 15 minutes or refrigerated.

EVALUATION

1. Assessed client's urine culture and sensitivity report.

2. Observed specimen for contaminants.

3. Asked client to describe procedure.

4. Identified unexpected outcomes.

RECORDING AND REPORTING

1. Recorded date and time specimen collected in nurses' notes.

2. Recorded characteristics of urine and signs and symptoms of infection in nurses' notes.

3. Notified physician of significant abnormalities.

Student _____   Date _____

Instructor _____   Date _____

PERFORMANCE CHECKLIST 43-2 **COLLECTING A TIMED URINE SPECIMEN**

	S	U	NP	Comments
ASSESSMENT				
1. Determined purpose and time period for specimen.	—	—	—	_____
2. Assessed if test required fluid or dietary requirements or medication administration.	—	—	—	_____
3. Determined if client is taking correct diet.	—	—	—	_____
4. Assessed client's ability to collect specimen independently.	—	—	—	_____
5. Assessed client's or family's understanding of purpose of test and reason for timed collection.	—	—	—	_____
6. Referred to agency policy for specimen collection procedure.	—	—	—	_____
NURSING DIAGNOSIS				
1. Developed appropriate nursing diagnoses based on assessment data.	—	—	—	_____
PLANNING				
1. Developed individualized goals for client based on nursing diagnoses.	—	—	—	_____
2. Identified expected outcomes.	—	—	—	_____
3. Instructed client to drink 2-4 glasses of fluids ½ hour before test began.	—	—	—	_____
4. Instructed client and/or family to save all urine during time period; notify nurse when client voids; keep feces and toilet tissue out of specimens; begin and end test with voiding; begin test at precise time.	—	—	—	_____
IMPLEMENTATION				
1. Provided privacy for client.	—	—	—	_____
2. Wore gloves when handling urine.	—	—	—	_____
3. Discarded first random urine specimen obtained and noted time for beginning of test.	—	—	—	_____
4. Provided client with required liquid or medication (as appropriate).	—	—	—	_____
5. Placed signs in client's room indicating time collections occurred.	—	—	—	_____
6. Measured volume of urine voided if client on I&O.	—	—	—	_____

	S	U	NP	Comments
7. Placed all voided urine into collection bottle.	—	—	—	_____
8. Kept urine refrigerated during collection period (if appropriate).	—	—	—	_____
9. Discarded gloves after each collection and washed hands.	—	—	—	_____
10. One hour before end of collection, instructed client to drink fluids.	—	—	—	_____
11. Encouraged client to void during last 15 minutes before end of collection period.	—	—	—	_____
12. Sent specimen to laboratory at end of collection period with appropriate requisition.	—	—	—	_____
13. Removed room signs after specimen collected.	—	—	—	_____

EVALUATION

	S	U	NP	Comments
1. Intermittently assessed client's compliance with saving all urine during collection period.	—	—	—	_____
2. Inspected urine for contaminants.	—	—	—	_____
3. Compared results of client's urinalysis with normal laboratory values.	—	—	—	_____
4. Identified unexpected outcomes.	—	—	—	_____

RECORDING AND REPORTING

	S	U	NP	Comments
1. Recorded starting time of urine collection in client's chart.	—	—	—	_____
2. Recorded pertinent data at end of test.	—	—	—	_____
3. Discussed abnormal results with physician.	—	—	—	_____

Student _____   Date _____

Instructor _____   Date _____

PERFORMANCE CHECKLIST 43-3 COLLECTING A STERILE URINE SPECIMEN FROM AN INDWELLING CATHETER

	S	U	NP	Comments

ASSESSMENT
1. Assessed client's or family's understanding of need for specimen.
2. Assessed client for signs and symptoms of urinary tract infection.
3. Checked catheter for presence of sampling port.

NURSING DIAGNOSIS
1. Developed appropriate nursing diagnoses based on assessment data.

PLANNING
1. Developed individualized goals for client based on nursing diagnoses.
2. Identified expected outcomes.
3. Explained reason for clamping catheter before specimen collection.
4. Explained procedure to client.

IMPLEMENTATION
1. Washed hands.
2. Clamped drainage tubing near catheter for 30 minutes.
3. Informed client when ready to collect specimen.
4. Washed hands and applied gloves.
5. Positioned client for easy access to catheter.
6. Cleansed entry port with disinfectant swab.
7. Inserted needle at 30-degree angle into catheter just above attachment to drainage tube or into sampling port.
8. Collected appropriate amount of urine.
9. Transferred urine into proper container.
10. Placed lid tightly on container.
11. Unclamped catheter and allowed urine to flow into drainage bag.

	S	U	NP	Comments

12. Disposed of soiled supplies; removed and discarded gloves. Washed hands.

_____ _____ _____ _____

13. Securely attached label to container and affixed requisition.

_____ _____ _____ _____

14. Sent specimen immediately to laboratory or placed in refrigerator.

_____ _____ _____ _____

EVALUATION

1. Compared client's laboratory results with normal laboratory values.

_____ _____ _____ _____

2. Observed characteristics of urine.

_____ _____ _____ _____

3. Observed urinary drainage system.

_____ _____ _____ _____

4. Identified unexpected outcomes.

_____ _____ _____ _____

RECORDING AND REPORTING

1. Recorded collection procedure time, date, and appearance of urine in nurses' notes.

_____ _____ _____ _____

2. Notified physician of changes in client's urine.

_____ _____ _____ _____

3. Documented unexpected outcomes.

_____ _____ _____ _____

Student _____   Date _____

Instructor _____   Date _____

PERFORMANCE CHECKLIST 43-4   **MEASURING SPECIFIC GRAVITY OF URINE**

	S	U	NP	Comments

ASSESSMENT

1. Assessed client's or family's understanding of need to test specific gravity.

2. Determined client's ability to collect specimen.

3. Assessed client's hydration status.

4. Assessed client's medical history.

NURSING DIAGNOSIS

1. Developed appropriate nursing diagnoses based on assessment data.

PLANNING

1. Developed individualized goals for client based on nursing diagnoses.

2. Identified expected outcomes.

3. Explained purpose of test to client and how specimen would be obtained.

IMPLEMENTATION

1. Washed hands and applied disposable gloves.

2. Poured specimen into glass cylinder until ⅔ to ¾ full.

3. Placed urinometer into glass cylinder and twirled stem.

4. Read calibrated scale at urine level and noted reading.

5. Discarded urine and cleaned equipment in cool water.

6. Removed and discarded gloves and washed hands.

EVALUATION

1. Observed specimen for contaminants.

2. Compared client's specific gravity with normal values.

3. Identified unexpected outcomes.

RECORDING AND REPORTING

1. Recorded specific gravity reading and noted character of urine in nurses' notes.

	S	U	NP	Comments
2. Recorded urine volume in I&O when appropriate.	___	___	___	_____
3. Reported abnormal values.	___	___	___	_____

Student _____   Date _____

Instructor _____   Date _____

PERFORMANCE CHECKLIST 43-5   **MEASURING CHEMICAL PROPERTIES OF URINE:
GLUCOSE, KETONES, PROTEIN, BLOOD, AND pH**

	S	U	NP	Comments
ASSESSMENT				
1. Determined why physician requested test.	—	—	—	_____
2. Assessed client's need to learn urine testing procedure.	—	—	—	_____
3. Assessed type of reagent test to use.	—	—	—	_____
4. Assessed client's knowledge of and compliance in obtaining double-voided specimen.	—	—	—	_____
5. Assessed medications client received for possible effects on reagent chemicals.	—	—	—	_____
6. Assessed for signs and symptoms of diabetes mellitus.	—	—	—	_____
7. Assessed client's ability to perform urine test.	—	—	—	_____
NURSING DIAGNOSIS				
1. Developed appropriate nursing diagnoses based on assessment data.	—	—	—	_____
PLANNING				
1. Developed individualized goals for client based on nursing diagnoses.	—	—	—	_____
2. Identified expected outcomes.	—	—	—	_____
3. Offered client fluids to drink before specimen collection.	—	—	—	_____
4. Explained procedure to client.	—	—	—	_____
IMPLEMENTATION				
1. Obtained double-voided urine specimen.	—	—	—	_____
2. Applied gloves.	—	—	—	_____
3. Performed glucose reagent tablet test correctly.	—	—	—	_____
4. Performed glucose ketone reagent strip test correctly.	—	—	—	_____
5. Performed ketone tablet test correctly.	—	—	—	_____
6. Used Multistix reagent test strip correctly.	—	—	—	_____
7. Washed hands after removing and discarding gloves.	—	—	—	_____
8. Discussed test results with client.	—	—	—	_____

	S	U	NP	Comments

EVALUATION

1. Compared test results with normal chemical levels.

2. Observed urine for contaminants.

3. Had client demonstrate testing and reading of results.

4. Identified unexpected outcomes.

RECORDING AND REPORTING

1. Recorded test results in nurses' notes or flowsheet.

2. Had client in home setting record results on flowsheet.

Student _____   Date _____

Instructor _____   Date _____

PERFORMANCE CHECKLIST 43-6 **MEASURING OCCULT BLOOD IN STOOL**

	S	U	NP	Comments
ASSESSMENT				
1. Assessed client's or family's understanding of need for stool test.	___	___	___	_____
2. Assessed client's ability to cooperate and collect specimen.	___	___	___	_____
3. Assessed medical history for evidence of bleeding or gastrointestinal disorder.	___	___	___	_____
4. Determined type of medications clients receives and their potential for causing bleeding.	___	___	___	_____
5. Checked physician's orders for medication or dietary restrictions before test.	___	___	___	_____
NURSING DIAGNOSIS				
1. Developed appropriate nursing diagnoses based on assessment data.	___	___	___	_____
PLANNING				
1. Developed individualized goals for client based on nursing diagnoses.	___	___	___	_____
2. Identified expected outcomes.	___	___	___	_____
3. Explained purpose of test and method by which client can assist.	___	___	___	_____
4. Initiated medication and dietary restrictions as ordered.	___	___	___	_____
IMPLEMENTATION				
1. Washed hands and applied disposable gloves.	___	___	___	_____
2. Obtained uncontaminated stool specimen.	___	___	___	_____
3. With tip of wooden applicator obtained small amount of feces.	___	___	___	_____
4. Performed Hemoccult slide test.	___	___	___	_____
5. Performed test using Hematest tablets.	___	___	___	_____
6. Wrapped wooden applicator in paper towel and disposed.	___	___	___	_____
7. Removed gloves and washed hands.	___	___	___	_____
EVALUATION				
1. Noted color changes in guaiac paper.	___	___	___	_____

	S	U	NP	Comments
2. Noted character of stool.	___	___	___	_____
3. Asked client to explain collection procedure.	___	___	___	_____
4. Identified unexpected outcomes.	___	___	___	_____

RECORDING AND REPORTING

	S	U	NP	Comments
1. Recorded test results in nurses' notes.	___	___	___	_____
2. Recorded unusual stool characteristics.	___	___	___	_____
3. Reported positive test results to nurse in charge or physician.	___	___	___	_____

Student _____   Date _____

Instructor _____   Date _____

PERFORMANCE CHECKLIST 43-7 **COLLECTING NOSE AND THROAT SPECIMENS FOR CULTURE**

	S	U	NP	Comments
ASSESSMENT				
1. Assessed client's understanding of procedure and ability to cooperate.	___	___	___	_____
2. Assessed condition of nasal mucosa and sinuses.	___	___	___	_____
3. Assessed client for symptoms of upper respiratory or sinus infection.	___	___	___	_____
4. Assessed condition of posterior pharynx.	___	___	___	_____
5. Assessed client for systemic signs of infection.	___	___	___	_____
6. Reviewed physician's orders for type of culture needed.	___	___	___	_____
NURSING DIAGNOSIS				
1. Developed appropriate nursing diagnoses based on assessment data.	___	___	___	_____
PLANNING				
1. Developed individualized goals for client based on nursing diagnoses.	___	___	___	_____
2. Identified expected outcomes.	___	___	___	_____
3. Planned to do culture before mealtime.	___	___	___	_____
4. Explained purpose for specimens and how client can assist.	___	___	___	_____
5. Explained common sensations felt during specimen collection.	___	___	___	_____
IMPLEMENTATION				
1. Washed hands and applied gloves.	___	___	___	_____
2. Assisted client to sit correctly in bed or chair.	___	___	___	_____
3. Placed swab and tube in accessible spot.	___	___	___	_____
4. Collected throat culture.	___	___	___	_____
5. Collected nose culture.	___	___	___	_____
6. Collected nasopharyngeal culture.	___	___	___	_____
7. Removed and discarded gloves and washed hands.	___	___	___	_____
8. Securely attached label to culture tube and affixed requisition.	___	___	___	_____

	S	U	NP	Comments

9. Sent specimen immediately to laboratory or refrigerated.   ___ ___ ___ _____

EVALUATION

1. Checked laboratory record for test results.   ___ ___ ___ _____

2. Observed that specimen was not contaminated.   ___ ___ ___ _____

3. Inspected client's nose for evidence of bleeding.   ___ ___ ___ _____

4. Asked client to describe need for collection.   ___ ___ ___ _____

5. Identified unexpected outcomes.   ___ ___ ___ _____

RECORDING AND REPORTING

1. Recorded specimen collection in nurses' notes.   ___ ___ ___ _____

2. Described appearance of nasal and oral mucosa in nurses' notes.   ___ ___ ___ _____

3. Reported unusual test results to physician or nurse in charge.   ___ ___ ___ _____

Student _____   Date _____

Instructor _____   Date _____

PERFORMANCE CHECKLIST 43-8 **OBTAINING VAGINAL OR URETHRAL DISCHARGE SPECIMENS**

	S	U	NP	Comments

ASSESSMENT

1. Assessed client's understanding of need for specimen and ability to cooperate.

2. Assessed condition of external genitalia.

3. Assessed client for symptoms of urinary or vaginal infection.

4. Collected sexual history of client when appropriate.

5. Referred to physician's orders for type of culture.

NURSING DIAGNOSIS

1. Developed appropriate nursing diagnoses based on assessment data.

PLANNING

1. Developed individualized goals for client based on nursing diagnoses.

2. Identified expected outcomes.

3. Explained procedure to client.

4. Selected area where privacy ensured.

IMPLEMENTATION

1. Washed hands.

2. Closed bed curtains or room door and hung "do not enter" door sign.

3. Assisted client to proper position and draped.

4. Applied disposable gloves.

5. Directed light onto perineum.

6. Opened culture tube and held swab in dominant hand.

7. Instructed client to breathe slowly during procedure.

8. Obtained specimen(s) using proper procedure according to sex of client.

9. Returned swab(s) to culture tube and secured top.

	S	U	NP	Comments
10. Properly removed and discarded gloves.	——	——	——	_____
11. Squeezed ampule in bottom of tube and pushed swab tip into medium.	——	——	——	_____
12. Labeled and affixed requisition to each specimen.	——	——	——	_____
13. Sent specimen immediately to laboratory or refrigerated.	——	——	——	_____
14. Assisted client in returning to comfortable position, replaced gown, and removed drape.	——	——	——	_____
15. Washed hands.	——	——	——	_____

EVALUATION

	S	U	NP	Comments
1. Checked laboratory results for bacterial growth.	——	——	——	_____
2. Noted character of discharge.	——	——	——	_____
3. Observed specimen for presence of feces.	——	——	——	_____
4. Identified unexpected outcomes.	——	——	——	_____

RECORDING AND REPORTING

	S	U	NP	Comments
1. Recorded type of culture and date and time sent to laboratory in nurses' notes.	——	——	——	_____
2. Described character of discharge and appearance of vaginal orifice and urethra.	——	——	——	_____
3. Reported laboratory test results.	——	——	——	_____

Student _____ Date _____

Instructor _____ Date _____

PERFORMANCE CHECKLIST 43-9 COLLECTING SPUTUM SPECIMENS

	S	U	NP	Comments
ASSESSMENT				
1. Reviewed physician's orders for specimen collection.	—	—	—	_____
2. Assessed client's understanding of procedure.	—	—	—	_____
3. Assessed client's ability to cough and expectorate.	—	—	—	_____
4. Determined if client required assistance in producing specimen.	—	—	—	_____
5. Assessed client's respiratory status.	—	—	—	_____
NURSING DIAGNOSIS				
1. Developed appropriate nursing diagnoses based on assessment data.	—	—	—	_____
PLANNING				
1. Developed individualized goals for client based on nursing diagnoses.	—	—	—	_____
2. Identified expected outcomes.	—	—	—	_____
3. Explained procedure to client.	—	—	—	_____
4. Assisted client in rinsing mouth before collecting expectorated specimen.	—	—	—	_____
IMPLEMENTATION				
1. Washed hands.	—	—	—	_____
2. Provided client privacy.	—	—	—	_____
3. Positioned client correctly.	—	—	—	_____
4. Assisted client in splinting painful area as needed.	—	—	—	_____
5. Collected expectorated or suctioned specimen correctly.	—	—	—	_____
6. Secured tops of container or sputum trap correctly.	—	—	—	_____
7. Cleaned outside of container with disinfectant as needed.	—	—	—	_____
8. Offered client facial tissues.	—	—	—	_____
9. Removed and disposed of gloves.	—	—	—	_____
10. Provided client mouth care as desired.	—	—	—	_____

	S	U	NP	Comments
11. Washed hands.	——	——	——	_____
12. Correctly labeled specimen.	——	——	——	_____
13. Placed specimen in appropriate bag or container.	——	——	——	_____
14. Sent specimen to laboratory or refrigerated.	——	——	——	_____

EVALUATION

	S	U	NP	Comments
1. Observed client's respiratory status during procedure.	——	——	——	_____
2. Noted presence of anxiety or discomfort.	——	——	——	_____
3. Observed character of sputum.	——	——	——	_____
4. Noted laboratory results.	——	——	——	_____
5. Asked client to describe/demonstrate procedure.	——	——	——	_____
6. Identified unexpected outcomes.	——	——	——	_____

RECORDING AND REPORTING

	S	U	NP	Comments
1. Recorded method of collection, date and time sent to laboratory, type of test ordered.	——	——	——	_____
2. Described characteristics of sputum in nurses' notes.	——	——	——	_____
3. Described client's tolerance of procedure.	——	——	——	_____
4. Reported unusual sputum characteristics.	——	——	——	_____
5. Reported abnormal test results.	——	——	——	_____

Student _____   Date _____

Instructor _____   Date _____

PERFORMANCE CHECKLIST 43-10 **OBTAINING GASTRIC SPECIMENS**

	S	U	NP	Comments

ASSESSMENT

1. Reviewed physician's orders before collecting specimen.

2. Determined presence of nasogastric tube or obtained order for inserting tube.

3. Assessed client's understanding of procedure.

4. Assessed medications and foods client received.

5. Determined if any dietary or medication restrictions required before test.

6. Assessed client for symptoms of gastrointestinal alterations.

NURSING DIAGNOSIS

1. Developed appropriate nursing diagnoses based on assessment data.

PLANNING

1. Developed individualized goals for client based on nursing diagnoses.

2. Identified expected outcomes.

3. Instituted ordered dietary or medication restrictions.

4. Explained procedure to client.

IMPLEMENTATION

1. Washed hands.

2. Applied disposable gloves.

3. Positioned client in high Fowler's position.

4. Provided privacy by closing curtains or door.

5. Inserted nasogastric tube, if indicated.

6. Obtained specimen correctly.

7. Applied 1 drop gastric sample to pH paper.

8. Read pH results correctly after 30 seconds.

9. Applied 1 drop gastric sample to Gastrooccult test paper.

10. Applied 2 drops of developer solution over sample and 1 drop to performance monitors.

	S	U	NP	Comments
11. Read test results correctly within 60 seconds.	—	—	—	_____
12. Explained results to client.	—	—	—	_____
13. Disposed of soiled supplies correctly.	—	—	—	_____
14. Reconnected nasogastric tube to drainage or clamped as ordered (removed tube if appropriate).	—	—	—	_____
15. Removed and disposed of gloves.	—	—	—	_____
16. Returned client to comfortable position and provided oral hygiene.	—	—	—	_____
17. Washed hands.	—	—	—	_____

EVALUATION

	S	U	NP	Comments
1. Assessed quantity and character of gastric secretions.	—	—	—	_____
2. Measured emesis for pH and blood.	—	—	—	_____
3. Compared test findings with normal expected results.	—	—	—	_____
4. Asked client about purpose of test.	—	—	—	_____
5. Identified unexpected outcomes.	—	—	—	_____

RECORDING AND REPORTING

	S	U	NP	Comments
1. Recorded test, source of specimen, and results in nurses' notes.	—	—	—	_____
2. Described characteristics of gastric contents.	—	—	—	_____
3. Reported abnormal results.	—	—	—	_____

Student _____   Date _____

Instructor _____   Date _____

PERFORMANCE CHECKLIST 43-11   **OBTAINING WOUND DRAINAGE SPECIMENS**

	S	U	NP	Comments
ASSESSMENT				
1. Assessed client's understanding of purpose of culture and ability to cooperate.	—	—	—	_____
2. Assessed condition of wound using sterile gloves.	—	—	—	_____
3. Assessed client for systemic signs of infection.	—	—	—	_____
4. Determined character of pain at wound site.	—	—	—	_____
5. Reviewed physician's orders for culture.	—	—	—	_____
NURSING DIAGNOSIS				
1. Developed appropriate nursing diagnoses based on assessment data.	—	—	—	_____
PLANNING				
1. Developed individualized goals for client based on nursing diagnoses.	—	—	—	_____
2. Identified expected outcomes.	—	—	—	_____
3. Determined client's need for analgesic before dressing change or specimen collection and administered correctly.	—	—	—	_____
4. Explained procedure to client.	—	—	—	_____
5. Explained that client may feel tickling sensation when wound swabbed.	—	—	—	_____
IMPLEMENTATION				
1. Washed hands.	—	—	—	_____
2. Provided privacy.	—	—	—	_____
3. Removed and disposed of soiled dressings, wearing disposable gloves.	—	—	—	_____
4. Cleansed wound edges with antiseptic.	—	—	—	_____
5. Disposed of antiseptic swab and gloves.	—	—	—	_____
6. Opened culture tube kits and sterile dressing supplies, keeping items sterile.	—	—	—	_____
7. Applied sterile gloves.	—	—	—	_____
8. Collected cultures, aerobic or anaerobic, correctly.	—	—	—	_____
9. Placed each specimen on appropriate label.	—	—	—	_____

	S	U	NP	Comments

10. Asked staff member to label and affix requisitions and send specimens to laboratory immediately.

11. Cleaned wound as ordered and applied new sterile dressing.

12. Disposed of gloves and soiled supplies.

13. Secured dressing.

14. Assisted client to comfortable position.

15. Washed hands.

EVALUATION

1. Checked laboratory report for culture results.

2. Assessed character of wound and wound drainage.

3. Asked client about purpose of culture.

4. Identified unexpected outcomes.

RECORDING AND REPORTING

1. Recorded specimen type, source, and date and time sent to laboratory in nurses' notes.

2. Described appearance of wound and drainage.

3. Reported evidence of infection to nurse in charge or physician.

Student _____   Date _____

Instructor _____   Date _____

PERFORMANCE CHECKLIST 43-12 **COLLECTING BLOOD SPECIMENS BY VENIPUNCTURE**

	S	U	NP	Comments
ASSESSMENT				
1. Determined client's understanding of procedure.	___	___	___	_____
2. Determined if special conditions needed to be addressed before collection.	___	___	___	_____
3. Determined client's risk for venipuncture.	___	___	___	_____
4. Determined client's ability to cooperate with procedure.	___	___	___	_____
5. Identified site contraindications for venipuncture.	___	___	___	_____
6. Reviewed physician orders for type of test(s).	___	___	___	_____
NURSING DIAGNOSIS				
1. Developed appropriate nursing diagnoses based on assessment data.	___	___	___	_____
PLANNING				
1. Developed individualized goals for client based on nursing diagnoses.	___	___	___	_____
2. Identified expected outcomes.	___	___	___	_____
3. Explained procedure to client.	___	___	___	_____
IMPLEMENTATION				
1. Washed hands.	___	___	___	_____
2. Placed equipment at client's bedside.	___	___	___	_____
3. Provided for privacy.	___	___	___	_____
4. Positioned bed at appropriate working height.	___	___	___	_____
5. Assisted client to appropriate position.	___	___	___	_____
6. Had another staff member help to immobilize venipuncture site.	___	___	___	_____
7. Applied disposable gloves.	___	___	___	_____
8. Properly applied tourniquet.	___	___	___	_____
9. Palpated distal pulse.	___	___	___	_____
10. Kept tourniquet on no longer than 1 or 2 minutes.	___	___	___	_____
11. Instructed client to open and close fist.	___	___	___	_____
12. Inspected extremity for best venipuncture site.	___	___	___	_____
13. Palpated selected vein.	___	___	___	_____

	S	U	NP	Comments
14. Selected venipuncture site.	——	——	——	_____
15. Correctly obtained blood sample by syringe or Vacutainer method.	——	——	——	_____
16. Applied pressure over venipuncture site with gauze until bleeding stopped.	——	——	——	_____
17. With syringe method, transferred specimens to tubes.	——	——	——	_____
18. Rotated all blood tubes containing additives.	——	——	——	_____
19. Inspected puncture site for bleeding and applied gauze.	——	——	——	_____
20. Assessed tubes for external contamination with blood and cleansed with 70% alcohol if necessary.	——	——	——	_____
21. Assisted client to comfortable position.	——	——	——	_____
22. Labeled each tube and affixed proper requisition.	——	——	——	_____
23. Disposed of all equipment in proper receptacle. Did not recap needles.	——	——	——	_____
24. Removed gloves.	——	——	——	_____
25. Washed hands.	——	——	——	_____
26. Sent specimens to laboratory.	——	——	——	_____

EVALUATION

	S	U	NP	Comments
1. Reinspected venipuncture site.	——	——	——	_____
2. Determined if client remained anxious or fearful.	——	——	——	_____
3. Checked laboratory results.	——	——	——	_____
4. Asked client to explain purpose of test.	——	——	——	_____
5. Identified unexpected outcomes.	——	——	——	_____

RECORDING AND REPORTING

	S	U	NP	Comments
1. Recorded procedure in nurses' notes.	——	——	——	_____
2. Described venipuncture site and client's response.	——	——	——	_____
3. Reported "stat" test results to physician.	——	——	——	_____
4. Reported any abnormal findings to physician.	——	——	——	_____

Student _____   Date _____

Instructor _____   Date _____

PERFORMANCE CHECKLIST 43-13 MEASURING BLOOD GLUCOSE LEVEL AFTER SKIN PUNCTURE

	S	U	NP	Comments
ASSESSMENT				
1. Assessed client's understanding of procedure.	—	—	—	_____
2. Determined if specific conditions needed to be met before procedure.	—	—	—	_____
3. Determined risks for performing procedure.	—	—	—	_____
4. Assessed area of skin to be used as puncture site.	—	—	—	_____
5. Reviewed physician's order.	—	—	—	_____
6. Assessed diabetic client's ability to handle skin puncture device.	—	—	—	_____
NURSING DIAGNOSIS				
1. Developed appropriate nursing diagnoses based on assessment data.	—	—	—	_____
PLANNING				
1. Developed individualized goals for client based on nursing diagnoses.	—	—	—	_____
2. Identified expected outcomes.	—	—	—	_____
3. Explained procedure to client.	—	—	—	_____
IMPLEMENTATION				
1. Washed hands.	—	—	—	_____
2. Instructed client to wash hands.	—	—	—	_____
3. Positioned client comfortably.	—	—	—	_____
4. Removed reagent strip from container and tightly sealed caps.	—	—	—	_____
5. Turned glucose meter on.	—	—	—	_____
6. Inserted strip into glucose meter.	—	—	—	_____
7. Removed reagent strip from meter and placed on clean, dry surface.	—	—	—	_____
8. Applied disposable gloves.	—	—	—	_____
9. Selected puncture site.	—	—	—	_____
10. Gently massaged finger to be punctured.	—	—	—	_____
11. Cleansed site with antiseptic swab and allowed to dry.	—	—	—	_____
12. Removed cover of lancet or blood-letting device.	—	—	—	_____
13. Correctly punctured finger.	—	—	—	_____

	S	U	NP	Comments

14. Wiped away first droplet of blood with cotton ball (or as manufacturer's directions describe).

15. Squeezed puncture site until droplet formed.

16. Lightly transferred drop of blood to reagent strip test pad. Prepared meter and reagent strip per manufacturer's instructions.

17. Applied pressure to skin puncture site.

18. Noted glucose reading on display.

19. Turned meter off and disposed of test strip and cotton balls.

20. Removed disposable gloves and disposed of properly.

21. Washed hands.

22. Shared test results with client.

EVALUATION

1. Compared glucose meter reading with normal levels.

2. Inspected puncture site for bleeding or tissue injury.

3. Determined if client had any questions or concerns.

4. Asked client to describe/demonstrate procedure.

5. Identified unexpected outcomes.

RECORDING AND REPORTING

1. Recorded procedure and glucose level in nurses' notes or special flowsheet as well as action taken for abnormal range.

2. Recorded administration of insulin or carbohydrate as ordered.

3. Described client's response and appearance of puncture site.

4. Described any explanations or teaching provided for client.

5. Reported abnormal blood glucose levels to physician.

Student _____ Date _____

Instructor _____ Date _____

PERFORMANCE CHECKLIST 43-14 **MEASURING ARTERIAL BLOOD GASES**

	S	U	NP	Comments
ASSESSMENT				
1. Identified need to obtain sample.	___	___	___	_____
2. Identified factors that could alter sample.	___	___	___	_____
3. Performed physical assessment of thorax and lungs.	___	___	___	_____
4. Reviewed criteria for choosing site for sample collection.	___	___	___	_____
5. Assessed arterial sites.	___	___	___	_____
6. Determined client's baseline arterial blood gases.	___	___	___	_____
7. Determined client's knowledge of procedure.	___	___	___	_____
NURSING DIAGNOSIS				
1. Developed appropriate nursing diagnoses based on assessment data.	___	___	___	_____
PLANNING				
1. Developed individualized goals for client based on nursing diagnoses.	___	___	___	_____
2. Identified expected outcomes.	___	___	___	_____
3. Prepared heparinized syringe.	___	___	___	_____
4. Explained procedure to client.	___	___	___	_____
IMPLEMENTATION				
1. Washed hands and applied gloves.	___	___	___	_____
2. Selected and palpated arterial site.	___	___	___	_____
3. Stabilized artery appropriately.	___	___	___	_____
4. Cleansed area with alcohol swab.	___	___	___	_____
5. Held swab with fingers to palpate artery.	___	___	___	_____
6. Kept fingertip on artery.	___	___	___	_____
7. Correctly performed arterial stick.	___	___	___	_____
8. Stopped advancing needle when blood noted.	___	___	___	_____
9. If open needle used, attached syringe securely.	___	___	___	_____
10. Used swab to catch any spilled blood.	___	___	___	_____
11. Drew sample slowly.	___	___	___	_____

	S	U	NP	Comments

12. Removed needle holding swab over site.   ___ ___ ___ _____

13. Applied pressure over site.   ___ ___ ___ _____

14. Maintained pressure for 5 to 10 minutes as indicated.   ___ ___ ___ _____

15. Inspected site for signs of bleeding.   ___ ___ ___ _____

16. Palpated artery.   ___ ___ ___ _____

17. Expelled air bubbles from syringe.   ___ ___ ___ _____

18. Removed and disposed of gloves and washed hands.   ___ ___ ___ _____

19. Prepared syringe for laboratory according to agency policy using common principles such as:

   a. Labeled syringe properly.   ___ ___ ___ _____

   b. Placed sample on ice.   ___ ___ ___ _____

   c. Prepared laboratory requisition.   ___ ___ ___ _____

   d. Indicated client's FiO_2 on requisition.   ___ ___ ___ _____

   e. Sent sample to laboratory immediately.   ___ ___ ___ _____

EVALUATION

1. Inspected area distal to puncture site for complications.   ___ ___ ___ _____

2. Reviewed results as soon as possible.   ___ ___ ___ _____

3. Obtained client's respiratory rate.   ___ ___ ___ _____

4. Identified unexpected outcomes.   ___ ___ ___ _____

RECORDING AND REPORTING

1. Recorded puncture site and disposition of specimen to laboratory in nurses' notes.   ___ ___ ___ _____

2. Reported results to physician.   ___ ___ ___ _____

3. Included FiO_2 and any ventilator settings in report.   ___ ___ ___ _____

4. Recorded test results and condition of puncture site in nurses' notes.   ___ ___ ___ _____

Student _____   Date _____

Instructor _____   Date _____

PERFORMANCE CHECKLIST 44-1   **ASSISTING WITH ABDOMINAL PARACENTESIS**

	S	U	NP	Comments
ASSESSMENT				
1. Assessed contraindications.	—	—	—	_____
2. Assessed vital signs.	—	—	—	_____
3. Assessed client's bladder for distention or time of last void.	—	—	—	_____
4. Determined whether client was allergic to local anesthetic or antiseptic solution.	—	—	—	_____
5. Weighed client. Assessed abdomen and correctly measured abdominal girth of client with ascites.	—	—	—	_____
6. Assessed respiratory status.	—	—	—	_____
7. Assessed client's knowledge regarding procedure.	—	—	—	_____
8. Checked institution's policy on written informed consent.	—	—	—	_____
NURSING DIAGNOSIS				
1. Developed appropriate nursing diagnoses based on assessment data.	—	—	—	_____
PLANNING				
1. Developed individualized goals for client based on nursing diagnoses.	—	—	—	_____
2. Identified expected outcomes.	—	—	—	_____
3. Organized equipment.	—	—	—	_____
4. Explained procedure and had client void.	—	—	—	_____
5. Administered preprocedure medication.	—	—	—	_____
IMPLEMENTATION				
Nurses' Responsibility				
1. Washed hands.	—	—	—	_____
2. Set up sterile tray or opened sterile supplies.	—	—	—	_____
3. Prepared fluid to be used for lavage; attached to IV tubing.	—	—	—	_____
4. Assisted client through procedure.	—	—	—	_____
5. Assessed vital signs before, during, and after procedure.	—	—	—	_____
6. Implemented fluid instillation for lavage.	—	—	—	_____

	S	U	NP	Comments

7. Opened tubing clamp to allow drainage of peritoneal lavage fluid.

8. Collected laboratory specimens in sterile containers.

9. Assessed client's tolerance of procedure, vital signs, pain, and sensorium.

10. Disposed of equipment, removed gloves, washed hands.

EVALUATION

1. Evaluated client's status.

2. Observed client for signs of discomfort.

3. Identified unexpected outcomes.

RECORDING AND REPORTING

1. Recorded procedure, type of dressing, presence of drainage, and client's tolerance in client's chart.

2. Recorded changes in abdominal girth and weight and characteristics of peritoneal fluid.

3. Reported unexpected outcomes to physician.

4. Reported to oncoming staff.

Student _____   Date _____

Instructor _____   Date _____

PERFORMANCE CHECKLIST 44-2 ASSISTING WITH ANGIOGRAPHY (ARTERIOGRAPHY)

	S	U	NP	Comments

ASSESSMENT

1. Assessed client's knowledge of procedure.

2. Assessed vital signs, including peripheral pulses. Auscultated heart and lungs and obtained weight for cardiac catheterization.

3. Determined type of arteriogram to be performed.

4. Assessed need for signed informed consent.

5. Assessed time of last ingested fluid or food.

6. Determined if client is allergic to iodine dye and notified appropriate physician.

7. Assessed laboratory results.

8. Reviewed physician's orders.

NURSING DIAGNOSIS

1. Developed appropriate nursing diagnoses based on assessment data.

PLANNING

1. Developed individualized goals for client based on nursing diagnoses.

2. Identified expected outcomes.

3. Prepared client for procedure.

IMPLEMENTATION
Nurse's Responsibility

1. Washed hands and applied gloves.

2. If client is having cardiac catheterization, provided IV access using large-bore cannula.

3. Measured vital signs, obtained weight, palpated peripheral pulses.

4. Assisted client in assuming comfortable position on x-ray table.

5. Provided support throughout procedure.

6. Told client sensation that may be felt during dye injection.

7. Ensured monitoring of levels of sedation and consciousness for client receiving IVCS.

	S	U	NP	Comments

8. Noted tendency of clients to cough when catheter placed into pulmonary artery.

   — — — _____

EVALUATION

1. Evaluated client's status.

   — — — _____

2. Observed for signs of discomfort.

   — — — _____

3. Identified unexpected outcomes.

   — — — _____

RECORDING AND REPORTING

1. Recorded in client's chart type of procedure and how client tolerated procedure.

   — — — _____

2. Recorded change in vital signs, peripheral pulses, and laboratory values.

   — — — _____

3. Followed specific postangiography orders according to agency guidelines.

   — — — _____

4. Recorded type of dressing, type and amount of drainage, and presence of pain.

   — — — _____

5. Reported unexpected outcomes to physician immediately.

   — — — _____

6. Reported pertinent data to oncoming shift.

   — — — _____

Student _____ Date _____

Instructor _____ Date _____

PERFORMANCE CHECKLIST 44-3   **ASSISTING WITH BONE MARROW ASPIRATION/BIOPSY**

	S	U	NP	Comments

ASSESSMENT

1. Assessed client's knowledge of procedure.

2. Assessed client's ability to assume position required for procedure.

3. Assessed vital signs to obtain baseline data.

4. Assessed client's coagulation status.

5. Determined purpose of procedure.

6. Ascertained presence of signed consent form.

7. Determined whether client was allergic to antiseptic and anesthetic solutions.

NURSING DIAGNOSIS

1. Developed appropriate nursing diagnoses based on assessment data.

PLANNING

1. Developed individualized goals for client based on nursing diagnoses.

2. Identified expected outcomes.

3. Explained steps to client.

IMPLEMENTATION
Nurse's Responsibility

1. Washed hands.

2. Set up sterile tray or opened supplies for physician.

3. Assisted client in maintaining correct position; reassured client while explaining procedure.

4. Assessed client's condition during procedure.

5. Noted characteristics of bone marrow aspirate.

EVALUATION

1. Monitored vital signs.

2. Inspected dressing over puncture site.

3. Observed client's level of comfort.

4. Identified unexpected outcomes.

	S	U	NP	Comments

RECORDING AND REPORTING

1. Recorded pertinent data in nurses' notes or on client's chart.

2. Reported unexpected outcomes to physician.

3. Reported results of procedure to oncoming shift.

Student _____ Date _____

Instructor _____ Date _____

PERFORMANCE CHECKLIST 44-4 **ASSISTING WITH BRONCHOSCOPY**

	S	U	NP	Comments
ASSESSMENT				
1. Assessed client's knowledge regarding procedure.	—	—	—	_____
2. Assessed vital signs to obtain baseline data.	—	—	—	_____
3. Assessed respiratory function.	—	—	—	_____
4. Determined purpose of procedure.	—	—	—	_____
5. Assessed need for signed consent form.	—	—	—	_____
6. Determined whether client was allergic to local anesthetic.	—	—	—	_____
7. Assessed need for preprocedure medication.	—	—	—	_____
8. Assessed time client last ingested food.	—	—	—	_____
9. Assessed vital signs and oxygen saturation if using IVCS.	—	—	—	_____
NURSING DIAGNOSIS				
1. Developed appropriate nursing diagnoses based on assessment data.	—	—	—	_____
PLANNING				
1. Developed individualized goals for client based on nursing diagnoses.	—	—	—	_____
2. Identified expected outcomes.	—	—	—	_____
3. Explained procedure to client.	—	—	—	_____
4. Assisted client to maintain position.	—	—	—	_____
5. Removed and stored client's eyeglasses, contact lenses, and/or dentures.	—	—	—	_____
6. Made sure that client remained NPO 8 hours before procedure.	—	—	—	_____
IMPLEMENTATION *Nurses' Responsibility*				
1. Assisted client in maintaining position.	—	—	—	_____
2. Instructed client not to swallow local anesthetic; provided emesis basin.	—	—	—	_____
3. Assisted client through procedure by explanations.	—	—	—	_____
4. Assessed client's respiratory status during procedure.	—	—	—	_____

	S	U	NP	Comments

5. Noted characteristics of suctioned material.   ___ ___ ___ _____

6. Wiped client's nose to remove lubricant after bronchoscope was removed.   ___ ___ ___ _____

7. Did not allow client to eat or drink until tracheo-bronchial anesthesia had worn off.   ___ ___ ___ _____

EVALUATION

1. Monitored vital signs.   ___ ___ ___ _____

2. Observed sputum production.   ___ ___ ___ _____

3. Observed respiratory status.   ___ ___ ___ _____

4. Assessed for return of gag reflex.   ___ ___ ___ _____

5. Asked client to describe postprocedure normal and abnormal symptoms.   ___ ___ ___ _____

6. Identified unexpected outcomes.   ___ ___ ___ _____

RECORDING AND REPORTING

1. Recorded pertinent data in nurses' notes or on client's chart.   ___ ___ ___ _____

2. Reported unexpected outcomes to physician immediately.   ___ ___ ___ _____

3. Reported results of procedure to oncoming shift.   ___ ___ ___ _____

Student _____   Date _____

Instructor _____   Date _____

PERFORMANCE CHECKLIST 44-5   ASSISTING WITH ELECTROCARDIOGRAM

	S	U	NP	Comments
ASSESSMENT				
1. Determined rationale for ECG.	___	___	___	_____
2. Determined if client has chest pain.	___	___	___	_____
3. Assessed client's knowledge regarding procedure.	___	___	___	_____
4. Obtained baseline vital signs.	___	___	___	_____
5. Obtained previous ECG tracings.	___	___	___	_____
NURSING DIAGNOSIS				
1. Developed appropriate nursing diagnoses based on assessment data.	___	___	___	_____
PLANNING				
1. Developed individualized goals for client based on nursing diagnoses.	___	___	___	_____
2. Identified expected outcomes.	___	___	___	_____
3. Prepared client for procedure.	___	___	___	_____
IMPLEMENTATION				
1. Washed hands.	___	___	___	_____
2. Provided privacy.	___	___	___	_____
3. Cleansed and prepared client's skin.	___	___	___	_____
4. Applied electrode paste and attached leads.	___	___	___	_____
5. Obtained tracing.	___	___	___	_____
6. Disconnected leads, cleansed skin, and washed hands.	___	___	___	_____
7. Delivered ECG tracing to appropriate laboratory or heart station.	___	___	___	_____
EVALUATION				
1. Assessed client's response to procedure.	___	___	___	_____
2. Measured vital signs.	___	___	___	_____
3. Identified unexpected outcomes.	___	___	___	_____
RECORDING AND REPORTING				
1. Recorded pertinent data in nurses' notes.	___	___	___	_____
2. Reported any unexpected outcomes.	___	___	___	_____

Student _____ Date _____
Instructor _____ Date _____

PERFORMANCE CHECKLIST 34-1 ASSISTING WITH ELECTROCARDIOGRAM

	S	U	NP	Comments
ASSESSMENT				
1. Determined rationale for ECG.				
2. Determined if client has chest pain.				
3. Assessed client's knowledge regarding procedure.				
4. Obtained baseline vital signs.				
5. Obtained previous ECG tracings.				
NURSING DIAGNOSIS				
6. Developed appropriate nursing diagnoses based on assessment data.				
PLANNING				
1. Developed individualized goals for client based on nursing diagnoses.				
2. Identified expected outcomes.				
3. Prepared client for procedure.				
IMPLEMENTATION				
1. Washed hands.				
2. Provided privacy.				
3. Cleansed and prepared client's skin.				
4. Applied electrode pads and attached leads.				
5. Obtained tracing.				
6. Disconnected leads, cleansed skin, and washed hands.				
7. Delivered ECG tracing to appropriate laboratory or heart station.				
EVALUATION				
1. Assessed client's response to procedure.				
2. Measured vital signs.				
3. Identified unexpected outcomes.				
RECORDING AND REPORTING				
1. Recorded pertinent data in nurse's notes.				
2. Reported any unexpected outcomes.				

Student _____   Date _____

Instructor _____   Date _____

PERFORMANCE CHECKLIST 44-6 **ASSISTING WITH ENDOSCOPY**

	S	U	NP	Comments
ASSESSMENT				
1. Assessed client's knowledge regarding procedure.	—	—	—	_____
2. Assessed vital signs.	—	—	—	_____
3. Determined presence of GI bleeding.	—	—	—	_____
4. Determined purpose of procedure.	—	—	—	_____
5. Assessed need for signed consent form.	—	—	—	_____
6. Verified that client was NPO for at least 8 hours.	—	—	—	_____
7. Verified that client did not have esophageal diverticulum.	—	—	—	_____
8. Reviewed physician's orders for preprocedure medication and IVCS.	—	—	—	_____
NURSING DIAGNOSIS				
1. Developed appropriate nursing diagnoses based on assessment data.	—	—	—	_____
PLANNING				
1. Developed individualized goals for client based on nursing diagnoses.	—	—	—	_____
2. Identified expected outcomes.	—	—	—	_____
3. Prepared client for procedure.	—	—	—	_____
IMPLEMENTATION				
Nurse's Responsibility				
1. Washed hands and applied gloves.	—	—	—	_____
2. Removed dentures and partial bridges.	—	—	—	_____
3. Assisted client in maintaining proper position.	—	—	—	_____
4. Ensured IV line patency for IVCS.	—	—	—	_____
5. Assisted client through procedure.	—	—	—	_____
6. Placed tissue specimens in proper containers.	—	—	—	_____
7. Suctioned if client began to vomit or accumulated saliva.	—	—	—	_____
8. Maintained client's NPO status until gag reflex returned.	—	—	—	_____
9. Provided oral hygiene when gag reflex returned.	—	—	—	_____

	S	U	NP	Comments
10. Assisted client to comfortable position. Washed hands.	—	—	—	_____

EVALUATION

1. Assessed client to determine response to endoscopy.	—	—	—	_____
2. Asked client to state postprocedure dietary and activity limitations.	—	—	—	_____
3. Identified unexpected outcomes.	—	—	—	_____

RECORDING AND REPORTING

1. Recorded pertinent data in nurses' notes.	—	—	—	_____
2. Reported unexpected outcomes to physician.	—	—	—	_____
3. Reported pertinent findings to nurse in charge.	—	—	—	_____

Student _____ Date _____

Instructor _____ Date _____

PERFORMANCE CHECKLIST 44-7 **ASSISTING WITH LUMBAR PUNCTURE**

	S	U	NP	Comments
ASSESSMENT				
1. Assessed client's ability to understand and follow directions.	—	—	—	_____
2. Assessed client's ability to assume correct position.	—	—	—	_____
3. Assessed degree of cooperativeness of client to remain in position.	—	—	—	_____
4. Examined medical record for contraindications.	—	—	—	_____
5. Determined whether client was allergic to medication to be used in procedure.	—	—	—	_____
6. Ascertained presence of signed consent form.	—	—	—	_____
7. Assessed client's knowledge regarding procedure.	—	—	—	_____
8. Assessed client's vital signs and neurologic status of legs.	—	—	—	_____
NURSING DIAGNOSIS				
1. Developed appropriate nursing diagnoses based on assessment data.	—	—	—	_____
PLANNING				
1. Developed individualized goals for client based on nursing diagnoses.	—	—	—	_____
2. Identified expected outcomes.	—	—	—	_____
3. Explained procedure to client.	—	—	—	_____
4. Had client empty bladder and bowels before procedure.	—	—	—	_____
5. Positioned client correctly.	—	—	—	_____
IMPLEMENTATION				
Nurse's Responsibility				
1. Explained to client need to remain in position.	—	—	—	_____
2. Held client's arms and legs in flexed position.	—	—	—	_____
3. Cautioned client not to cough and to breathe slowly and deeply.	—	—	—	_____
4. Explained each step that might produce discomfort.	—	—	—	_____
5. Applied gloves in preparation for handling body fluids.	—	—	—	_____

S   U   NP   Comments

6. Properly labeled tubes.

7. Assisted with placement of direct pressure and bandage.

8. Removed gloves and washed hands.

9. Assisted client in assuming comfortable position.

10. Asked client to maintain supine or dorsal recumbent position.

11. Provided client with medication if ordered.

12. Observed client's response to procedure.

13. Encouraged client to force PO fluids if not contraindicated.

EVALUATION

1. Assessed needle insertion site for drainage.

2. Assessed level of consciousness, vital signs, pupils, respiratory status, numbness or tingling in legs.

3. Asked client to describe postprocedure positioning and activity restriction.

4. Identified unexpected outcomes.

RECORDING AND REPORTING

1. Recorded pertinent data in nurses' notes.

2. Recorded and reported pertinent findings to nurse in charge and physician.

Student _____   Date _____

Instructor _____   Date _____

PERFORMANCE CHECKLIST 44-8 **ASSISTING WITH MAGNETIC RESONANCE IMAGING**

	S	U	NP	Comments

ASSESSMENT

1. Assessed client's knowledge of procedure.

2. Assessed stability of client's medical condition.

3. Assessed need for signed informed consent.

4. Assessed client's weight.

5. Assessed client for cardiac pacemaker, aneurysm clips, or history of valve replacement (implantable metal objects).

6. Assessed client for claustrophobia.

7. Assessed client for pregnancy.

8. Assessed client's ability to remain still throughout procedure.

9. Assessed for allergies to dye and contrast medium.

NURSING DIAGNOSIS

1. Developed appropriate nursing diagnoses based on assessment data.

PLANNING

1. Developed individualized goals for client based on nursing diagnoses.

2. Identified expected outcomes.

IMPLEMENTATION
Nurse's Responsibility

1. Showed client picture of magnetic resonance imaging (MRI) machine, if possible, and encouraged questions.

2. Removed all metallic objects from client.

3. Had client void and put on hospital gown.

EVALUATION

1. Evaluated client's status after procedure.

2. Identified unexpected outcomes.

	S	U	NP	Comments

RECORDING AND REPORTING

1. Recorded in client's chart date, time, place MRI performed, if contrast medium used, and client's tolerance of procedure. ___ ___ ___ _____

2. Reported duration of procedure and client's response to nurse in charge or oncoming shift. ___ ___ ___ _____

Student _____   Date _____

Instructor _____   Date _____

PERFORMANCE CHECKLIST 44-9   ASSISTING WITH THORACENTESIS

	S	U	NP	Comments

ASSESSMENT

1. Assessed client's knowledge of procedure.

2. Assessed client's ability to assume correct position.

3. Assessed vital signs.

4. Determined presence of possible thrombocytopenia.

5. Assessed respiratory function.

6. Determined purpose of procedure.

7. Assessed need for signed consent form.

8. Determined whether client was allergic to antiseptic or anesthetic solutions.

9. Assessed need for preprocedure pain medication.

NURSING DIAGNOSIS

1. Developed appropriate nursing diagnoses based on assessment data.

PLANNING

1. Developed individualized goals for client based on nursing diagnoses.

2. Identified expected outcomes.

3. Prepared client for procedure.

4. Explained sensations that may be felt during procedure.

IMPLEMENTATION
Nurse's Responsibility

1. Washed hands.

2. Set up sterile tray or opened supplies for physician.

3. Assisted client in maintaining correct position.

4. Assisted client through procedure.

5. Assessed client's pulse and respiratory status during procedure.

6. Assisted client in assuming comfortable position in bed.

	S	U	NP	Comments

EVALUATION

1. Noted characteristics of pleural fluid.

2. Monitored vital signs.

3. Monitored client for complications.

4. Noted presence of drainage on chest dressing.

5. Followed up on postthoracentesis chest x-ray.

6. Asked client to describe postprocedure limitations and positioning.

7. Identified unexpected outcomes.

RECORDING AND REPORTING

1. Recorded pertinent data in nurses' notes.

2. Reported unexpected outcomes to physician immediately.

3. Reported to oncoming staff.

Student _____   Date _____

Instructor _____   Date _____

PERFORMANCE CHECKLIST 45-1   **CARE OF THE BODY AFTER DEATH**

	S	U	NP	Comments

ASSESSMENT

1. Assessed for presence of family or significant others and whether they have been informed of client's death. Asked if family wished to view the body.   __ __ __ _____

2. Allowed time for family or significant others to ask questions.   __ __ __ _____

3. Assessed client's religious preference or cultural heritage and determined if family wished to have minister or priest at bedside.   __ __ __ _____

4. Determined general condition of body.   __ __ __ _____

5. Reviewed agency policy for preparation of the body; determined if autopsy planned.   __ __ __ _____

NURSING DIAGNOSIS

1. Developed appropriate nursing diagnoses based on assessment data.   __ __ __ _____

PLANNING

1. Developed individualized goals for client and family.   __ __ __ _____

2. Identified expected outcomes.   __ __ __ _____

3. Explained to family about time period needed to prepare body for viewing.   __ __ __ _____

4. If another client is in the room, explained what has happened and offered opportunity to leave room.   __ __ __ _____

5. Prepared needed equipment.   __ __ __ _____

IMPLEMENTATION

1. Washed hands.   __ __ __ _____

2. Applied disposable gloves and gown or protective devices if applicable.   __ __ __ _____

3. Provided privacy.   __ __ __ _____

4. Correctly identified client.   __ __ __ _____

5. Correctly positioned client.   __ __ __ _____

6. Placed small pillow under head or elevated head of bed slightly.   __ __ __ _____

7. Gently held eyelids closed for a few seconds.   __ __ __ _____

	S	U	NP	Comments

8. Inserted client's dentures into mouth.

9. Removed all collection devices and tubes not needed for autopsy examination.

10. Clamped or cut tubes to remain in body and secured with tape.

11. Removed soiled dressings and replaced with clean gauze dressings.

12. Washed soiled body parts.

13. Placed absorbent pad under client's buttocks.

14. Brushed and combed client's hair.

15. Removed all jewelry unless otherwise requested by family.

16. Placed clean gown on body.

17. Accounted for all valuables remaining in client's room.

18. Placed client's clothing and shoes in labeled bag.

19. Completed identification tags and placed on client according to policy.

20. If family requested viewing, placed sheet or blanket over client with shoulders and head exposed.

21. Remained at bedside with family and allowed time to view body privately.

22. After family left, removed all linen and client's gown. Placed body in body bag or applied shroud.

23. Secured shroud with tape.

24. Attached label to outside of body bag.

25. If client had transmissible infection, applied special labeling as indicated.

26. Arranged for transportation of body.

27. Carefully transferred body to stretcher.

28. Closed other client's doors and arranged for transport to be as inconspicuous as possible.

29. Removed remaining items and linens from client's room.

30. Washed hands.

EVALUATION

1. Observed family's response to loss of loved one.

Student _____   Date _____

Instructor _____   Date _____

	S	U	NP	Comments
2. Offered family opportunity to ask questions and express feelings.	—	—	—	_____
3. Assisted family in making necessary calls to other family members.	—	—	—	_____
4. Noted appearance and condition of client's skin during body preparation.	—	—	—	_____
5. Identified unexpected outcomes.	—	—	—	_____

RECORDING AND REPORTING

	S	U	NP	Comments
1. Recorded date and time of death and pertinent data in nurses' notes.	—	—	—	_____
2. Documented any marks, bruises, or wounds on body.	—	—	—	_____
3. Documented handling of valuables and personal belongings.	—	—	—	_____